D0900936

DRIVING LESSONS
Exploring Systems That Make Traffic Safer

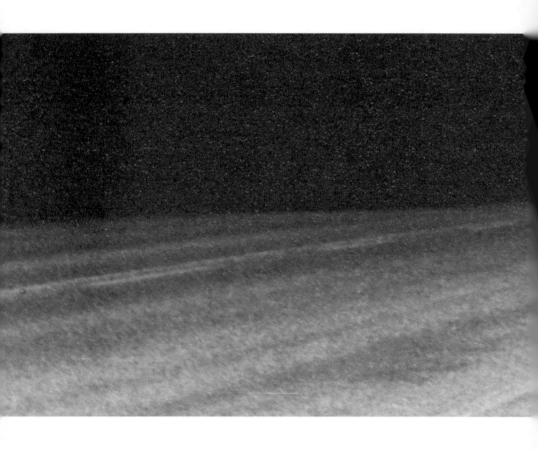

The University of Alberta Press

Foreword by ROB TAYLOR, *Mission Possible*

DRIVING LESSONS

LESSONS

Exploring Systems That Make Traffic Safer

J. PETER ROTHE

editor

Published by
The University of Alberta Press
Ring House 2
Edmonton, Alberta T6G 2E1

in association with
Alberta Centre for Injury Control and Research
and
Mission Possible: Traffic Safety in Action

National Library of Canada Cataloguing in Publication Data

Main entry under title:
Driving lessons

    Includes bibliographical references and index.
    ISBN 0-88864-370-5

    1. Traffic safety. 2. Traffic accidents. I. Rothe, J. Peter (John Peter), 1948-
HE5614.M68 2002   363.12'5   C2001-911481-8

Printed and bound in Canada by Houghton-Boston, Saskatoon, Saskatchewan.
∞ Printed on acid-free paper.
Proofreading by Lisa LaFramboise.
Publication assistance by Tara Taylor.

The University of Alberta Press acknowledges the financial support of the Government of Canada
through the Book Publishing Industry Development Program for its publishing activities. The Press
also gratefully acknowledges the support received for its program from the Canada Council for
the Arts.

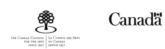

THE CANADA COUNCIL | LE CONSEIL DES ARTS
FOR THE ARTS | DU CANADA
SINCE 1957 | DEPUIS 1957

Canadä

Contents

CONTRIBUTORS

ROBERT M. ARTHUR is a PhD Candidate in the Department of Geography at the University of Calgary.

WALTER BARTA works for the Alberta Motor Association in Edmonton, Alberta.

MIKE BOYES teaches in the Department of Psychology at the University of Calgary.

GARY D. BRINKER is Assistant Professor in the Department of Sociology and Anthropology at Southwest Missouri State University. He also serves as Associate Director of the Center for Social Sciences and Public Policy Research (formerly the Center for Social Research).

LOUIS HUGO FRANCESCUTTI teaches in the Department of Public Health Sciences at the University of Alberta and is the Director of the Alberta Centre for Injury Control and Research.

JORGE FRASCARA teaches in the Department of Art and Design at the University of Alberta.

PETER E.S. FREUND teaches in the Department of Sociology at Montclair State University.

MOHAMMED NASEEMUL HOQUE is a medical student at the University of Alberta.

LEON JAMES is Professor of Psychology at the University of Hawaii.

JOANNE JARVIS is the National Victim Services Manager for Mothers Against Drunk Driving (MADD) Canada and works at the National Office.

CLAY LAFLEUR teaches at the Ontario Institute for the Study of Education, University of Toronto.

PHIL LITKE teaches in the Department of Psychology at the University of Calgary.

LAWRENCE P. LONERO is a partner with Northport Associates working in road-safety research.

DAVID MACGREGOR teaches in the Department of Sociology at King's College, University of Western Ontario.

GEORGE T. MARTIN teaches in the Department of Sociology at Montclair State University.

JEFFREY E. NASH is Professor and Head of the Sociology and Anthropology Department at Southwest Missouri State University.

DONALD A. REDELMEIER, MD, works at Sunnybrook Hospital, University of Toronto.

J. PETER ROTHE is a Senior Associate with the Alberta Centre for Injury Control and Research (ACICR) and Assistant Professor in Public Health, University of Alberta.

SERGIO L. SCHMIDT is Professor at the State University of Rio de Janeiro.

ROBERT J. TIBSHIRANI teaches at Sunnybrook Hospital, University of Toronto.

NIGEL WATERS teaches in the Department of Geography at the University of Calgary. He is also the Director of the Master's in Geographic Information Systems program.

SANY ZEIN is the president of Hamilton-Finn Road Safety Consultants, based in Calgary, and consults on road-safety engineering around the world.

FOREWORD

THE *SHINKANSEN*, OR BULLET TRAIN, darts across the picturesque Japanese landscape at more than 270 kph, one of 130 similar trains operating simultaneously throughout the densely populated network. During peak hours, trains arrive and depart Tokyo Station every three and a half minutes. In total, roughly 1,000 high-speed trains travel daily between Tokyo and Hakata, carrying the equivalent of 4,000 fully loaded 747s.

In the 37 years since the Central Japan Railway Company introduced the Super Express, these high-speed trains have been on time within 30 seconds, with no collisions or derailments—a marvel of transportation-system management. How has the railway been able to sustain its impeccable scheduling and safety record? Since 1992, complexity science has been a large part of the solution. The railway's COMTRAC (computer-aided traffic control) system incorporated a complexity simulator to deal with unpredictable bottlenecks in the schedule, such as snow delays. This faster-than-real-time system, running on 9 Macintosh computers, allows 1,000 train agents to interact with 2,000 track-segment agents and reroute around potential disruptions. This complexity-based solution proved so effective that the railway has been able to increase train frequency and speed while maintaining a perfect safety record and making schedules more flexible.

The *shinkansen* is perhaps the ultimate example of a systems approach to transportation safety. It is hard to resist comparing its safety record—no system failures in 37 years—with the road transportation system in Alberta, which, like many jurisdictions in North America, has a mean time between failures (MTBF) of about five minutes. Of course, the comparison of an open system like road transportation with a quasi-closed system like the Central Japan Railway is more than a little unfair, but the miraculous success of this system gives the lie to the view that collisions, or "accidents," are somehow an inevitable consequence of mobility.

The book *Driving Lessons: Exploring Systems That Make Traffic Safer* is an outcome of the Traffic Safety Summit held in Kananaskis, Alberta, in 1998. The Summit was a collaborative effort conceived under the Mission Possible Traffic Safety Initiative. One of the more ambitious objectives of the Summit was to promote a systems approach to managing road safety—a concept central to the Mission Possible Initiative—and to stimulate exploration of the potential of applying non-linear science—system dynamics, complexity and chaos theory—to this intransigent problem. Dr. Peter Rothe was originally commissioned by the Alberta Motor Association and the Alberta Centre for Injury Control and Research to assemble the conference proceedings, but after some thought he counter-proposed a more ambitious project that would extend the central themes of the Summit by inviting new submissions from presenters and other experts in related disciplines. The proposal was accepted and this book is the result.

While the non-linear sciences of complexity and chaos theory are well developed in disciplines such as quantum physics, cellular biology, computing sciences and meteorology, their application to transportation studies is very much in its infancy. Nonetheless, there is growing recognition that road transportation is a complex adaptive system. Some interesting work is beginning to emerge on topics like the thresholds of chaos in traffic, dynamic wave theory (how the amplification of small inputs produces major disruptions in traffic streams—see, for example, Chapter 9, "Sugar Bear in the Hot Zone," for a fascinating analysis of the aftermath of catastrophic system failure), and simulations using cellular automata to predict self-organizing behaviours in traffic. Increasingly we see examples of cross-fertilization between traditional disciplines—guidance-system software for "smart" missiles based on genetic algorithms, for example. The next decade should see some significant breakthroughs in our understanding of road-system safety through the application of these new tools.

One exciting feature of this book is the exploration of the sub-systems that overlap and interact with the road-transportation system: the political, legal, economic, psychological, sociological and cultural subsystems, to mention a few. There is huge potential for quantum improvement through collaborations between neuropsychologists and engineers; between human factors specialists, designers and collision reconstructionists; between anthropologists, human ecologists and social marketers. Through multidisciplinary and, more importantly, interdisciplinary inquiry and collaboration, we will come to an improved understanding of the dynamics of the system and how human performance affects—and is affected by—other elements of the road-transportation system.

Interestingly, many of the disciplines mentioned are experimenting with their own applications of complexity science. Rae Blackerby's *Application of Chaos Theory to Psychological Models* (1998) is a brilliant case in point. Malcolm Gladwell's *The Tipping Point* (2000), which advances a theory of social epidemics, provides numerous fascinating examples of how carefully selected small inputs can produce large scale social change—a classic demonstration of chaos theory.

At a less esoteric level, the systems approach can be as simple as an acknowledgement that collisions and traffic phenomena are systemic in nature. This is a promising departure from traditional approaches to traffic safety that have been dominated by reductionist Cartesian/Newtonian thinking. The *modus operandi* has been to break the system into component parts and address problem symptoms in a linear, cause-and-effect manner. This simplistic and symptomatic approach has produced some gains, but it has also produced numerous perverse effects. When we ignore the systemic nature of the problem, we discover, to our dismay, that anti-lock brakes—a multi-million dollar improvement in automotive design—not only did not provide a safety benefit but produced a 24-percent increase in single-vehicle crashes. There is significant research that suggests that marking crosswalks, a presumed safety enhancement, actually increases injuries. In both cases, the human factors—the ergonomics of the enhancement—were ignored: a failure to take a systems approach.

Anyone with an interest in traffic or system safety should find this book an interesting theoretical romp. I would like to thank Peter Rothe for the thematic concept of the book and for assembling a stimulating collection.

ROB TAYLOR
Mission Possible
Alberta Motor Association

BEFORE YOU DIVE INTO *Driving Lessons: Exploring Systems That Make Traffic Safer*, I would like to explain the context of this book's development. The articles presented here reflect a loose design-systems theory that served as the original theoretical underpinnings of a Mission Possible traffic-safety conference, Traffic Safety Summit '98. The object of the conference was to challenge traditional roles and thinking, and to build new knowledge by sampling current research in multiple disciplines. By synthesizing this knowledge into understanding through discussion, participants hoped to develop a coordinated action plan.

Speakers from around the world shared their messages, which collectively served as the launch pad for the book you now hold. When the conference sponsors proposed a book to reflect the heart of the conference, I recognized the great potential for such a project to broaden the horizons of traffic safety while staying faithful to the conference, its sponsors and speakers. Furthermore, key conference organizers and I agreed that a book should reach beyond the conference itself and ask noteworthy scholars and practitioners to submit articles on relevant, creative and non-traditional topics that complemented the ideas of the Summit. All submissions were critically reviewed and arranged in an order that corresponds to second-generation cybernetics. The product was intended to be more helpful to traffic-safety professionals than the typical conference proceedings that does little more than compile presentations as submitted.

This book is a compilation of articles that are a part of, yet apart from, the conference. The articles do not negate the principles of the conference; rather, they lend a greater coherence to the person–community–society design.

Collectively, they promote debate and encourage intervention or prevention strategies, opening new doors to familiar issues and proposing ways to address new issues.

I have tried, as far as possible, to present divergent thinking within a loose cybernetic model, and to illustrate how such thinking has potential for action on traffic safety. Hence, this work is a book of alternative thinking, framed within recent cybernetic theory, to explore venues outside the various traffic-safety traditions. It should motivate readers to search deeper, look farther and expect better. It is consistent with my belief that we must put ourselves outside the ordinary range of tradition to find creative solutions.

ACKNOWLEDGEMENTS

WITH A BOOK LIKE THIS ONE, it is difficult to single out specific people and thank them for their extraordinary involvement in the many steps that eventually produced the manuscript. But I shall try. First to be thanked are Mr. Rob Taylor, Director of Mission Possible, and Ms. Joanne Vincenten, Executive Director, Alberta Centre for Injury Control and Research, for their trust in my abilities to carry off such a project, their financial assistance and their support of the concept and ideas. Were it not for these two wonderful people, this book would definitely not have seen the light of day.

Second, I must acknowledge all the authors who contributed their time and energy and who articulated perspectives on the topic. They are Robert Arthur, Walter Barta, Mike Boyes and Phil Litke, Louis Francescutti and Naseem Hoque, Jorge Frascara, Peter Freund and George Martin, Leon James, Joanne Jarvis, Clay Lafleur, Larry Lonero, David MacGregor, Jeffrey Nash and Gary Brinker, Donald Redelmeier and Robert J. Tibshirani, Sergio Schmidt, Nigel Waters and Sany Zein.

Because of unforeseen medical difficulties, Liza Sunley stepped in at the final stages of completion and did a super job. Thank you, Liza. Further, I wish to extend my thanks to Leslie Vermeer, managing editor at the University of Alberta Press. Her support and sense of professional camaraderie added depth and breadth to the completed product.

Finally, I wish to thank the many people behind the scenes, the colleagues who offered their opinions and the clerks and aides who helped assemble the articles. Your help was invaluable.

INTRODUCTION

J. PETER ROTHE

LET ME BEGIN THIS BOOK with the familiar truism that we all suffer, or as Taylor and Watson (1989, p. 1) wrote, "Suffering, psychological or physical, is universal in scope."

There is little new in this observation. In fact, it may sound a little pretentious for the opening of a book on traffic safety. It is designed to be so. Let me expand on the issue of suffering by asking several provoking questions. Has the introduction of the automobile and its many uses exacerbated our suffering? If so, how? Or has the automobile filled a personal, social and economic void, providing more pleasure and fulfillment than it does suffering? These questions, although slightly esoteric, serve as the foundation for new ways in which to define traffic safety.

Over the years we have sought a deep understanding of traffic-safety-related factors like roadway-user behaviour, medical results from crashes, vehicle ergonomics and road engineering. The analysis of these topics has gone a long way toward improving the safety of roadway users. But it has also created a paradox. With extraordinary attention focussed on the mind, body, vehicle and roadway, there evolved a tendency to avoid exploring other vital perspectives like culture, economics, politics and social behaviour. Our assumptions, research methodologies, language for sense-making, research tools and prevention strategies kept us from exploring a range of experiences and interests that contribute to daily driving and safety.

Traffic safety is a complex phenomenon, and it changes with each new generation. Hence, we as traffic-safety incumbents need to change to accommodate such developments as road rage, photo-radar cameras and aging drivers, just to name a few examples. This book was developed to help address such changes.

Driving Lessons: Exploring Systems That Make Traffic Safer begins with a description of the second-generation cybernetic perspective and how it serves as the conceptual thread that binds the different articles together. Second-generation cybernetics frames events according to intersections among different yet related phenomena. This framework helps reduce the complexity of traditions, provides a fuller account of traffic-related phenomena and attends to social changes. It helps us move closer to a broad-based understanding of the topic and thereby better plan and orchestrate preventive measures. The organization of the book is intended to defeat critical responses to old cybernetic theories that are standardized according to tightly controlled feedback loops. Second-generation cybernetics moves beyond these tight controls, adopting a framework that captures the community pulse.

The rest of the book is divided into three sections, organized around personal, institutional and technical sub-systems. In Section One, Sergio Schmidt discusses neuro-behavioural research and traffic behaviour, while Leon James explains how personal stress affects the psychological sub-system. Louis Francescutti, Naseem Hoque and Peter Rothe look at the health sub-system as it relates to traffic safety. The social sub-system is explored in Jeffrey Nash and Gary Brinker's chapter about family and friends, Peter Rothe's chapter about the differences between urban and rural drivers, and Mike Boyes and Phil Litke's chapter about lifespan and driving identities. The last chapter in this section, by Peter Freund and George Martin, examines mobility, social space, movement and consciousness.

To open Section Two, David MacGregor turns his discussion toward the political sub-system as it interacts with roadways. The economic sub-system of the roadway is illustrated in Peter Rothe's article about the economics of traffic dispatch and in Walter Barta's chapter about practising traffic safety in the workplace. The legal subsystem is examined in Joanne Jarvis' discussion of drunk driving and voluntary court monitoring. Jorge Frascara explores the media sub-system in his look at communications and traffic safety. Larry Lonero describes driver training and education in terms of licensure and entry into the world of automobility, while Clay LaFleur's chapter studies the possibilities of action research and traffic safety.

Technology is a mediary that crosses all sub-systems and influences the entire roadway system, and hence, Section Three explores technical sub-systems. Nigel Waters and Rob Arthur discuss the process of analyzing geographic information systems (GIS) in two related papers. Sany Zein extends the discussion into the engineering integration framework. The last two papers look at specific technological introductions that have had a profound effect on traffic safety: cellular phones and red-light cameras. Donald Redelmeier and Robert Tibshirani review recent research on cellphones and their impact on the roadway system, while Peter Rothe discusses the pros and cons of red-light cameras at intersections. The volume concludes with some further thoughts about the complexity of human issues in traffic safety and roadway systems.

At a basic level, this book is intended to explore directions that are contributing to the changing reality of traffic safety. Scholars and practitioners have brought their experiences to bear on the driving situation, defining it according to a more total perspective. Thus, the book is a departure, sometimes radically so, from the past. I hope it helps to open the door for greater opportunities to address serious traffic-safety problems.

1 THE CYBERNETIC FRAMEWORK

J. PETER ROTHE

Traveler, your footsteps are
The road, and nothing more;
Traveller, there is no road;
It is made as you walk.

—ANTONIO MACHADO

THE TRADITIONAL EMPHASIS of cybernetics is on communication and control, as exemplified in Wiener's (1961) early writings. However, this book is structured according to more recent conceptual developments by such exemplars as Maturna (1987). In brief, according to cybernetics, society is composed of a number of systems—such as health, education, the law, economics and the family—that are themselves built on interrelated sub-systems. As it is understood in this book, cybernetics focusses on the interrelationships of the sub-systems and on the patterns of behaviour within sub-systems (Rothe, 2000).

A comprehensive system links many sub-systems (Dym, 1987), forming a cybernetic web. To illustrate, let's compare traffic safety to medicine. Research has linked physical illness to psychological states of stress and personality type, and to social behaviour states of interpersonal relationships and loneliness (Fabrega, 1974). Unmitigated stress and unresolved conflicts have been correlated with the onset of streptococcal infection (Meyers & Hagerty, 1962), heart disease (Watzlawick et al., 1974) and cancer (Cousins, 1983). Further, the course of diseases like asthma has been shown to be influenced by personality patterns (Dym, 1987). Similarly, the onset, course and treatment of major injuries

I

sustained in a car crash have great influence on individual patients, family members, health workers, lawyers and the courts, and emergency personnel; and less influence on civil engineers, driver trainers, teachers and the media.

With the plethora of research findings and perspectives comes the need for theoretical frameworks that can organize and give direction to the emergence of holistic traffic safety. Too many research projects and intervention programs have a narrow focus; they examine only one or two variables, such as the correlation between graduated licenses and the reduction of crashes or between the type of risk and the severity of crashes. Although some traffic-safety initiatives have taken a broader view of the problem, two hurdles remain. First, they imply a linear version of causality, like an account that states that the driver's age is a significant factor causing crashes. (One need only go to the many traffic-safety research conferences to hear presentations that end with the timely conclusion, "The best we can establish is that the major factor causing crashes among the young drivers is their age.") The second hurdle is that traditional frames of research narrow the field of inquiry. For example, many researchers claim that teenagers are risky drivers. According to cybernetic theory, many factors—such as family relationships or supports, education, peer influence and risk-taking in recreational activities—play a role in a teen's driving habits (Rothe, 1990).

Driving is located in an ongoing interaction among the ecological context (exemplified in civil engineering and roadway design); psychological sensitivities (neuro-psychological features, cognition and perception); social factors; economic, political and legal interests; the media; and education. To succeed, the framework should not be cumbersome, but rather simple and accessible.

■ The Framework as Evolving Cybernetics

Unlike traditional approaches to research, in which efforts are made to maintain scientific objectivity, the cybernetic approach is designed to promote understanding of traffic safety not as a compilation of isolated variables but as an interactive process, set about by systematic relationships. Some influences are directly observable while others are unnoticed but profound.

Our view of cybernetic theory is loosely focussed around the concept of adaptation, which refers to the features that compensate for changing overall conditions by making coordinated changes in the sub-systems. Since no system can survive without patterns and structure, the pulse of the system includes regularities, rules and frameworks that organize the system and maintain its efficient workings when significant deviations occur. From a cybernetic point of view, patterns of driver behaviour are adaptive responses to changes, both subtle and gross, in infrastructure (Erchak, 1984). A dynamic system like traffic continually adjusts to both internal changes (such as developmental crises in individual drivers) and external changes (such as poorly constructed intersections that create high mortality rates). For example, economic stress on truckers (produced by transportation industry officials) combined with psychological variables (e.g., personal pressure) and situational factors (e.g., congested traffic) increase the likelihood of altered patterns of driving. Our challenge is to develop a design that recognizes the need for adaptation to change. It requires our attention to constantly changing factors, patterns of stability and adjustments that adapt to the roadway pattern.

I agree with anthropologist Lévi-Strauss (1973) when he stressed that a state of continuing death and injury is a systemic product rather than the product of individual pathology. That means traffic is considered according to the following principles:

- understanding how the parts of traffic relate to each other and constitute the whole of the roadway as a self-organizing process;
- understanding the interactive processes between different sub-systems;
- understanding the likely effects in the whole of roadway-user behaviours, and vice versa;
- understanding the language and emotions most likely to produce stable sub-systems; and
- understanding situational complexity in traffic. (Espejo, 1994, p. 210)

From a cybernetic point of view, recursive cycles focus on relationships among sub-systems like the environmental (roadway conditions during different seasons), psychological (driver anxiety), social (family relationships), economic (cost of attending to crashes), legal (charges and violations) and educational (new training methods for emerging technology like ABS brakes). So, for example, assertive driving by one driver might be followed by either submissive driving or equally aggressive, retaliatory driving by another. Without mitigating factors, like penalties, there is a danger of systemic breakdown and runaway escalation of submission or assertion (Bateson, 1973). Certain circumstances must be introduced so that the drivers and other roadway users are held together by some form of common interest (fear, status, penalty, awareness or a return to a status quo) to establish what has gone wrong and solve the problem. If the situation continues, the actions of both drivers may become even more bizarre. One may tailgate, cut the other off, communicate insults through hands or words, and engage in road rage. Traffic-safety researchers and practitioners need to understand the interconnected factors to avoid a twisted sequence of regenerative feedback. Troublesome driving by one driver expands to other, different driving situations, drawing other drivers into the malaise.

Cybernetics is a multidisciplinary approach that helps to distill and clarify ideas and conceptual patterns, opening new pathways of understanding in traffic safety. It serves as a tool for the analysis of sub-system interactions when dealing with a problem. It assists traffic-safety personnel to elaborate complementary descriptions of traffic events, descriptions that lead to the formation of questions that require traffic-safety researchers to shape many-sided descriptions of events.

■ Towards a Cybernetics of the Observer

Since its inception 40 years ago, cybernetics has had numerous technological and conceptual applications. Wiener (1948) originally described cybernetics as the study of control and communication in person and machine. Examples of technological applications were industrial robots and computers. Since then, ybernetics has been successfully applied to understanding the patterned development of roles in political science, psychology and administration.

Cybernetics originally focussed on observed systems as a control theory applicable to the study of behaviour and organizations (Edwards, 1992). More recent discourse, found in other bodies of knowledge, has been evolving and transforming the original concepts. There has been a shift from simply observing systems to understanding that the world as we know it is constructed by us (Von Glaserfeld, 1984).

We cannot separate traffic phenomena from our systems of knowing. Furthermore, the system must be seen in a new way. To understand a phenomenon, we must look at a situation not as a passive event of input leading to output, but rather as an active event that is internally coherent and organizationally more open than closed (Maturana, 1978). Everyday traffic situations are turned into well-organized and meaningful units (Kampis, 1991, p. 222). Accordingly, the roadway system does not have an independent existence; instead, it is constituted as we interact with each other. It is through these interactions that relationships are formed, in a given space and time.

A system is a way of looking at the world. It is a mental construct of a whole for which it is possible to establish a set of interrelated parts. Its identity, parts and relationships are nothing more than a construct of an observer; and different observers in different contexts and with different purposes make different distinctions. In this sense, the definition of a system is viewpoint-dependent.

In everyday language we talk about health, legal or education systems, making reference to perceived wholes in the real world. We appear to refer to well-defined interactive networks (of humans and other resources) as if they had an objective existence. How often have we heard that the health system is suffering? When I pose this question, I am not only asking as an observer of the health organization but also assuming that other people will share, and make sense, of my construct. I assume that others will ascribe the same purpose to this organization; otherwise, my question is meaningless.

A common assumption is that the parts reflect the nature of the whole, since they take their specific shape at any one time in relation to the contingencies and problems arising in the total situation. For instance, when trouble occurs on the roadway, it is typically seen as "someone else's problem," since those using the roadway often do not know, care about or have the authority to deal with the situation. Remedial action must be initiated and controlled from elsewhere. A degree of passivity and neglect is built into the system.

The system has five major component parts that require clarification. The first is called *redundancy of parts*. Each part is designed to perform specific functions, such as maintaining a sense of self-organization, providing enough room for different people to manoeuvre, maintaining ongoing affairs through interacting parts, and helping to control other parts. Examples of redundancy of parts are police officers who spend their time ensuring that drivers operate within the limits of the law, emergency teams who stand by for crashes and roadway maintenance crews who respond to roadway problems like fallen trees and potholes.

For maximum effect, people operating within various sub-systems add operating functions, so that each part is able to engage in a range of functions rather than just perform a single, specialized activity. For example, police officers engage in traffic-safety programs as school instructors or program facilitators, contribute to seat-belt surveys and get involved in traffic-safety project planning; they acquire these multiple skills so they can perform more jobs. Firefighters learn EMS skills and operate the Jaws of Life to help save motorists. But at any one time, the new skills are not always being used for the job at hand.

The second major part is *redundant functions*. This part suggests that the whole is built into the parts. For example, police officers, traffic authorities, truckers, efficiency experts and road users have fixed roles to perform. The whole is the sum of pre-designed parts. Redundant functions operate where the nature of a person's role is set by the changing pattern of the demands with which s/he is dealing. It is more holistic and all-absorbing. The question for traffic safety is how much redundancy should be built into any given part. It is impossible for everybody to be skilled and knowledgeable about everything. So what do we do?

The third part is *requisite variety*. This part suggests that the internal diversity of any system must match the variety and complexity of its environment if it is to deal with the challenges posed by that environment. A system like the law has policing functions that must be as varied and complex as the traffic environment being controlled. Requisite variety means that all the elements of the law should embody critical dimensions of traffic that police have to deal with, so that they can cope with the demands they are likely to face.

Requisite variety embraces proactive engagement in all its diversity. For example, the roadway system can be developed in a cellular manner around self-organizing, multidisciplinary groups that have the requisite skills and abilities to deal with the environment in a holistic and integrated way. But very often practitioners do the reverse, reducing variety in order to achieve greater consensus.

The fourth part of a system is *minimum critical specification*. It means that practitioners adopt primarily a facilitating and orchestrating role, creating "enabling conditions" that allow a system to find its own form. For example, the more the police attempt to specify or pre-design behaviours, the more those prescriptions erode personal flexibility. Minimum specification helps to preserve flexibility by suggesting that, in general, we should specify no more than is absolutely necessary for a particular activity. In other words, the police should define only those behaviours that directly affect safety, not on convenience, political expediency or economic gain.

The fifth principle of a system is *learning to learn*. In this part, roles are allowed to change and evolve according to circumstances. Hierarchical organization is replaced by a heterarchical pattern, in which the dominant element at any given time depends on the total situation. Learning to learn is intended to design and manage enabling conditions—to create a context that fosters a kind of shared identity and learning orientation. Specialized personnel, educators and self-learning contribute to the functions needed for people to share in the system patterns.

■ Avoiding Noxiants

When we pursue a specific goal, we orient ourselves to a fixed point of reference. When we do so, relationships within systems can usually be seen and manipulated in an instrumental way. We try to create conditions that help achieve targets. In this process, independent and often conflicting lines of action combine to make achieving desired goals increasingly difficult. And when a goal has successfully been reached, another goal soon becomes apparent and the scramble begins again.

A strategy often introduced in traffic safety is the avoidance of noxiants or potential harms. It involves a choice of limits and constraints rather than a choice of ends, creating degrees of freedom that allow meaningful direction to emerge. This cybernetic principle underpins many aspects of social life. Most of our great codes of behaviour are framed in terms of "thou shalt not"; whether we examine the Ten Commandments or contemporary legal systems, we find principles of avoiding noxiants defining a space of acceptable behaviours within which individuals can self-organize. As new noxiants are identified, or old ones deemed less of a threat, they are typically added to or removed from the list, thus modifying the space of action.

■ The Roadway System as a Living System

A living system makes continuous adjustments to maintain its balance, like a race car driver zeroing in on the finish line in stormy weather. With each effort comes new information, and with new information comes better or more appropriate driving (Bateson, 1972). A feedback loop is created or stable, and regular patterns of adjustment (recursive cycles) are invoked (Dym, 1987). Recursive cycles are always changing, although most of the changes are slight, such as a small turn of the wheel for better vision in the rain.

Let's look at an extended example of recursive cycles in the roadway system. George, an intercity trucker, has a problem with drinking alcohol. His safety supervisor warns him about the dangers of his habit. The warning is given in the warehouse office, causing tension in a public space; other truckers leave the office area to escape the tension. George becomes increasingly anxious as the safety supervisor adds a warning letter to his file. He loses his Christmas bonus for the upcoming holidays.

George feels guilty, alone and vengeful. The next day he drinks, the safety supervisor warns him of a suspension and the recursive cycle continues. George then gets caught by the police for drinking and driving, and loses his job driving a truck. A relationship exists among the various system levels: the biological (George's health), the psychological (George's lack of confidence), the social (George's loneliness), the economic (George's loss of Christmas bonus and future income) and the legal (George's charge of impaired driving) all co-evolve. Each may be said to set the stage for the other.

This example shows that the definition of George's predicament encompasses a series of factors. Physical, psychological, social, legal, economic and other aspects are all integral to the situation; they interconnect to provide a whole. When does a drinking problem begin? Does the onset of drinking come from personal pressure or workplace stress? Are the various factors hierarchical or do they form linear logic? Do they interact at strategic junctures to form a system of interplay? Concentrating solely on one element, no matter how important it might be, distorts the problem.

■ Cybernetics with Respect to This Book

Cooperation is the name we may give to the overall interrelationships of things (Burneko, 1991). These interrelationships are more dynamic than static. Everything in this process is itself, by virtue of its interaction with others, mutually constituting one another's being. Such interaction is reality. The mind emerges in the dynamic of an evolving universe. So it is in traffic safety.

The cybernetic framework presented in this book consists of a series of vibrant, changing sub-systems that interpenetrate one another at key junctures. They are inextricably engaged with one another in dynamic cooperation to form a changing system that seeks stability amid all its changes. In the process, one sub-system triggers the workings of the next one. According to Dym (1987), such a system is like the transmission of electrical messages through the nervous system. The firing occurs when the activity in one nerve reaches certain electrical potential. In the process, patterns of interaction are developed as recursive measures.

The version of cybernetics embraced by this book is based on the complementary relationship between change and stability (Keeny, 1983). That is, driving systems maintain their form throughout various processes and instances of change. The point for the book is to signify that events traditionally labeled as cause or contributing factor and those labelled as effect have reciprocal relationships (Dym, 1987). These factors co-evolve during the course of the problem and become ingredients of change in the recursive cycle to maintain stability over time. A complex, unified field like a trucking company, at a given time, can be represented in a simple form, sensitive to both internal and external change.

Traffic safety can be divided into a number of major areas. The first area is the psychological self as driver, followed by physical well-being or health. A third aspect is the social—family and friends. The fourth element includes physical environment and engineering: roadway design. The fifth area is the legal arena—police and the courts—while the sixth is politics. Economics and industry form the seventh area, while the eighth is driver training. The ninth and tenth are education and media. Cutting across these sub-systems is technology, a mediary that forms junctures at each sub-unit, creating change and impact.

For the present purposes, I define the course of traffic as the shifting design of recursive cycles as they move through the geo-psycho-social field, changing in order to remain stable and positive. Throughout, intervention imitates this cybernetic model, as it attempts to force adjustments of the system so that specific issues are no longer integral parts. Rather, the parts change to form stability through many adjustments made to the different levels of the systems.

SECTION ONE
PERSONAL SUB-SYSTEMS

WHAT RESOURCES MUST DRIVERS HAVE in order to operate a vehicle comfortably and safely in a stressful social and physical environment? Psychologists see driving health as the driver's ability to cope with the mental processing of the traffic environment, other road users, and personal levels of confidence, skill and problem-solving. Drivers must use their internal resources to function successfully in traffic.

If they possess highly developed psychological resources, drivers can deal with great traffic complexities and still maintain the integrity of their personalities. In some cases, drivers' internal adaptive mechanisms can be redeveloped so that they can compensate in the face of driving stress (Becker, 1966). Good mental health for drivers means a capacity to adapt to changing roadway circumstances, events and moods without fleeing from them, becoming physically or emotionally ill, or taking precipitous action that does harm to the driver or other roadway users. Chapters 2 and 3 examine how personal psychology interacts with driving and traffic safety.

■ The Health Sub-System

Without good health, people are destined to suffer or die prematurely. But health is multidimensional. The World Health Organization (WHO) defines health as a complete state of physical, mental and social well-being and not merely the absence of illness. The promotion of health and our response to injury form a vital system that affects people's everyday life.

According to Shah (1994, p. 4), health not only focusses on the integrity of the body but also encompasses social and political concerns and the relationship of individuals to their environment. Health directly affects traffic and the many sub-systems that support the traffic context. Thus, the health system demands inclusion as a dominant unit in the cybernetic analysis of traffic. Chapter 4 looks at an innovative, community-based model for responding to traffic-safety issues.

■ The Social Sub-System

Human beings are essentially social beings. It is in the presence of others and in cooperation with others that we discover ourselves, learn appropriate social roles, act out social expectations and come to experience the world in a shared way.

We need not stray too far to appreciate how social behaviour on its grand scale is directly applicable to the roadway. Families, peers, coworkers, organizations and institutions all influence roadway users before, during or after engaging in driving, biking or walking. Social study of the roadway system is inevitably the study of society itself, and it reproduces the controversies, challenges and strengths experienced by society generally. It embodies the folk wisdom, truisms and clichés that make up a significant part of people's everyday knowledge about the world. The world in which roadway users live entails a meaning of traffic that is maintained, threatened or recreated in face-to-face relations with other people, the most important of which is the micro-world of family. Chapters 5 and 6 examine the formation of social roles, behaviours and responsibilities in the context of driving.

■ The Cultural Sub-System

The fundamental structures in which social experience takes place are seldom questioned: they appear to us as natural and self-evident features of life. For example, the social experience of driving is taken for granted as a familiar routine regardless of where the drivers live. While we are on the road, we presume similar backgrounds, experiences, needs, values and patterns of behaviour. Chapter 7 looks at some of the assumptions we hold about rural versus urban drivers, while Chapter 8 considers the automobile within a culture of space.

The driving experience occurs in a varied and complex environment. Yet if we stand back and observe our actions, and the reasoning behind those actions, we can discern patterns, trends and adaptations that reflect our situatedness in the world. If, however, something happens to interrupt routine behaviour, we are more likely to become aware of our patterns and reflect on their influence on our behavior. The chapters in this section look at the possibilities for change within personal sub-systems.

2

NEURO-BEHAVIOURAL VARIABLES AND TRAFFIC SAFETY

SERGIO L. SCHMIDT

■ **The Importance of Neuropsychology and Higher Brain Functions**

NEUROPSYCHOLOGY COVERS the most advanced and complex aspects of cognition and behaviour. The domain of neuropsychology includes such functions as memory, attention, language, perception, planning and decision-making, personality and social behaviour; its focus is on disorders of these functions. To test higher-order behaviour, the neuropsychologist has access to testing procedures that allow quantification of complex functions such as attention and memory.

Clinical neuropsychology is an applied science concerned with the behavioural expression of brain dysfunction. Specialists often consult not only in departments of neurology, neurosurgery and psychiatry but also in emergency (e.g., patients with traumatic brain injury), oncology (e.g., CNS tumours), infectious disease (e.g., AIDS), cardiology (e.g., to evaluate patients who have suffered strokes) and rehabilitation departments. Neuropsychologists are widely accepted as necessary members of multidisciplinary teams that deal with assessment, care and treatment of brain-damaged patients. Further, recent technological advances in structural and functional neuroimaging technologies (e.g., functional magnetic resonance imaging) have provided support for the validity of several neuropsychological instruments.

Neuropsychology continues to change. Whereas before, the first large-scale demand for neuropsychology was the need for screening and diagnosis of behaviourally disturbed servicemen during war time, today neuropsychological assessments help identify candidates for military services who may have behavioural problems. In addition, functional neuroimaging data clarified the relationship between brain activity and behaviour in normal subjects, usually described as people without structural brain lesions. It is well established that neuropsychological data provide sensitive indices of mental efficiency. Demands on attention, visuo-spatial abilities and information-processing make driving a complex cognitive task (Hunt et al., 1993, 1997). Thus, it is conceivable that a neuropsychological examination could answer questions about a person's ability to drive a car.

The first part of this chapter describes how neuropsychological examination can be used for the improvement of medical and psychological screening for selecting drivers. Consideration is given not only to potential contributions to screening systems but also potential contributions that translate into viable benefits for mobility. The second part of this chapter discusses neuropsychological explanations of human errors in complex systems. This analysis focusses on the need for engineering methods to support or constrain fallible human behaviour. Finally, I discuss the contribution of social and cultural experiences, and how economic pressures, personal demands and lifestyle can affect important neuropsychological variables.

■ Neuropsychology and Screening Systems

Driver selection by medical and psychological tests is primarily intended to protect people from risks created by dangerous drivers. Good health has generally been considered a precondition for driving ability. In many countries, the medical examination is an obligatory part of the initial screening. In some jurisdictions, drivers forty-five and older must pass a medical examination every five years or so, depending on age (Kroj & Utzelmann, 1997). Clearly, license-related health controls imply costs. So far, however, no corresponding benefits have been clearly demonstrated. Moreover, it has been reported that only a superficial check-up may be included in screening exams.

However, medical intervention cannot be imposed on people if its usefulness has not been clearly demonstrated. In addition, when people's mobility is limited, especially in the elderly, their health may decline, leading to increased costs for institutional care. Therefore, unsatisfactory screening systems are unacceptable from both ethical and economical points of view. Even if we assume that the medical exam is not a superficial check-up, a question still remains. Does an examination of general health and vision fulfill the criteria of specificity and sensitivity? This question must be answered on the basis of solid scientific evidence (Drachman, 1988). This is where neuropsychological research can contribute. Neuropsychological research has helped to define testing methods to identify subgroups of older drivers who actually have a higher-than-acceptable crash risk.

While driving promotes independence for the elderly, studies have reported that accident and fatality rates for senior drivers are significantly higher than those for other age groups (Evans, 1988). In this regard, age-associated illness that affects cognition, such as Alzheimer's disease, is expected to impair driving ability. Accordingly, investigators have demonstrated that individuals with dementia are more likely to be involved in motor-vehicle traffic crashes than healthy age-matched controls (Parasuraman & Nestor, 1991). However, it is possible to speculate that not all persons in the earliest stages of dementia of the Alzheimer type (DAT) are unsafe drivers. This hypothesis is supported by the fact that driving represents a highly automated skill and some automatic tasks are well preserved in DAT. This issue was addressed by a prospective study involving patients with DAT and healthy controls that were assessed using a standardised road test. Hunt et al. (1997) found that dementia affects driving performance even in its mild stages. They proposed that functional assessment of driving ability should include performance-based road tests that examine cognitive behaviours. More recently, Ducheks et al. (1998) examined performance on various neuropsychological measures in relation to driving, in order to better identify screening measures that predict unsafe driving in DAT patients. The researchers found that general cognitive status may be useful but that measures of visual attention better differentiate safe from unsafe drivers in the DAT population. They pointed out that the assessment of visual attention processing, which relies on the ability to select relevant information in the stimulus environment and inhibit irrelevant information, is the best predictor of driving performance in mildly DAT or otherwise demented drivers (Ducheks et al., 1998).

Although drivers suffering from dementia may be responsible for a significant number of vehicle crashes among the older driver population, it is still important to find adequate routine screening measures that can predict unsafe driving in healthy senior drivers. In this regard, Owsley et al. (1998) made an important discovery that will likely influence how older drivers will be screened for licensing. Their prospective study found that those who performed poorly on a test of visual attention were 2.2 times more likely to be involved in a car crash during a 3-year follow-up period. Further, the study showed that visual attention in healthy older drivers is more closely associated with car crashes than any other variable, including conventional ophthalmologic tests.

From the above discussion it is clear that, for both older healthy drivers and those who suffer from age-associated illness, neuropsychological assessment of visual attention should be incorporated into routine screening. There is solid scientific evidence that a careful exam of visual attention is better than conventional mental-status batteries (Owsley et al., 1998). More important is the fact that this finding would force a departure from the current reliance on conventional visual tests, such as visual acuity and visual field, which have not been predictive of crashes. As mentioned before, the arbitrary restriction of driving privileges for seniors who are still safe drivers limits their mobility and represents a bigger health risk than crash rates (Hakamies-Blomqvist, 1997). Therefore, medical exams that cover only general health and vision do not fulfil the criteria of specificity and sensitivity needed for a valid and reliable screening of drivers.

The finding that disturbances of visual attention affect driving performance in older drivers may explain the excess risk factors for this age group. Elderly drivers demonstrate excess risk for factors such as inattention, improper turning and collisions at intersections (Zhang et al., 1998). In contrast, risk factors for young drivers include alcohol and illicit drug use, fatigue and falling asleep, and speeding (Robertson, 1981). This is particularly important because the distribution of the incidence and mortality rates associated with vehicle crashes depends on age: young and elderly drivers have a higher risk of being involved in fatal crashes than have middle-aged drivers. This finding leads us to another question: can neuropsychology improve the screening system for young drivers?

■ An Improved Screening System

Considering the risk factors associated with young drivers, a highly relevant issue is the extent to which the driver's personality is an underlying causal factor. To address the problem properly, we must look at the phenomenon of sensation-seeking, typically defined as "the need for varied, novel, and complex sensations and experiences and the willingness to take physical and social risks for the sake of such experiences" (Hilakivi & Veilahti, 1989; Stacy et al., 1991). As expected, there is a positive relationship between sensation-seeking and risky driving. The ability to screen for the sensation-seeking predisposition has implications for traffic safety that may be explored by further neuropsychological research. It is also worth mentioning that individuals with a higher disposition to sensation-seeking have different levels of norepinephrine and dopamine than do individuals with a low disposition to sensation-seeking. According to Zuckerman (1983), the differences between low and high sensation-seeking subjects may occur in the part of the brain's denominated limbic system, which provides rewards and punishments. This finding opens up many possibilities for future research on the relationship between the brain and driving.

Another point of interest is the assessment of patients who wish to return to driving after suffering an acute disease. Let's focus on stroke patients. In certain countries, stroke patients who wish to return to driving must pass a medical-psychological exam or be evaluated in a driving centre (Nouri & Lincoln, 1992). Depending on how they perform on driving assessments, they may or may not be advised to drive. According to some authors (e.g., Nouri & Lincoln, 1992), the advice is normally based on subjective criteria, which may be inconsistently adopted. However, simple and easily administered cognitive tests may be reliably used as indicators of driving performance. Although cognitive tests may be useful, we hypothesize that a careful examination of visual perception is better than mental status batteries, which contain insufficient measures of visual perception. This hypothesis is based on two facts. First, perceptual problems are common following strokes: right cerebral hemisphere lesions give rise to deficits in visual spatial tasks, while left cerebral hemisphere lesions cause difficulties in more complex spatial tasks, such as route finding (Edmans, 1987). Second, visual perception problems in stroke patients may be responsible for the phenomenon of "looking without seeing" that has been reported as an important cause of vehicle crashes. In other words, patients' problems in visual perception of objects and space may impair recognition of the "target" and the appropriate reaction (for instance, making the appropriate response after looking at a red light). However, we must admit that while such relationships can easily be hypothesized, they are much more difficult to demonstrate empirically. Thus, neuropsychological research is needed to give scientific support to defining valid testing methods that could be used to identify who among stroke patients actually has a higher-than-acceptable crash risk.

The analysis of the relationship between the brain and driving has provided scientific support for the use of neuropsychological tests in driver assessment. Driving is a complex cognitive task. Drivers "see" with their brain, which is why "looking without seeing" or driving without paying close attention to the task is a common contributory factor to vehicle crashes. The ophthalmologic exam, covering visual field and visual acuity, is an outdated practice that cannot predict vehicle crashes, and must be replaced by neuropsychological assessments of visual attention and perception. Although neuropsychology is essential for the improvement of the screening system, it is also necessary to extend the analysis of the relationship between brain and driving to better facilitate the task for drivers. For example, because we know that older drivers face visual attention problems, it is important for traffic engineers and neuropsychologists to re-design the driving task, to the extent possible, to make it easier for the older operator (e.g., reducing visual "intrusion" in intersections).

■ Supporting Fallible Human Behaviour

It is now clear that neuropsychologists and engineers must work together to facilitate the driving task and find ways to support fallible human behaviour. Let's look at two specific topics: drowsy driving and alerting devices, and handedness (that is, the fact that we have unequal skills in our hands and most people are right-handed).

I would like to stress at the onset of the discussion of drowsy driving that sleep is a neurobiological need. The sleep–wake cycle is governed by homeostatic and circadian factors (Carskadon & Dement, 1981). The term *homeostasis* refers to the biological processes that keep body variables within a fixed range. In the context of the need for sleep, the longer the period of wakefulness, the more difficult it is to resist sleeping. *Circadian* comes from the Latin words *circum* (about) and *dies* (day); an endogenous circadian rhythm is thus a self-regulated rhythm that lasts about a day. Homeostatic mechanisms control circadian factors to regulate the timing of sleeping and waking. The practical implication for those who sleep at night is that there is a predictable pattern of two peaks of sleepiness, which commonly occur during the afternoon (i.e., about twelve hours after the mid-sleep period) and before bedtime (at night) (Carskadon & Dement, 1987). Moreover, the sleep–wake cycle is not a pattern we can decide to ignore. Sleepiness can cause motor-vehicle crashes because it impairs performance (reaction time, vigilance, attention and information-processing) and can lead to the inability to resist falling sleep at the wheel (Brown, 1994; Horne & Reyner, 1995). Untreated or unrecognized sleep disorders, such as sleep apnea syndrome and narcolepsy, and sleep loss are two factors that are definitively associated with increased risk of drowsy driving. In sleep apnea syndrome, individuals are unable to breathe while sleeping. Poor sleep often leads to daytime sleepiness. Narcolepsy also causes daytime sleepiness, and patients exhibit approximately fifteen-minute involuntary naps at three-hour intervals throughout the day (Dinges, 1995). However, sleep loss is by far the primary cause of drowsy driving. Because we now recognize sleepiness as a serious problem for traffic safety, we have begun to develop countermeasures and alerting devices. For example, engineers have developed rumble strips for the shoulder of roads. American reports on the effectiveness of rumble strips have shown that they reduce crashes due to driving off the road by nearly 40 percent (National Sleep Foundation, 1997). There are also many devices designed to detect and evaluate driver sleepiness. These developments clearly illustrate the impact of the knowledge of the brain mechanisms involved in the driver task and its association with the development of traffic engineering methods intended to support fallible human behaviour.

The second issue is handedness. Handedness is a remarkable human charac-teristic, with 90 percent of people being right-handed (Oldfield, 1971). It is now clear that handedness must be taken into account in neuropsychological assessments because right-handers show greater manual asymmetries than left-handers in several motor and visual-motor tests (Schmidt et al., 2000 a, b). This finding is vital for screening drivers since adequate norms depend on handedness. Even though left-handers have motor skills equal to or better than right-handers, they are nearly twice as likely to have car crashes and nearly four times as likely to die in car crashes than are right-handers. Epidemiologists have argued that true death rates for left-handers can only be ascertained by measuring the percentage of left-handers who die relative to the percentage of the general population. However, there are physiological differences between right-handers and left-handers that may lend theoretical support to the claim that left-handers are more prone to die in motor-vehicle crashes (Coren, 1992). In a test of startle and defence reflexes, it was found that left-handers raised their right hand higher than their left hand. Right-handers exhibited the opposite pattern. Thus, it was speculated that this response could make it more likely for startled left-handed drivers with both hands on the steering wheel to swerve left—into oncoming traffic (Coren, 1992). In terms of traffic engineering, it is suggested that gearshifts on cars are more hazardous for left-handers if they drive on the left as usually happens in many countries (Great Britain is an exception). Further research is needed to verify whether these hypotheses are true. However, traffic-engineering methods need to consider fallible behaviour in left-handers.

■ Social and Cultural Experiences

In future, the evaluation of neuropsychological data must take into account the contribution of social and cultural experiences and attitudes to test perform-ance. Society places specific demands on people that may interfere with basic neuropsychological processes required for safe driving. The best example is the economic pressure to work instead of sleep. Many people do not get the sleep they need because their schedules do not allow adequate time for it. Neuropsychological research on cognitive demands related to driving makes clear that sleep cannot be seen as a luxury, since we cannot "decide" to ignore the sleep–wake cycle.

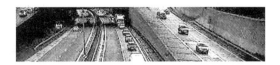

ALTHOUGH I HAVE FOCUSSED on the brain mechanisms involved in the driving task, traffic behaviour must be seen as a systemic product rather than a product of individual behaviour. A full description of traffic safety can be made only if we use a wide context. Thus, I propose that neuropsychology is indispensable for those interested in traffic safety.

3

DEALING WITH STRESS, AGGRESSION AND PRESSURE IN THE VEHICLE

Taxonomy of Driving Behaviour as Affective, Cognitive and Sensorimotor

LEON JAMES

DRIVING IN TRAFFIC routinely involves events and incidents. Events are normal sequential manoeuvres such as stopping for lights, changing lanes and braking. Incidents are frequent but unpredictable events. Some incidents are dangerous and frightening, like near-misses, while others are merely annoying or depressing, like missing one's turn or being insulted by a motorist. Driving events and incidents are the source of psychological forces capable of producing powerful feelings and irrational thought sequences. Driving is a highly dramatic activity that millions of people perform daily. The drama stems from high risk and unpredictability.

Driving has two conflicting structural components: predictability and unpredictability. Both are present all of the time. Predictability, like maintaining steady speed in one's lane, creates safety, security and usually escape from disaster. Unpredictability, like impulsive lane changes without signalling, creates danger, stress and frequently crashes. For many people, driving is linked to freedom of locomotion. On the one hand they get into cars and drive off where they please, the very symbol of freedom and independence. But on the other hand, they encounter restrictions and constrictions that prevent them from driving as they wish.

The following list identifies fifteen widely known aspects of driving that act as stressors. They pose emotional challenges that may provoke hostility and aggressiveness on the road.

1. IMMOBILITY: During driving, most of the body remains still and passive, unlike walking, in which the entire body exerts effort and remains continuously active. Tension tends to build up when the body is physically restricted and constricted.

2. CONSTRICTION: Motor vehicles are restricted to street lanes and narrow bands of highway. In congested traffic, one's progress is inevitably blocked by other cars. Being thwarted when you expect to go forward arouses feelings of restriction and constriction, and, concurrently, anxiety and the desire to escape the constriction. This anxiety and avoidance prompts drivers to perform risky or aggressive manoeuvres that may cause accidents.

3. REGULATION: Driving is a regulated activity, which means that government agencies and law enforcement officers tell drivers where, how and how fast to drive. Cars and trucks have powerful engines capable of going much faster than is permitted. Drivers are punished for violating these regulations, which they are responsible for knowing and obeying. This imposition, although lawful and necessary, arouses a rebellious streak in many people, which prompts them to disregard whatever regulations seem contrary to their mood or wrong at a given moment.

4. LACK OF CONTROL: Traffic follows the laws that govern flow patterns like rivers, pipes, blood vessels or streaming molecules. In congested traffic, flow depends on the available spaces around the cars, as can be ascertained from the view of a traffic helicopter or from a bridge above the highway. When one car slows down, hundreds of other cars behind run out of space and must tap their brakes to slow down or stop altogether. No matter how we drive, it's impossible to beat the traffic waves, which originate miles from where we are. This lack of control is frustrating and stress-producing, and tends to lead to drivers' venting their anger on whoever is around—another driver, or a passenger, pedestrian, construction worker or government official.

5. BEING PUT IN DANGER: People love their cars. But even a scratch can be stress-producing because it reduces the car's value and is expensive to repair. Congested traffic, filled with impatient and aggressive drivers, numerous hair-raising close calls and hostile incidents within moments of each other, produces real physiological stress, along with many negative emotions: fear, resentment, rage, helplessness, moodiness and depression. For many motorists, driving becomes a dreaded, daily drudge, an emotional roller coaster and a source of danger and stress.

6. TERRITORIALITY: The symbolic portrayal of the car is tied to individual freedom and self-esteem, promoting an attitude of defensiveness and territoriality. Motorists consider the space inside the car to be a castle and the space around the car their territory. As a result, they feel repeatedly insulted or invaded while they drive, leading them to a hostile mental state. Some drivers adopt warlike postures and aggressive reactions to routine incidents, which are perceived as skirmishes, battles or duels between drivers.

7. DIVERSITY: There are about 200 million licensed drivers in North America today, representing a diversity of drivers who vary in experience, knowledge, ability, style and purpose for being on the road. These social differences reduce our sense of predictability because drivers with different abilities and purposes don't behave according to our expected norms. Our peace and confidence are shaken by traffic events that are unexpected, and driving becomes more complex, more emotionally challenging. Diversity or plurality increases stress because it creates more unpredictability.

8. MULTI-TASKING: The increase in dashboard complexity and in-car activities, like eating, talking on the phone, and checking voice mail and e-mail, challenge people's ability to remain alert and focussed behind the wheel. Drivers become more irritated at each other when their attention seems to be lacking due to multi-tasking behind the wheel. Multi-tasking without adequate training increases stress by dividing attention and reducing alertness.

9. DENYING OUR MISTAKES: Driving is typically performed through automatic habits acquired over years, which means that much of it occurs outside people's conscious awareness. Drivers typically tend to exaggerate their own "excellence," overlooking their many mistakes. When passengers complain or when other drivers are endangered by these mistakes, there is a strong tendency to see complaints as unwarranted and deny the mistakes. Denial allows drivers to feel self-righteous and indignant at others, enough to want to punish and retaliate, adding to the general hostility and stress level on highways.

10. CYNICISM: Many people have learned to drive under the supervision of parents and teachers who are critical and judgemental. We don't just learn to manipulate the vehicle; we also acquire an over-critical mental attitude towards it. As children we are exposed to the constant judge-

mental behaviour of the adults who drive us around; it is reinforced in movies portraying drivers behaving badly. This culture of mutual cynicism among motorists promotes an active and negative emotional life behind the wheel. Negative emotions are stress-producing.

11. LOSS OF OBJECTIVITY: Driving incidents are not neutral: someone is always thought to be at fault. We tend naturally to want to attribute fault to others rather than to ourselves, and we lose objectivity and right judgement when a dispute arises. This self-serving bias even influences the memory of what happened, slanting the guilt away from self and placing it on others. Subjectivity increases stress by strengthening the feeling that one has been wronged.

12. VENTING: Part of our cultural heritage is the process of venting anger by reciting the details of another individual's objectionable behaviour. The nature of venting is such that it increases by its own logic until it breaks out into overt hostility and even physical violence. People need motivation and training to bring venting under control before it explodes into the open. Until it is brought under conscious control, we feel venting as an energizing "rush" that promotes aggressiveness and violence. Nevertheless, this seductive feeling is short-lived and is accompanied by a stream of anger-producing thoughts that impair our judgement and tempt us into rash and dangerous actions. Repeated venting takes its toll on the immune system and acts as physiological stress with injurious effects on the cardio-vascular system (Williams & Williams, 1993).

13. UNPREDICTABILITY: The street and highway create an environment of drama, danger and uncertainty. In addition, heat, noise and odours act as physiological stress and aggravate feelings of frustration and resentment. Competition, hostility and rushing further intensify negative emotions. The driving environment has become tedious, brutish and dangerous, difficult to adjust to on the emotional plane.

14. AMBIGUITY: Motorists don't have an accepted or official gestural communication language. There is no easy way of saying "Oops, I'm sorry!" as we do in a bank line, and this inability allows for ambiguity to arise: "Did he just flip me off or was that an apology?" It would no doubt help if vehicles were equipped with an electronic display allowing drivers to flash pre-recorded messages. Lack of clear communication between motorists creates ambiguity, which contributes to stress.

15. LACK OF EMOTIONAL INTELLIGENCE: Driver education was traditionally conceived of as a way to acquaint students with some general principles of safety, followed by a few hours of supervised hands-on experience behind the wheel or on a driving simulator. Developing sound judgement and emotional self-control was not part of the training, even though these goals were mentioned as essential. Most drivers today are untrained, or under-trained, in cognitive and affective skills. Cognitive skills are good habits of thinking and judgement. Affective skills are good habits of attitude and motivation. Drivers thus lack the necessary coping abilities such as how to cool off when angered or frustrated, or how to cooperate with, and not hinder, the traffic flow. This lack of training in emotional intelligence (Goleman, 1995) creates high stress conditions for most drivers.

It is common to relate aggressiveness to social and environmental factors, in addition to individual personality factors. For instance, congestion on highways and anonymity in cars interact with faulty attitudes and inadequate coping skills to produce aggressive traffic behaviour under certain identifiable critical conditions. These apparent triggering conditions are unpredictable and involve symbolic meaning for the dignity or self-worth of the interactants who may later report having felt that they were insulted or threatened. It is part of popular psychology to call these provocative and dramatic conditions "triggers," as in, "It's not my fault. He provoked me. It's his fault. He made me do it." The trigger theory of anger serves to absolve the perpetrator from some or all of the responsibility for the aggression or violence. The attackers construct themselves as the victims through self-serving speech acts by which they escape culpability and opprobrium (Searle, 1969). It is common for road-ragers to show no remorse for their assaults, judging what they did as justified and deserved.

■ Road Rage and Aggressive Driving
Driving places millions of people in a position of experiencing health and economic risks, daily hassles and possible tragedies. The roadway environment appears to have become more hostile and dangerous, leading to more traffic and transportation regulations. A dozen US states have passed aggressive driving bills that change what were merely citations and vehicle checks to misdemeanors or felonies, accompanied by mandatory classes that help offenders better manage their traffic emotions.

Law enforcement initiatives against aggressive drivers are called "aggressive initiatives." Federal agencies are promoting the use of integrated action between several police forces, including helicopter support. The evidence of aggressive driving appears to be growing in the media and on the World Wide Web, where numerous activist groups promote citizen involvement in monitoring and reporting the license plates of aggressive drivers. Such drivers are usually depicted as dangerous people, like car thieves or bank robbers.

However, personal research on what drivers think and feel behind the wheel has convinced me that aggressive driving is a cultural norm, not a deviant behaviour. We acquire hostile driving norms in childhood as passengers and adults; we practice these norms and pass them on to our children. Still, individual differences, in terms of frequency and modality of expressing hostility, remain. These differences are conditioned by social factors such as gender, education, age, personality style, demeanor and conduct. For instance, we would expect gender differences in driving aggressiveness to be consistent with cultural norms for family or workplace violence: men are commonly more aggressive than women.

The likelihood of more men participating in aggressive driving was evident in the results of a study I recently completed (James, 1998). Data collection of a Web survey of 2010 respondents was completed in 1998. Participants were invited to respond to itemized lists of driving behaviours often considered aggressive and illegal. By checking items, respondents were making confessions or self-witnessing reports like "I sometimes engage in this behaviour." Tabulating the results in terms of demographic variables allowed us to explore various cultural influences on specific forms of aggressive driving. For example, Table 3.1 displays findings established by gender.

More men report engaging in aggressive driving behaviours than do women; the percentage differences are statistically significant for all items. These results confirm what earlier surveys have found: men drive more aggressively than women and manifest road-rage symptoms more regularly. However, popular surveys show that a growing number of women are engaging in aggressive driving behaviour and are involved in a higher rate of non-fatal collisions than men (Woman Motorist, 1999). The greater aggressiveness of men drivers and the increasing aggressiveness of women drivers are cultural trends that reflect an expanding permissiveness towards the expression of anger behind the wheel. Some of the rise in women's aggressive driving is attributed to the increased presence of women in the workplace. There are 88 million licensed women drivers in the US today. The proportion of women in the driver population rose from 43 percent in 1963 to 50 percent in 1999. More women are stuck in congested traffic, experiencing the stress and frustration men have endured for decades. Additionally, women have more stops to make while they cart children to school, sports and lessons, as well as driving to work, running errands, shopping and banking. Women are forced to drive

TABLE 3.1
Self-reported aggressive driving behaviour

	% of Men	% of Women
making illegal turns	18	12
not signalling lane changes	26	20
following very close	15	13
going through red lights	9	7
swearing, name-calling	59	57
speeding 15 to 25 mph	46	32
yelling at another driver	34	31
honking to protest	39	36
revving engine to retaliate	12	8
making an insulting gesture	28	20
tailgating dangerously	14	9
shining bright lights to retaliate	25	13
braking suddenly to punish	35	29
deliberately cutting off	19	10
using car to block the way	21	13
using car as weapon to attack	4	1
chasing a car in hot pursuit	15	4
getting into a physical fight	4	1

under time pressure during congestion. As a result, auto insurance rates for young women are now closer to that of inexperienced young men, who are still being charged 185 percent above the base rate (MSN MoneyCentral, 1999).

Health professionals generally attribute part of the increase in driving pugnacity to social factors such as swelling congestion, urbanization, dual-income families, workplace downsizing that increases crowding, family discord, job dissatisfaction and physical illness. The connection between stress and illness has long been established in medicine, and new research shows that driving-related stress is no different from life stress in the way it affects our health (APA Monitor, 1996). The overt expression of anger and hostile behaviour is normally "inhibited" or kept under wraps because we are directly or indirectly punished for it in various ways. In the past decade, public schools have implemented conflict-resolution and peer-mediation programs to help children acquire the habit of resolving disagreements non-physically, non-violently (Goleman, 1995). The key element of this civilized conduct is the skill of inhibiting the physical expression of anger or fear, so it doesn't come out in provocative or violent behaviour. When a neighbor encroaches on our territory, normally we don't start shooting or suing. We first find out what's going on, why it's happening and what we can do about it peacefully and lawfully through discussion or submission of a formal complaint. This principle of non-aggressiveness has been overtaken by a cynicism on the highways. As educators and change agents, we must find ways to restore it.

One of the major reasons that highways have become more unsafe is people's unwillingness to scrutinize their own conduct; they prefer to blame other drivers. Surveys consistently show that most people have an inflated self-image of their motoring ability, rating the safety of their own driving as much better than the average motorist's and underestimating or dismissing their own faults. For instance, two out of three drivers (67 percent) rate themselves almost perfect drivers (9 or 10 on a 10-point scale), while the rest consider themselves above average (6 to 8). Surveys typically show that 70 percent of drivers report being a victim of an aggressive driver, while only 30 percent admit to being aggressive drivers (James, 1998). One way to examine this finding is to compare the aggressiveness of the two-thirds majority of drivers who rate themselves as near perfect with the one-third minority that see themselves "above average, but with some room to improve" (James, 1998).

The difference is dramatic. The drivers who consider themselves near perfect or excellent, with no room for improvement, also confess to significantly more aggressiveness than drivers who see themselves as still improving. Despite their self-confessed aggressiveness, the respondents still thought of themselves as near-perfect drivers with little room to improve. This egocentric phenomenon can be seen in specific forms of aggressive behaviour. For example, those who see themselves as near-perfect drivers admit to twice as much chasing of other cars compared to those who see themselves as less perfect; the difference, 15 percent vs. 8 percent, is statistically significant (James, 1998). The fact is clear: part of being an aggressive driver is to deny the need to improve. This is what I call resistance to change.

■ Why Intervention Hasn't Worked
In North America, cars have been mass-produced for more than 100 years; there are now 177 million licensed drivers in the United States alone. Driving

is the most dangerous activity for the majority of people in an industrialized society. Road crashes have killed millions of people since 1900, and the number of crashes increases in proportion to the number of drivers and the total number of miles driven in a jurisdiction. Although still high, traffic-related deaths and serious injuries in North America have reduced as a result of several developments:

- *more and better roads:* safer roads with better traction, visibility and maintenance;
- *better-designed cars:* cars equipped with safety devices and crash-proof designs that save lives—safety belt, air bag, child-restraint car seats, shock absorption and controlled collapse, crash tests with dummies;
- *better emergency medical services and infrastructure on highways and streets:* more survivors after crashes;
- *better law enforcement:* more personnel, use of electronic surveillance devices on highways and key intersections, legislation to facilitate the conviction of guilty drivers, greater involvement of courts in remedial driver training for offenders;
- *mandated driver and safety education in schools:* graduated licensing and other special provisions for elderly and handicapped drivers;
- *more sophisticated transportation-management systems:* computer-controlled traffic lights, traffic-calming devices, re-routing schemes, high-occupancy vehicle (HOV) lanes, alternative transportation initiatives; and
- *economic incentives:* higher insurance premiums for accident-prone drivers, increased incentives or lower insurance premiums for drivers who remain accident-free, special benefits accruing for enrolling in refresher courses and other self-improvement activities.

It is important to note that despite these definite and significant improvements, the rate of traffic deaths and injuries remains relatively constant when viewed over a long-term perspective of years and decades. For instance, in the 1950s the annual fatality rate due to driving accidents was around 50,000, while in the 1990s it has been around 40,000. There is certainly a reduction, but the curve has quickly levelled off and remains above 40,000 deaths and over 5 million injuries annually in the US (NHTSA, 1999).

There seem to be two opposing forces operating. On the one hand, there are external environmental forces for greater safety and thus less risk, as described above. On the other hand, there are internal individual forces for maintaining high risk (less safety):

- the widespread acceptance of a competitive norm that values getting ahead of other drivers;
- the daily pressure of time and its mismanagement through rushing and disobeying traffic laws;
- the weakness of driver-education programs that provide inadequate training in emotional self-control;
- the portrayal in the media of aggressive driving behaviours as fun; and
- the psychological tendency to maintain a preferred level of risk, so that increased risks are taken when environmental improvements are introduced (also called "risk homeostasis," see Wilde, 1994, 1988).

Scientists and safety officials attribute the resistance to accident reduction to the attitude and behaviour of drivers who respond by engaging in more dangerous driving.

A critical aspect of driving is the driver's ability to balance risk with safety. Driving risk is largely under the control of drivers. They decide at every moment which risks to take and which to inhibit or avoid. Risk-taking varies greatly between drivers and with the same driver at different times. Thus, if a road is made safer by straightening it or by moving objects that interfere with visibility, drivers will compensate for greater safety by driving faster—the so-called risk homeostasis phenomenon. The result is the maintenance of a constant subjective feeling of risk that is the normal habitual threshold for particular drivers. In such a driving environment, the rate of deaths or injuries tends to remain high, despite safety improvements.

The legal institution's response to the stalemate between safety and risk tolerance has been to increase enforcement activities like traffic monitoring, ticketing motorists and jailing hundreds of thousands of drivers. Nevertheless, the number of deaths and injuries has remained nearly steady, year after year. Besides law enforcement, there has been an increase in litigation due to aggressive driving disputes between drivers, as well as more psychotherapy and counselling services, including anger-management clinics and workshops, and community initiatives (James & Nahl, 2000). These are but scattered attempts and have been unable to alter basic driving patterns.

■ From Traffic Safety to Driving Psychology

Driver training continues to focus on imparting a minimum knowledge of safety principles and of vehicle operation and manipulation. Courses and manuals generally include a brief section on "driver attitude" and "driver error." This inclusion acknowledges that instruction should address personality habits.

My research has addressed this behavioural component, and to allow specific recognition of this subject in driver education, I have proposed the phrase "driving psychology" to represent this new driver instruction area. The basic principles of driving psychology are as follows:

1. Driving is a complex of behaviours acting together as cultural norms.
2. Driving norms exist in three domains: affective, cognitive and sensorimotor.
3. Driving norms are transmitted by parents, other adults, books, movies and television.

The primary affective driving norms for this generation include valuing territoriality, dominance, and competition as a desirable driving style; condoning intolerance of diversity (in needs and competencies of other drivers); supporting retribution ethics (or vigilante motives with desire to punish or amend); accepting impulsiveness and risk-taking in driving; and condoning aggressiveness, disrespect, and the expression of hostility. These affective norms are negative and anti-social. Socio-cultural methods must be used to reduce the attractiveness of these aggressive norms and to increase the attractiveness of positive and cooperative driver roles.

The primary cognitive driving norms include inaccurate risk assessment, biased and self-serving explanations of driving incidents, lack of emotional intelligence as a driver, and low or underdeveloped level of moral involvement (dissociation and egotism). These norms are inaccurate and inadequate. Self-training and self-improvement techniques must be taught so that drivers can better manage risk and regulate their own emotional behaviour.

The primary sensorimotor driving norms include automatic habits (e.g., unself-conscious or unaware of one's style and risk), errors of perception (e.g., distance, speed, initiating wrong action) and lapses in one's attention or performance due to fatigue, sleepiness, drugs, boredom, inadequate training or preparation. These norms are inadequate and immature. Lifelong driver self-improvement exercises are necessary to reach more competent driving habits.

Driving is a semi-conscious activity. Much of it depends on automatic habits acquired through culture and experience over several years. Obtaining a driver's license cannot be considered the end of driver training, and continued driver education, in the form of guided, lifelong self-improvement activities, is essential for acquiring new skills. Driving also involves taking risks, making errors and losing emotional self-control. Thus, drivers need to be trained in risk-taking, error recovery and emotional control under conditions of emergency or provocation.

Driving norms and behaviour can be changed by socio-cultural management techniques that make the driver want to change, by weakening negative norms and strengthening positive norms of driving. Since driving is a habit in three domains of behaviour, driving self-improvement is possible. Specific elements in each domain must be addressed, because driving consists of thousands of individual habits or skills, each of which can be identified, tested and improved on a long-term basis. However, self-assessment is not objective or accurate until the driver is trained in objective self-assessment procedures.

Drivers strongly resist externally imposed restrictions and regulations, so these methods alone are insufficient to create real changes in driver behaviour; instead, socio-cultural methods of influence must be used. Driving psychology adopts socio-cultural methods as change agents. For example, quality driving circles (QDCs) are informal groups whose function is to exert a long-term or permanent socio-moral influence on the driving quality of its members. The QDC curriculum is created through the principles of driving psychology, as approved by designated safety officials or agencies on a regional or national basis. Group activities focus explicitly on drivers' resistance to change; theory is put into conscious practice through follow-up self-witnessing activities behind the wheel. Members exert a positive influence on each other when they adhere to QDC standards.

Of course, the standard QDC curriculum must be updated regularly. Updates focus on technology developments in vehicles and on roads, all of which require drivers to acquire new skills, such as managing car-audio devices, reading maps on-screen, using computers, note-taking, talking on phone or radio and keeping to a schedule. Driving psychology refers to the knowledge drivers need to accumulate throughout their career as drivers—between six and seven decades for most North Americans. This knowledge focusses on self-instructional methods as reflected by a new paradigm called the Lifelong Driver Self-Improvement Program, consisting of a driving-psychology curriculum for kindergarten through grade 12 followed by lifelong membership in a quality driving circle (James & Nahl, 2000).

Driving psychology is a behavioural engineering tool. Research in driving psychology uses the self-witnessing approach, defined as a method of generating objective data on oneself as a driver (James, 1996). The driver operates in three separate but interacting behavioural domains. It takes the motive of a goal destination (affective domain) to keep the car moving, as well as a variety of related motives (affective) such as the desire (affective) to avoid a collision or the emotion of anger (affective) at another driver. It also takes knowledge (cognitive domain) of vehicle operation and traffic regulations to make judgements (cognitive) about other motorists' intents. Further, it takes the coordinated execution or performance (sensorimotor domain) of hand, foot and eye movements in appropriate response to the motive and the judgement. These three behavioural domains jointly and interactively constitute driving behaviour. Lifelong driver self-improvement training has the purpose of empowering drivers to take charge of their habit structures in these three behavioural areas (James & Nahl, 2000).

The new and the older traffic psychologies represent distinct paradigms in the study of driver behaviour. For example, input-output relations and those involving internal states differ (Michon, 1985). Input-output models use taxonomies or inventories based on task analyses, as well as functional control models of a mechanistic nature. Internal state models use trait analyses of drivers and their motivational-cognitive context. Michon considers the input-output models "behavioural" while the internal states models are "psychological." However, driving psychology considers the affective and cognitive domains to be behavioural areas, just as the sensorimotor domain is. Although inventories of driver tasks have been based on external observation and description of driving performance, the self-witnessing approach is a way of obtaining internal behavioural data, sometimes called "private data" (McKnight & Adams, 1970).

Driving psychology is the study of the social-psychological forces that act upon drivers. Situations are analyzed through external as well as internal methods of data gathering. For example, almost all drivers, when provided with the opportunity, will turn right on red, but a significant number of drivers fail to make a complete stop or yield to pedestrians before turning (ITE Journal, 1992). In another study, drivers spoke their thoughts into a tape recorder, giving their perceptions and reactions to traffic events and incidents. It was found that the average trip from home and work is filled with many incidents that arouse feelings of hostility and thoughts of mental violence (James, 1987). This is an instance of the driver's internal behaviour.

A driver's style of coping with traffic stress is related to personality and character. Acts, thoughts and feelings interact in an integrated system. A driving trip typically involves a dominant motive such as rushing or the desire to outplay other drivers by getting in front of them. The dominant motive (affective domain) is a character tendency that expresses itself in other settings as well. For example, a person may experience hostile thoughts (cognitive behaviour) towards others wherever competition occurs, whether in a bank line, a restaurant or switching traffic lanes (sensorimotor domain). Data on drivers' private world show that frustration begets anger, which leads to feelings of hostility that are elaborated in mental violence and ridicule, and finally acted out in aggressive behaviour (James, 1987). Aggressive behaviour is an outward consequence of an inner interplay between negative feeling and its conscious justification or legitimization. This threefold aspect of driving behaviour is at the centre of driving psychology.

The topics of driving psychology often overlap with traffic psychology or applied psychology, but the method of generating data is distinct; an example is the study of risk-taking in driving (Wilde, 1994). Few traffic situations are without risk, and drivers are constantly involved with risk. Incidents occur consistently, and the threat involved is experienced as stress. Reduction of traffic stress is a major concern for both driving psychology and applied traffic psychology. In the old paradigm, methods include extending traffic-safety education to children, providing driver education for adolescents and continuing driver education for adults through courses, legislation and public media campaigns. Driving psychology adds a major new component to these methods, namely the idea that driver training is lifelong self-training. It involves developing our emotional habits in traffic, paying attention to our thinking habits behind the wheel and recognizing overt actions for which we are legally and socially responsible.

■ Driver Self-Witnessing

Educators and test makers have used think-aloud verbalizations with college students to study student problem-solving abilities (Bloom, 1956). Meichenbaum and Goodman (1979) and Watson and Tharp (1985) used silent verbalizations in the form of self-regulatory sentences that mediate and control the overt performance of students and clients in need of greater self-control of their behaviour in different areas of life (Luria, 1961). Abelson (1981) proposed script analysis as a method of reconstructing the cognitive activities that underlie routine behaviours like ordering food in a restaurant. Ericsson and Simon (1984) described their means of protocol analysis, which involves audio-taping study participants' think-aloud routines while they are engaged in problem-solving activities like solving chess problems. The findings allowed Simon to create the first chess-playing computer program by rendering each thought sequence into a program line. More recently, the MIT media lab has created computer programs that not only model human cognitive processes but also affective processes (Picard, 1997). These efforts represent significant advances in the scientific study of individuals' private worlds.

I designed the self-witnessing technique to obtain reliable data on events in the private world of drivers. The method was initially used in the analysis of self-witnessing reports written by students while engaged in library research or using Internet search engines (Nahl, 1997, 1998; Nahl & James, 1996). The method is readily meaningful to people since they report on the activities (what they did, who was there) and mental focus (what they thought at the time, what they felt) in their daily lives. When people are asked to introduce themselves as drivers in writing, they spontaneously mention aspects of themselves such as driving experience, kinds of cars driven (e.g., gear shift or automatic), driving effects on everyday life (e.g., costs, dangers, frustrations, stress), projected images as drivers (e.g., power, status, lifestyle), assessments of being good or bad drivers, common reactions to routine driving situations, their mood changes as a result of driving episodes, assessments of traffic and particular trips, their driving records (e.g., traffic tickets, accidents, near misses) and others. These ingredients constitute dimensions of discrimination along which drivers spontaneously monitor themselves; they feature a driver's self-image.

Interviews with drivers and written self-assessments by drivers yield retrospective data in which the respondents' recollection of facts is mixed with their self-image as drivers. By contrast, self-witnessing reports yield data that are present, on-going and concurrent. The driver speaks out loud into a recorder at the moment the emotions, thoughts, perceptions and actions arise, concurrent with the act of driving. Later analysis of the transcripts displays patterns of feelings, thoughts and perceptions that accompanied particular driving episodes. This method provides a sample "online transaction log" that demonstrates the driver's affective states and cognitive processes. The adequacy of the sample still needs to be evaluated theoretically and practically, but the initial effort in driving psychology has been to develop a taxonomy of driving behaviour so that there might be a theoretically justified classification system capable of listing driver behaviours in the three domains and at relative levels of attainment or development.

■ The Driver's Threefold Self

In its modern version, behaviorism is committed to a unified theory that tries to deal with external and internal aspects of the self (Staats, 1975; Mischel, 1991). For instance, personality is defined in terms of built-up repertoires of basic habits. These are actually skills and errors that can be modified through further learning. This acquisition process occurs in three distinct domains of the person's activity: affective, cognitive and sensorimotor. All skills at any level of expertise contain affective, cognitive and sensorimotor features. The following transcript from a driver's self-witnessing record illustrates the three-fold nature of driving behaviour.

Oh, no, there's a police car coming up from behind. I hope he didn't see me driving fast. Besides, I'm not the only one who is driving fast. If he pulls me over to the side, he has to pull everyone else over too. I'll be so embarrassed if he pulls me over. Everyone will know that I was breaking the law.

Content analysis focusses on the "speech act" value of the components of verbalizations (Searle, 1969; Nahl, 1993). For instance, "Oh, no" and "I hope" indicate the affective involvement of the driver whose emotions form an integral part of the driving act. The comment "Besides, I'm not the only one" hints at this individual's feelings of guilt or self-justification for going over the speed limit. The statement "I'll be so embarrassed ... Everyone will know ..." indicates the driver's affective involvement with self-image or reputation. A little later this same driver displays affections of condemnation or disapproval when another car cuts in front: "Careless and pushy drivers always do things like that." In another episode, the driver expresses anxiety and fear:

> I almost sideswiped a car, which had been traveling in my blind spot. As I was turning back into the middle lane I was in a state of mild anxiety. Thinking about what could've happened made me scared.

Expressing fear in a driving incident and showing disapproval of another driver are instances of affective driving behaviour. An individual's internal dialogue can be used as an index of the affective states and cognitive processes that constitute the internal component of any outward behaviour. For example,

> I should cut down on how fast I'm driving and maintain the required speed limit. I'm in the middle lane and yet I'm driving like an aggressive person in the left lane. I could be increasing my chance of becoming a victim on the road. If the police pull me over and give me a ticket it's nobody else's fault but my own. I should follow the rules. I don't want others to get a bad impression of me and think that I'm a speed demon.

Reasoning about propriety is evident ("I should maintain the proper speed limit," "I'm driving like an aggressive person"), which also indicates self-evaluation. Propriety and morality are involved in the driver's reasoning of error attributed to the self ("It's nobody else's fault but my own"), while the comment "I don't want others to get a bad impression of me" reveals the speaker's image-management techniques.

In the following entry, the driver seems to be overwhelmed by the reasoned consequences of his action:

I'm thinking to myself I could have killed the guy back there. I'm so careless. He must be swearing at me and saying what an idiot I am. I could've smashed up my brother's car.

Note that this self-analysis includes an imagining of what the others are thinking, feeling or saying ("He must be swearing ..."). Witnessing and describing one's reasoning about a driving situation, or attributing an error to oneself, provides data on the driver's cognitive behaviour.

In the next segment the driver gives some details on sensorimotor behaviour, including the sensation of getting warmer:

I'll drive at the required speed limit and get to my destination safely. I'm leaning slightly forward in my seat rather than my normal slightly reclined position. I have both hands on the steering wheel rather than my normal one hand. And I can feel my temperature rising. My stomach feels queasy.

Some of this sensory information might be available through use of special data-collection procedures like well-placed cameras or observer ride-alongs. However, the meaning of driver acts would remain obscure without the concurrent self-witnessing report. For example, the comment "I am leaning slightly forward in my seat ... rather than my normal slightly reclined position" indicates a perception of abnormality in the sensation which would require enormously sophisticated instrumentation for support data. Witnessing and describing sensations or motor actions provide data on the driver's sensorimotor behaviour.

■ The Mental Health of Drivers

The cumulative research, using the self-witnessing reports of hundreds of drivers, reveals an agitated inner driving world that is replete with extreme emotions and impulses seemingly triggered by little acts. Ordinary drivers display maniacal thoughts, violent feelings, virulent speech and physiological signs of high stress:

Right now I feel scared, anxious, fearful, panic-stricken, agitated, bothered, irritated, annoyed, angry, mad. I feel like yelling and hitting. I'm thinking, Oh, no what's he doing. What's happening. How could he do that. And I hear myself saying out loud, "Asshole. Stupid jerk!" I'm breathing fast, gripping the wheel, perspiring, sitting up straight and slightly forward, my eyes are open and watching straight ahead.

This incident involved a car cutting into the lane and forcing the driver to slam on the brakes, causing a chain reaction. Fortunately, no collision occurred. Drivers' self-witnessing reports routinely contain scary incidents like this in which near misses occur. Hence, it has become normal for drivers to experience stress, even panic, under everyday traffic conditions.

The following is a summary of the variety of negative reactions routinely mentioned in driver self-witnessing reports.

EXTREME PHYSIOLOGICAL REACTIONS: Heart pounding, momentary stoppage of breathing, muscle spasms, stomach cramps, wet hands, pallor, faintness, trembling, nausea, discoordination, inhibition, visual fixation, facial distortion, back pain and neck cramp.

EXTREME EMOTIONAL REACTIONS: Outbursts of anger, yelling, aggressive gestures, looking mean and glaring, threatening with dangerous vehicle manipulation, fantasies of violence and revenge, panic, incapacitation, distortion, regressive rigid pattern of behaviour, fear, anxiety and delusional talk against non-present drivers and objects.

EXTREME IRRATIONAL THOUGHT SEQUENCES: Paranoiac thinking that one is being followed or inspected, addressing other drivers who are not within earshot, script-writing scenarios involving vengeance and cruelty against "guilty" drivers, denial of reality and defensiveness when a passenger complains of a driver's error, and psychopathic interactions as when two drivers alternately tailgate each other dangerously at high speed.

These findings raise an important public issue: the mental health of the nearly 200 million licensed drivers in North America. Demographic sampling research with the self-witnessing method could assess the generality of early findings. We need to create behavioural maps of drivers under varying social and psychological conditions in order to construct a comprehensive theory of driving behaviour within the language of drivers, not the language of scientists. Managing the future of driving in our society requires a knowledge of driving psychology because it provides the content needed by instructors, safety officials, law enforcement and other regulatory agencies that administer roads, cars and drivers. An appropriate phrase is "driving informatics" (Nahl, 1999): it covers the entirety of information sources society now needs to manage its expanding driving and automotive environment.

To supply the information needed for driving informatics, future research may investigate the conditions that foster greater internalization of compliant driving behaviour. This information may be collected by having drivers provide self-witnessing reports under various independently manipulated situations, such as driving in the right lane vs. the left lane; driving to work regularly (going with the traffic) vs. driving while watching the speedometer and staying within posted speed limits; driving alone vs. driving with one or more friends; driving in heavy traffic vs. light traffic; driving while in a hurry or after a quarrel with someone vs. driving under other mental states; driving on specific roads, with days and times contrasted; driving contrasted by demographic variables (age, experience, gender, religion, political views, geographic location, education, vehicle driven); and driving contrasted by individual variables (experience, training, driving record, personality characteristics). Such independently manipulated environmental and experiential contrasts reveal how drivers' feelings, thoughts, perceptions, verbalizations and actions (the dependent conditions or variables) are influenced by roadway conditions like traffic density and driver aggressiveness or by mental states such as driver feelings of pressure versus feelings of happiness (the independent conditions or variables). In one project, I compared the self-witnessing reports of students in which the intervention treatment (or independent manipulation) was to drive within speed limits for one week; the dependent measures were self-witnessing reports for the affective, cognitive and sensorimotor domains of their driving behaviour (threefold self). During the week of self-imposed driving within speed limits, students commonly reported extreme paranoiac feelings and thoughts, e.g., "Everybody is giving me the stink eye for holding them up. They are going to attack me, ram me off the road" (Student Reports, 1999). These thoughts did not appear on the baseline records that described students' regular driving patterns. The baseline-intervention design is flexible and productive when coupled with random assignment of subjects to predefined conditions. It also allows statistical tests of significance.

■ Taxonomy of Driving Behaviour

The development of a comprehensive driving theory based on self-witnessing reports makes it possible to construct a classification scheme or taxonomy that can help identify the components of driver behaviour from the perspective of the driver. Such an inventory may be useful for driver assessment and driver education and can provide norms or expectations of driving skills and errors in the affective, cognitive and sensorimotor domains. For instance, a driver's self-witnessing report may be analyzed by counting the presence of affective errors (e.g., "I was so mad I didn't care if I was going to hit him or not!"), cognitive errors (e.g., "I figured there is no speed limit in this parking lot 'cause I don't remember seeing any speed limit signs here") and sensorimotor errors (e.g., "I lowered my window and yelled at him, 'You stupid idiot!'"). A driver's error score can be obtained to evaluate the effect of various intervention programs for driver self-improvement. Error patterns may be correlated with demographic or psychological characteristics of drivers (e.g., men vs. women, contrasting age groups). Such data are valuable for developing models of driver behaviour, especially those involving higher-control mechanisms that include motivational and trait-related features (Picard, 1997). As Michon (1985, p. 488) has argued, driver research should go cognitive (and I would add, affective) since human mobility is embedded in a psychosocial environment as well as a technological environment. Feelings, thoughts and perceptions are as much traffic and transportation issues as road conditions and traffic flow.

Table 3.2 shows the beginning iteration of the taxonomy in its general form and structure. Driving behaviour is represented as a collection of skills and errors within the three behavioural domains of the self. Skills receive a (+) symbol while errors are noted by a (-) symbol. Entries within each behavioural area are self-witnessing units culled from drivers' self-reports. Categorization of an item is a matter of common sense, following speech act rules known by ordinary speakers (Searle, 1969). Although all drivers were able to report their emotions, thoughts and actions in traffic, individual differences were observed in detail, focus, comprehensiveness and clarity. As driver self-witnessing becomes a generational norm and cultural practice for all drivers, the richness and depth of the accumulating data will increase, giving us the ability to construct even better driving theories and self-training procedures.

The second iteration of the taxonomy (shown in Table 3.3) introduces three levels of development or driver competence (1, 2, 3, etc.) within the three behavioural domains (A [Affective], C [Cognitive] S [Sensorimotor]) and the two skill orientations (+ vs. -). Three behavioural domains by three developmental levels yields a matrix of nine zones of possible driver behaviours. Adding a + or - orientation yields a total of eighteen behavioural zones.

The taxonomy will be described from bottom up to indicate that habits are built on top of habits, and that higher habits are acquired later in experience. Once established, higher habits exert a causative (downward) influence on lower habits. The three domains at Level 1 occupy Driver Competence Zones 1, 2, and 3, respectively, in relation to skills, and Zones 10, 11, and 12, for errors; Levels 2 and 3 are similar. Zones 1 through 9 represent skills, and their corresponding errors populate zones 10 through 18. Each "zone" of driving behaviour consists of habit structures that coalesce because of their similarity to the level and domain they belong to as a "zone" or area in one's driving personality. Since each zone of driving behaviour has a positive and negative form, there are eighteen zones in all. In the table, the nine competence zones receive a + sign while the corresponding error zones have a - sign.

The labelling of the three levels should be considered part of the theory. As research continues, evidence will evolve to allow more accurate representa-

TABLE 3.2

Driver behaviour as skills and errors in three behavioural domains

Skills (+)

Affective (+A)	Cognitive (+C)	Sensorimotor (+S)
I've got to be careful here. Don't want to cut anybody off.	This person looks like he's in a hurry to get in. I better let him in.	(Gesticulating and smiling) Go ahead. You go first.

Errors (-)

Affective (-A)	Cognitive (-C)	Sensorimotor (-S)
I wish I could give that guy a piece of my mind.	I don't think people like that should be allowed on the road.	(Yelling) You stupid idiot, why don't you watch where you're going!

TABLE 3.3

Classification scheme for the taxonomy of driver behaviour

	Affective	Cognitive	Sensorimotor
Level 3, Responsibility	+A3 = 7, -A3 = 16	+C3 = 8, -C3 = 17	+S3 = 9, -S3 = 18
Level 2, Safety	+A2 = 4, -A2 = 13	+C2 = 5, -C2 = 14	+S3 = 6, -S3 = 15
Level 1, Proficiency	+A1 = 1, -A1 = 10	+C1 = 2, -C1 = 11	+S1 = 3, -S1 = 12

tions of each level. For now, I present results of personally initiated studies. Level 1 driving behaviour is labelled "Proficiency" to represent the new driver's initial overriding focus on three proficiencies: staying calm and alert (affective proficiency), figuring out what happens around drivers (cognitive proficiency) and coordinating eyes, hands and legs to keep the vehicle from colliding (sensorimotor proficiency). Level 2 is labelled "Safety" to represent avoidance of trouble (affective safety) joined by problem-solving processes to identify trouble spots (cognitive safety) and taking prudent actions (sensorimotor safety). Level 3 is labelled "Responsibility" to represent the motive of remaining accountable for hurting others (affective responsibility). This motive creates prosocial rather than antisocial thought sequences and plans (cognitive responsibility) that eventuate in the quality of driving life (sensorimotor responsibility). The full taxonomy is shown in Table 3.4.

Labelling of each behavioural zone is part of the theory and needs additional confirmation by more extensive research. Every behavioural skill zone has a corresponding error zone. A driver may be represented as a collection of skills and errors, each of which is a habit that can be witnessed and modified with appropriate procedures. This process of habit self-modification occurring simultaneously in each of the eighteen zones is what I call the Lifelong Driver Self-Improvement Program. Therefore the Quality Driving Circle (QDC) curriculum is based on self-witnessing activities in the eighteen zones.

An illustration of how driver taxonomy can be used for planning and monitoring self-improvement activities is shown in Table 3.5. It is a radical overhaul of old habit structures—a driving personality makeover. The featured driver used the taxonomy to map out a self-modification plan that contained two stages: first, to do what it takes to avoid being an aggressive driver; and second, to do what it takes to become a supportive driver (the opposite of an aggressive driver). The driver decided to list for himself the behavioural objectives in the three domains, without keeping track of the level. He correctly decided that the first step is affective, in this case to "overcome his resistance to change," and picked several affective objectives that counteract his habitual aggressive driving motives and tap into his higher value system, which he believed he had in reserve. Under the prodding of this new motive, he picked several cognitive objectives that gave him practice in counteracting his lack of objectivity when thinking about driving situations. Finally, the new motive must actualize in civil behaviour or else it is only an imagined change. Thus, he had to pick relevant sensorimotor objectives to actualize the new persona. This he did, as shown in Table 3.5.

The second phase is the maturing stage. What the driver had to "force himself" to avoid doing in Stage 1, he now enjoyed doing in Stage 2. This is an example of a changeover. The supportive orientation involves a prosocial

TABLE 3.4
The eighteen behavioural zones of driving

Affective Responsibility in Driving A3 (+ or -)	Cognitive Responsibility in Driving C3 (+ or -)	Sensorimotor Responsibility in Driving S3 (+ or -)
(7) altruism and morality vs.	(8) positive dramatizations and mental health vs.	(9) enjoyment and satisfaction vs.
(16) egotism and deficient conscience	(17) negative dramatizations and insanity	(18) stress and depression

Affective Safety in Driving A2 (+ or -)	Cognitive Safety in Driving C2 (+ or -)	Sensorimotor Safety in Driving S2 (+ or -)
(4) defensive driving and equity vs.	(5) objective attributions vs.	(6) polite exchanges and calmness vs.
(13) aggressiveness and opportunism	(14) biased attributions	(15) rude exchanges and overreaction

Affective Proficiency in Driving A1 (+ or -)	Cognitive Proficiency in Driving C1 (+ or -)	Sensorimotor Proficiency in Driving S1 (+ or -)
(1) respect for regulations and self-control vs.	(2) knowledge and awareness vs.	(3) correct actions and alertness vs.
(10) disrespect for authority and deficient self-control	(11) untrained and faulty thinking	(12) faulty actions and inattention

driving persona that is balanced and objective in thinking, and non-competitive and helpful in behaving. It is associated with a maximum of safety and a minimum of stress while restoring the sense of fun and enjoyment to driving. Once such a plan is drawn up through self-study or instruction and counselling,

T A B L E 3.5

Two stages of a driving personality makeover plan

Stage 1: Avoid Being an Aggressive Driver

Affective Level	**Cognitive Level**	**Sensorimotor Level**
Overcoming my resistance to change	*Learning to do rational analyses of traffic incidents*	*Acting out civil behaviour*
• Committing myself to inhibit or mitigate states of anger and retaliation	• Reasoning against my attribution errors (it's always their fault; it's never my fault)	• Waving, smiling, signalling
• Making it acceptable for passenger to complain or make suggestions	• Counteracting my self-serving bias in how I view incidents	• Not crowding, not rushing in, not swearing
• Making it unacceptable for me to ridicule or demean other drivers	• Acquiring more socialized self-regulatory sentences I can say to myself	• Not aggressing against passengers
• Activating higher motives within myself such as love of order and fair play, public spiritedness, charity, kindness to strangers		• Pretending that I'm in a good mood even when not

its execution involves a strategy called the three-step program. Each item on the self-modification plan is practised singly per driving trip. To illustrate:

First step: Acknowledging that I have this particular negative habit (A);
Second step: Witnessing myself performing this negative habit (W);
Third step: Modifying this habit (M).

For example, the driver picked the item "feeling regret at my unfriendly behaviours and impulses" for one trip to work. This selection constitutes

TABLE 3.5 (CONT.)
Two stages of a driving personality makeover plan

Stage 2: Becoming a Supportive Driver *(presumes or contains Stage 1)*

Affective Level	Cognitive Level	Sensorimotor Level
Maintaining a supportive orientation towards other drivers	*Analyzing driving situations objectively*	*Behaving like a happy person*
• Feeling responsible for errors and seeking opportunities to make reparations • Feeling regret at my unfriendly behaviours and impulses • Feeling good about behaving with civility or kindness • Feeling appreciation when being given advice by passengers • Being forgiving of others' mistakes and weaknesses	• Acknowledging and knowing my driving errors • Planning and rehearsing the modification of those habits • Analyzing other drivers' behaviours objectively or impartially	• Anticipating the needs of other drivers and being helpful to them • Verbalizing nice sentiments • Enjoying the ride and relaxing

Step 1, because selecting the item is an act of acknowledgment. Then, the driver has to witness the behaviour during the trip. In other words, he stays alert, focussing on his emotions as he drives. As soon as he detects the presence of hostile feelings, he follows it up with sentiments of regret. The normal habit would be to give into initial hostile impulses, to magnify them, to rehearse them several times. All these habitual procedures are now interrupted and interfered with by means of the sentiments of regret interjected into the event in accordance with the plan. Now we have modification. When the three-step process is practised on repeated trips, the old habit sequence gradually weakens and is replaced by a new, positive habit sequence. The cyclical process is repeated item by item. Thus I conclude that self-improvement needs to go on a lifelong basis. Social support methods, like QDC groups, are needed to help drivers persist and not give up.

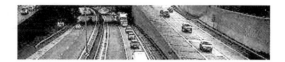

DRIVING PSYCHOLOGY is an applied field that creates a popular language of behavioural thinking about driving as a societal issue. This issue is complex and overlaps with technical and non-technical intellectual environments. The language and ideas in driving psychology are scientifically sound and accurate. However, driving psychology is not a basic science like psychology and does not follow its rigour in application. The theory and concepts of driving psychology can be freely borrowed from existing fields of study, as follows:

- social psychology (e.g., schemas, scripts, attribution error, territoriality, etc.);
- developmental psychology (e.g., stages of moral development, moral IQ, etc.);
- health psychology (e.g., resistance to compliance, addictive behaviours, lifestyle management);
- applied psychology (e.g., driving behaviour, risk homeostasis, ergonomics of errors, etc.);
- traffic psychology (e.g., driver management, pedestrian behaviour, traffic-safety education, etc.);
- clinical psychology (e.g., behaviour self-modification of maladaptive habits, etc.);
- traffic sociology (e.g., social conventions on highways, attitudes towards laws, etc.);
- automotive medicine (e.g., seat-belt and child-restraint use, effect of cars on health, etc.);
- transportation engineering (e.g., traffic calming devices, alternative transportation initiatives, etc.); and
- accident reconstruction.

The language of driving psychology is adapted to specific populations and purposes. Its principles and programs are cast in a popularized but scientific language that is suitable for people of different educational levels, age and experience. For driver-management programs to be effective, the drivers involved must be motivated to cooperate on their own. The desire for cooperation must stem from their understanding and acceptance. Understanding must be taught and acceptance must be won. Internal motivation for lifelong driver self-improvement is effective and dependable, but externally imposed rules are less effective and dependable.

The concepts and methods of driving psychology must be clear to the drivers involved. Driving psychology maintains an internal rhetoric of persuasion designed to empower drivers to overcome their spontaneous inner resistance to its principles. It is to be expected that drivers will experience feelings of resistance to the principles of driving psychology because it involves self-assessment and self-modification, both of which are painful to most people. There is a natural and predictable resistance to changing automatic habits in the sensorimotor domain, resistance to changing cognitive norms of evaluating and judging other drivers, and resistance to giving up affective norms of hostility, and self-assertiveness as a driver. Driving psychology predicts the forms of internal resistance and provides drivers with socio-cultural methods they can use to overcome their internal resistance to change, as the steps below demonstrate.

1. Encourage drivers to practise self-witnessing behind the wheel (self-observation and self-monitoring record keeping using a variety of tools such as data forms, trip logs and tape recordings).
2. Teach drivers how to apply self-modification principles (baseline/intervention techniques by drivers).
3. Teach the three-step program for driving personality makeovers.
4. Encourage drivers to maintain a driving log as way of promoting their long-term commitment to self-improvement.
5. Promote partnership driving arrangements to encourage friends or co-workers to assist drivers in self-improvement efforts.
6. Promote quality driving circles as a socio-cultural method for building up driver motivation to practise lifelong self-modification activities. Such promotion includes a national or regional program of incentives, awards and benefits for drivers who maintain their QDC activities, and also includes providing guidance through instructional materials such as TEE cards, Keeping-Track forms, logs or schedules that assist individuals in their driving exercises. These forms may also be made available anonymously to scientists who can use them as a continuous source of data for studying driver behaviour on a long-

term basis. Such research will help government agencies to continue the effective management of driving.

7. Increase people's awareness and focus public attention on the social implications of car society, car talk, car attitudes and behaviours, through content analysis of the accounts (or stories) drivers give when telling what happened; messages drivers write in electronic discussion groups; newspaper accounts of driving incidents and duels; public or media portrayals of drivers and driving (including books and advertising); and other sources that access the thoughts and feelings of people about driving. Analysis of Internet newsgroups about driving, with participants from North America, Britain, Australia and Singapore, has shown that aggressive and hostile attitudes among drivers is universal and transcends ethnic background (James, 2000), although the psychological mechanisms that justify this hostility may vary from culture to culture. It is therefore necessary to develop culture-specific methods of social influence to bring about a change in norms of competition and hostility.

8. Build inventories and taxonomies of affective, cognitive and sensori-motor driving behaviours to guide scientists and safety officials and to define the content of public instruction and other educational materials for self-improvement efforts. Current inventories of driving behaviours in North America have been obtained through various methods, including surveys or polls using driver-behaviour check lists (James, 1998); content analysis of driving accounts (personal stories and media reports) (James & Nahl, 2000); protocol analysis of transcripts of tape recordings made by drivers behind the wheel (self-witnessing method) (James, 1987); observations made by passengers and pedestrians; data gathered with specially equipped research vehicles; and data gathered from driving simulators.

9. Support and promote civic activism and social organizations that focus on driving and the car culture. Such organizations may include groups that focus on aggressive-driving prevention for children, citizen groups against drunk driving or speeding, designated-driver programs to fight alcohol-related driving fatalities and youth organizations against road rage. Other strategies may include public procedures for recognizing driver excellence (e.g., awards, certificates, nominations), the creation of positive driving roles and heroes (e.g., culturally integrated symbols of collectivist driving through music, drama and dance), and providing racing parkways and off-road driving in reserved areas to allow more acceptable alternatives to speeding and rough-driving enthusiasts.

10. Provide access to driving informatics facilities to satisfy people's driving information needs. Such facilities might include driving self-improvement workbooks and curricula; standard QDC curricula; accident recovery support organizations; automotive needs (maintenance, repair, sales) and travel information (maps, weather, traffic); insurance and legal services; training and licensing; aggressive-driving prevention programs for children; civic organizations (traffic control, safety education, impaired driving, legislation); car culture and history; and Internet activities (driving sites, newsgroups, organizations, conferences, initiatives and news).

4 | INNOVATIONS IN INJURY CONTROL

From Crash to
the Community

LOUIS HUGO FRANCESCUTTI,
MOHAMMED NASEEMUL HOQUE &
J. PETER ROTHE

CRASH! In milliseconds a car crash resulting in injury has changed a life, a family and a community. Multiple organizations, from emergency medical services (EMS) to the medical examiner's office, become involved in the crash investigation. EMS and emergency physicians collect data on patient injuries while police collision reconstructionists collect data on the how the crash occurred. Unfortunately, these organizations do not collectively study how the injury happened.

Motor vehicle-related injury is the leading cause of unintentional injury death in Canada, the US and many other parts of the world. For example, for the past 10 years motor-vehicle-related injuries have been the leading cause of death for people under age 25 in Alberta, Canada (Alberta Centre for Injury Control and Research, 1998). It seems intuitive that studying the mechanisms of injury would be the first step toward preventing them, or at least decreasing their severity.

This chapter describes the design and development of a collaborative injury-analysis program between University of Alberta injury-control epidemiologists, emergency medical services, police, trauma physicians and the medical examiner to study the causes of serious motor-vehicle injuries. The objective of this program is to move beyond traditional accident reconstruction to collaboratively investigate how motor-vehicle-collision injuries occur, so that injury-prevention strategies can more easily be devised.

■ Background to the Model

Understanding the mechanism of injury begins at the scene of a crash, where accurate data on crash velocity, angles of impact and directions of force can be collected. Expert collision reconstructionists gather and analyze this information while trauma physicians and surgeons treat and study the injuries. Facilitating between these groups, researchers can link the data and study the actual mechanisms of the injuries. As part of a feedback loop, the information can be disseminated to the community, where members of different community agencies can collaborate to devise and recommend better injury-prevention strategies, such as increased police enforcement, innovative vehicle design, more effective lobbying strategies and more relevant local policy recommendations.

The injury-based research approach uses primary data sources such as police reports, hospital charts and in-depth collision investigations. The following factors guided the model design (Dalkie, 1993):

- An appropriate analysis system must be in place;
- The research model must be feasible and sustainable; and
- The model must have general applicability.

The program we discuss in this article extended Dalkie's (1993) model for investigating road-safety issues. Central concepts from various medical, community development and observation frameworks have contributed to the design of an injury-analysis program that relies heavily on collaboration to study injury biomechanics. It maximizes the use of rich data being collected by police, hospitals and EMS personnel.

Our model was developed on the principle that the police share collision-reconstruction data analysis with us at the scenes of crashes. This information is passed on to emergency-room physicians so they can more easily identify possible mechanisms of injury before or as a patient arrives at the trauma centre. The practice helps optimize injury-control procedures by allowing physicians to establish starting points for investigation. In return, medical staff provide the injury-analysis team with valuable injury data for analysis.

Our collision-injury data model specifically targets the study of serious motor-vehicle-collision injuries. For example, in Edmonton, Alberta, the police's Traffic Section responds only to collisions involving serious injury as determined

Program development conceptual framework

(adapted from the University of Alberta Injury Prevention Centre, 1993)

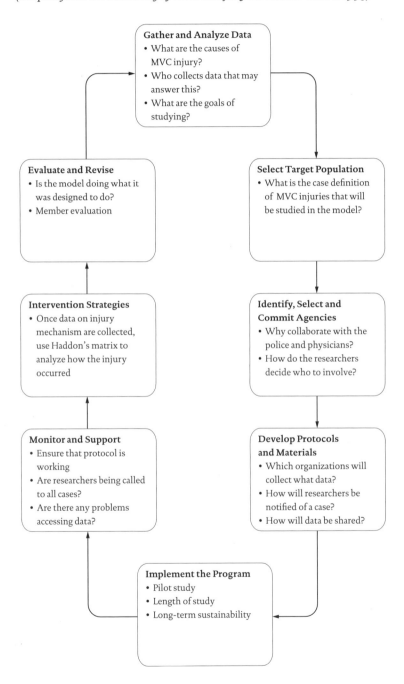

FIGURE 4.2

Model of collaborative injury biomechanics analysis and prevention implementation

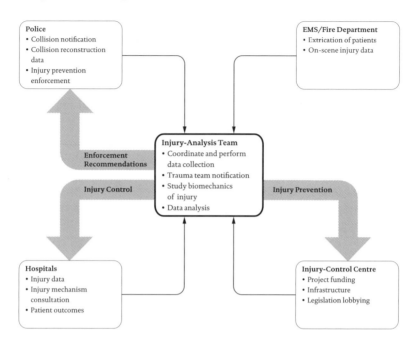

by the first patrol unit on scene. (For the sake of brevity, serious injury is defined as a pedestrian or vehicle occupant who sustains injury requiring EMS and transportation to a trauma centre.) The Traffic Section has members with Level 3 and Level 4 collision-reconstruction training, which allows in-depth collision reconstruction. By collaborating with police, researchers may obtain in-depth collision information such as vehicle compartment intrusions, vehicle speeds, angle of impact, driver and passenger position data, seatbelt use, type of collision, driver and pedestrian data, vehicle access, scene photographs, and other factors that may have caused injury.

☐ *Maximizing existing data sources*

By collaborating with police, the injury-analysis team may discover factors that caused a particular injury. The police are less concerned about articulating why injuries occurred, however: their primary interest is to discover why the collisions happened so that charges can be laid if necessary. Thus, an injury-analysis team requires collision and biomechanics reconstruction training to perform in-depth injury analysis in cooperation with the police investigation.

By collaborating with emergency physicians and trauma surgeons, the team has access to detailed patient injuries, medical interventions, emergency services and patient outcomes. These data are usually collected by or available to major hospitals. Having physicians participate in the model helps researchers who do not have the clinical skills to study injuries. Further, paramedic data, including extrication details, patient condition at the scene and stabilization procedures, are routinely collected by professional EMS staff, making the information easy for a injury-analysis team to collect, analyze and synthesize.

☐ *Putting appropriate analysis systems in place*
We encouraged expert collision reconstructionists to share their analysis with our researchers. Further, hospital chiefs of staff of emergency departments or trauma centres agreed to share injury data required by our team. The collaboration design was essential because when we analyzed patient admission forms to emergency rooms (ER), we found that, in many cases, "motor-vehicle accident" was listed as the only cause of injury. There was no mention of a mechanism of injury. Thus, our team developed a strategy to bridge collision reconstruction and injury investigation. Part of the model involves the electronic transfer of injury-causation data to the trauma room as soon as the team arrives at the scene. This transfer helps the trauma physicians to know what type of injuries to expect. Critical time is saved in the trauma room, which can mean the difference between life, disability and death.

☐ *Model sustainability*
From the Edmonton pilot project we learned that police and trauma physicians are willing to participate in this kind of injury-prevention research. We had little difficulty accessing injury data from the trauma centres. The police were always willing to share data required by the injury-analysis team, and in many cases expanded their investigation to facilitate the researchers. Both medical personnel and the police displayed interest in sustaining and expanding the program, assuring that sustainability through support is feasible, if not secure.

With appropriate injury-control infrastructures and with funding from injury control and research centres, our model can be sustainable. Many jurisdictions have injury control and research centres that could provide the office space and other infrastructure required to house an injury-analysis team. As well, injury control and research centres often lobby for safety policies. Having teams located at such sites helps assure that the findings from the team's research are implemented.

■ General Applicability of the Model

The injury-analysis program was designed to be applicable to any type of motor-vehicle crash injury investigation. If the resources are available and local officials have the will, the model can be appropriately deployed for both low- and high-severity injuries resulting from road crashes. The model has strong potential for ongoing collaboration between strategic agencies because the distributed information benefits everyone involved.

□ *Model's collaboration framework*

The National Committee on Injury Prevention and Control (NCIPC) (1989) states that a key step in preventing injuries is to involve the community. The NCIPC identifies possible collaborators for injury prevention such as police departments, hospitals, emergency medical services, epidemiologists and schools of public health. Cohen, Baer and Satterwhite (1991) developed an effective coalition-building framework for establishing coalitions. Based on community experiences in Contra Costa County, they published an updated version of the NCIPC framework. This model served as the benchmark for the collaboration component of our injury-analysis research program.

A coalition is a union of people and organizations working to influence outcomes on a specific problem. It is a "network," a group formed primarily for the purpose of resource and information sharing. An eight-point strategy was used to help construct a successful collaborative coalition for the model's pilot test in Edmonton:

1. Analysis of the program's objectives and determination of benefits for forming a coalition.
2. Recruitment of the right people.
3. Development of preliminary objectives and activities.
4. Plans to convene the coalition.
5. Anticipation of necessary resources.
6. Definition of the elements of a successful coalition structure.
7. Maintenance of coalition vitality.
8. Implementation of improvements based on evaluation results.

Thus, the Edmonton project involved organizations like the Royal Alexandra Hospital and University of Alberta Hospital emergency departments; the Edmonton Police Service, Traffic Section; the Royal Canadian Mounted Police; emergency medical services and the Office of the Chief Medical Examiner. For the purpose of our injury-analysis model, the injury-analysis team was located at the hub of the network. It served as the "lead agency," the unit that convened the coalition and assumed responsibility for its operation.

□ *Building the coalition*

Once the injury-analysis team formulated the design objectives, it was time to recruit participants. Our first contacts were the chiefs of staff at the Royal Alexandra Hospital and University of Alberta Hospital trauma centres. The meetings led to a participation agreement. Researchers were granted access to the trauma room to talk with physicians and collect data on injuries. The chiefs of staff were particularly interested in receiving data that may benefit patient treatment; as medical leaders, they recognized the impact such research would have on the health-care system.

The next step involved meeting the Superintendent and staff sergeants of Edmonton Police Services, Traffic Section. The police agreed to participate on the basis that their participation would benefit policing because it would help them evaluate their own traffic-injury control programs, such as seat-belt use and speed enforcement. Project data could reveal areas where enforcement might aid injury control, which could in turn guide police policy development. Members of the research team agreed not to interfere with crash scene investigations and to assist on the scene whenever officers requested it. To "learn the ropes" of police investigations, members of the research team initially went on regular ride-alongs with crash investigators. Ride-alongs allowed us to get to the crash scene quickly and they helped us to develop a good working relationship with members of the Traffic Section. After several months, we were paged when a crash happened and proceeded to the scene in our own vehicles.

Step three consisted of meetings with the Chief Medical Examiner and the Director of Emergency Medical Services. Both agreed to allow their personnel to share any data that would guide us in determining how an injury occurred.

Once everyone joined the network, we sought permission from the University Health Research Ethics Board to conduct the pilot study. The ethics board had concerns about patient confidentiality because researchers would be accessing patient charts. We explained that the only way to study how the injury occurred would be to correlate the injuries with vehicular and scene damage. Accessing patient charts and communicating directly with their health-care providers would be the most efficient way to gain this data.

□ *Case definition*

Subjects included in the pilot study were involved in motor-vehicle collisions attended by the Edmonton Police Service, Traffic Section. To be included in the study, patients had to require pre-hospital EMS and were transported to the emergency department of either the University of Alberta or Royal Alexandra hospitals. All injured persons, including drivers, passengers, and pedestrians, were documented and analyzed. Our research team studied collisions involving both injuries and fatalities. Twenty-three collisions were studied over a seven-month period.

☐ *Scene activities*

The police department's first priority was to proceed with the investigation of fault. Once fault was established, police participated in the research. While on site, members of the research team took precautions not to interfere with police investigations. As the study progressed, the relationship between the police collision investigators and the research team was one of cooperation. Over time, roles and functions were specified in relation to the research. For example, police activities in the research allowed us to access the scene and vehicles, measure the scene and vehicle damage, photograph the vehicles and scene, and calculate vehicle speeds and angles of impact. Our primary roles included assisting the police in documenting evidence (such as taking measurements at the scene of crashes as requested) and providing information gathered from the hospital information forms while maintaining patient confidentiality. The primary role of the emergency physicians was to provide team members with precise data about patient injuries. We reciprocated by providing data on the type of crash, information about the speed of vehicles and photos of the crash scene.

■ **Sensitivity and Specificity of the Model**

Sensitivity refers to the ability of a data-collection system to include all cases of a particular motor-vehicle collision injury. *Specificity* refers to the ability of the system to exclude other phenomena that may be mistaken for the one being studied (NCIPC, 1989). In this model, the researchers wanted to study only serious motor-vehicle crash injuries that required EMS care and transport to a trauma centre. However, there was a shortcoming to this decision. Some crashes were originally judged as producing low-severity injuries and thus were not investigated by the Traffic Section. However, the patient injuries were upgraded to severe or critical after the patient was examined in the trauma room. The researchers missed these types of cases in which acute injuries were evident only in the clinical investigation, not the on-site analysis.

The following procedures were used to investigate serious motor-vehicle-collision injuries occurring in the City of Edmonton with the cooperation of the police.

- Investigators arrived at the collision scene, which was investigated by the Traffic Section of the Edmonton Police Service.
- Investigators attended the collision investigation with police.

- Investigators assisted police in such tasks as vehicle and road measurements. All vehicles involved in the collision were inspected by police and investigators.

- Investigators inspected all hospital charts of injured patients, detailing injuries sustained and medical procedures performed. Investigators made estimates to identify the probable injury sources and mechanisms.

- For each case studied, a case narrative was completed, providing details of how the injury likely occurred. A scene diagram illustrated the vehicle kinematics. Photographs of the scene, vehicles and injuries were used for documentation, presentation of analysis and conclusion of possible injury-prevention measures.

■ Sample Case: Case 18, Mazda 626 LX vs. Light Post
□ *Collision summary*

At 15:51 on a clear and sunny day, a seventeen-year-old male driver was travelling at (police estimated) 100 kph entering eastbound into the City of Edmonton in the number-four lane of a one-way, four-lane road. The Mazda 626 he was driving approached a traffic-signal-controlled intersection for which, according to witness statements in the police report, the light was green for eastbound traffic. The driver began to change into the number-two lane but saw that there was a vehicle stopped at the intersection in that lane. The driver then attempted to get into the number-one lane, which is an exit southbound. The number-one lane merges away from the number-two lane and is separated by an island which also supports the traffic light. The driver of the Mazda was unable to negotiate the turn into the number-one lane, and the vehicle jumped the island and smashed head-on into the light pole.

There were four occupants in the vehicle including the driver. The driver and the seventeen-year-old male front passenger were both wearing seat belts. The driver was transported to the University of Alberta Hospital and the front passenger to Misericordia Hospital. The right-rear female passenger, a seventeen-year-old female and the left-rear passenger, an eighteen-year-old female, neither of whom were wearing seat belts, were both transported to the University Hospital.

The vehicle sustained severe frontal crush to the front-centre bumper and engine bay. The driver's side floor pan was pushed into the driver's seat. The whole left dash intruded into the passenger compartment. The left rocker panel at the driver's side was bent downward, corresponding with the intrusion of the floor pan. The steering column was bent downwards. The left-front roof over the driver's area was bent down into the occupant compartment.

The left-rear passenger died in hospital. The mechanisms of her injuries appear to be as follows:

The eighteen-year-old female first crashed into the right front passenger seat. The chair was bent forward and to the right. She then continued forward and smashed into the front windshield. The windshield had a spiral in it with hair evidence as well. There was a second spiral with hair evidence in front of the right front passenger, which corresponds to his head also striking the glass. The eighteen-year-old female sustained one more collision. A VCR sitting on the rear shelf of the back seat was thrown upon impact and hit the back of her head. The VCR had a dent in it the shape of the back of her head.

☐ *Injury-prevention measures*
The fatal injuries sustained by the eighteen-year-old female could have been prevented had she been wearing a lap and shoulder belt. The VCR on the back shelf was not properly contained and should have been kept in the trunk. Newton's First Law states that an object will continue in motion unless acted on upon by an external force. Sadly, in this case, it was the back of the passenger's head that stopped the VCR. A breakaway pole would have decreased the severity of the crash. This was the second fatal crash along this stretch of road in three months. Police are advised to monitor the location for traffic violations.

■ Outcome of the Pilot

This project was a collaborative process in which the researchers were responsible for combining data collected by police and emergency physicians. The researchers were at the centre of a network that transmitted data between the researchers, police and emergency physicians. We collected crash data from the police and shared it with the emergency physicians to elucidate possible injuries sustained by the patient; we then provided the injury data to the police so they could target enforcement for injury prevention.

An important element of the networking collaboration was the facilitation that members of the injury-analysis team provided between the police and emergency physicians. In cases where the police met with doctors, a researcher accompanied the officer into the trauma room to learn about the injuries. This accompaniment fostered an environment in which member organizations got to know each other on a personal level. It also showed the member organizations how they were contributing to community collaboration.

There were no turf issues because of the nature of the investigations carried out by collaboration members. The police conducted scene investigations. Our

TABLE 4.1
Patient injuries, left-rear passenger (18-year-old female)

Injury	AIS	ISS Body Region	Highest AIS	AIS^2
Closed head injury (diffuse axonal injury)	140628.5	Head/neck	5	25
Scalp laceration	110600.1	Head/neck		
Ventricular tachycardia				
Abrasions of ankles	810202.1	Extremities	1	1 AIS=25

TABLE 4.2

Patient injuries, driver (17-year-old male)

Injury	AIS	ISS Body Region	Highest AIS	AIS^2
Abrasions left cheek	212202.1	External	1	1
Abrasions left neck	310202.1	External		
L1 spinous process fracture	650618.2	Abdomen	2	4
L1 transverse process fracture	650420.2	Abdomen		
L2 spinous process fracture	650618.2	Abdomen		
L2 transverse process fracture	650618.2	Abdomen		ISS=5

TABLE 4.3
Haddon's matrix

Phase	Factor		
	Host	*Vehicle*	*Environment*
Pre-event	Driver speeding	Brakes in poor condition	Speed limit; No breakaway pole
Event	No seat-belt use by rear passengers	Speeding	Light post
Post-event	Age; Physical condition	VCR in rear struck occupant	911 emergency number; EMS; Trauma care systems; Rehabilitation systems

FIGURE 4.3
Outcome of model's pilot

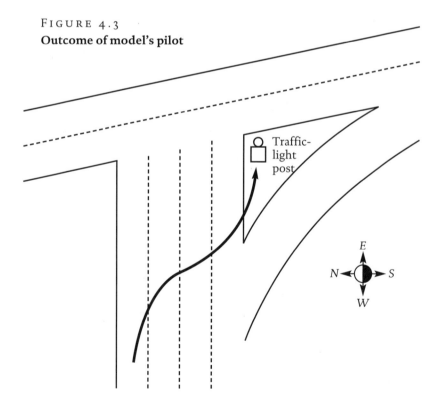

participation in the model did not change their work: when the researchers were on scene, the police were in charge. In the trauma room, the physicians were responsible for the clinical investigation of the injuries. Neither the researchers nor the police were involved in clinical investigations.

The future looks bright for expansion of this model. Members of the injury-analysis team are discussing the possibility of having EMS personnel conduct the injury investigations on site. The new direction makes sense because para-medics are usually the first to arrive on the crash scene, even before the police in some instances. EMS personnel can collect scene data pertaining to the injuries and extrication, and transmit scene photos to the emergency room before the patient arrives at the hospital. After the EMS team transports the patient to hospital, members can return to the scene of the crash to help police investigate the causes of injury. Such a process is feasible. In many cases, the EMS personnel have already transported the patient to the trauma centre before the police begin their investigation. Upon completing the scene investigation, the EMS personnel can return to the trauma centre to document the patient injuries.

The most efficient method for sending photos of the crash scene and extrication of the patient to emergency physicians is the use of digital technology. Photographing the scene with a digital camera and then electronically mailing the pictures to the emergency room by cellular phone supports this techno-logical innovation.

□ *Ascertaining causes of the crash*

The pilot study included in-situ interviews with drivers to gain insight into the reasons for the collision. Rothe (2000) has described interviewing strate-gies like unstructured, semi-structured, structured and focus group interviews that can be applied to injury-control research. Each style has its advantages and disadvantages and should be used according to the research situation. Two styles of questioning are particularly relevant to injury analysis: the funnel approach and the pyramid approach. In the funnel approach, questions are structured from general to specific (Rothe, 2000). Each succeeding question relates to the preceding one but has a narrower focus. The pyramid approach involves asking questions from specific to general, with each succeeding ques-tion related to the preceding one (Rothe, 2000).

Although the primary goal of the model is to understand how injuries occur, understanding why the collision occurred contributes substantially to the development of prevention strategies. Rothe's (2000) methodology allows the driver to provide extended and personally meaningful answers, allowing us to look for trends that would not be possible using quantitative methods. By combining data on the reasons that the crash occurred with the reasons that the injury occurred, prevention strategies can be more easily defined and presented to local agencies.

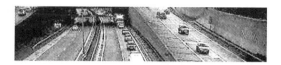

THIS RESEARCH WAS UNDERTAKEN to design a data-collection process so that researchers can understand how injuries occur and how findings can best be shared. As a unique perspective in public health, the collaboration component of the research process allowed researchers rapid access to information. The ultimate goal of the model is to help deal with severe injuries suffered in traffic collisions. The collaborative network, which allows information exchange between the police, emergency doctors and EMS professionals, is a shift in medical ideology and therefore requires further research and development. An impact on injury control would be a welcome achievement.

5

*How Intimate Social Life
Contributes to Risky Driving*

JEFFREY E. NASH &

GARY D. BRINKER

LEAVE IT TO THE NEUROLOGICAL SCIENTIST to explain how selective memory and attention function: how is it that a mind (the senior author's) transposes numbers according to some rule that operates independent of consciousness, yet recalls with vivid and accurate detail a crash witnessed twenty-two years ago? No doubt this witnessing altered the mind, for it now serves as the basis for a discussion of the interrelationships that can exist between being social and being a risky driver. Consider this recollection of the senior author.

I was driving my 1977 Volvo to pick up my two-year-old son from his Montessori school. I don't recall where my other son was or the where-abouts of my wife, and I doubt I had my lap belt fastened. I do remember the weather that day. It was cloudy and warm for early March, and the temperature was near freezing. The considerable snowfall of the winter had begun to melt. Water was puddled in low-lying areas. I was driving under the Interstate on a four-lane city street. There were traffic lights at both ends of the route that took me under I-90, but the distance from that first light travelling north to the next after coming up from the under-pass was nearly a quarter of a mile—plenty of room to get up some speed.

I was travelling in the inside lane downhill toward the bottom of the underpass, a vehicle just a few car lengths ahead of me in the outside lane. I looked in my rearview mirror. I saw a dark four-door sedan coming down the grade at high speed. I held my speed steady as the sedan passed me on the right and then the car in the outside lane on the left. In the next instant, the sedan reached the bottom of the underpass where there was a puddle of water, perhaps several inches deep. The sedan passed through the water and then began to skid, into a fishtail, and then back onto dry pavement that propelled the car straight across the low concrete divide separating the north from the southbound lanes. The sedan crashed head-on into a vehicle travelling south. I could see directly into the face of the driver in that small Honda car at the very moment of impact as I drove to the perfect position to see it all. The sound was very loud and the moment frozen in time. It was over in an instant. The sedan slid to the side of the little Honda car and rested, as dust settled around it.

One by one teenagers emerged from the sedan—one, two and then three of them (the driver was trapped behind the wheel), each dazed and immediately taking a seat on the embankment next to the road. By now I had stopped and gotten out of my car. I and another passerby ran to the small car hoping to see the driver alive. The door on the driver's side had flown open from the impact. The driver, a young woman, was slumped over to her right on the seat, a surprised look but no blood on her face (she was wearing a lap belt); there was no sign of life in her body, just the blank look of death. We could feel no pulse at her neck. Within minutes the paramedics and the police arrived. Names of witnesses were taken, and we were told to go to the police station to write out an accident report the next day. I got back in my Volvo and continued toward the Montessori school and the routine that was that day.

I read in the newspaper the next day about the fatal accident on Fairview at the underpass at I-90. I read about the victim, a twenty-two-year-old woman on her way home from the grocery store, whose aorta was severed by the impact of the crash, and the driver of the sedan, a high-school student who had skipped afternoon classes to cruise around town with three of his friends. He was from a well-known family, a family respected for their involvement in the community and their support of the high school their son attended. The teenager and his friends had not been drinking that afternoon (at least not yet). That afternoon, they were just out to have a good time, but something went terribly wrong. The passengers received minor injuries and the driver a broken foot. But the Honda driver—she was gone.

To understand what went wrong, we must recognize that a particular event, in this case a fatal crash, is more than a tragic accident. It is the outcome of a complex set of situations that make up an even more elaborate system that merges the act of operating an automobile with the meanings of everyday life. In this volume, Rothe refers to this approach to understanding traffic and related safety issues as cybernetics. We want to deconstruct the cybernetics of intimate social life and safety. The first step is to take apart the system by its principle components.

■ Intimate Social Life

A major sociological contribution to understanding social organization has been to recognize that distinctions between formal and informal (Homans, 1950), impersonal and personal (Nash & Calonico, 1996), everyday and bureaucratic (Hummel, 1998) can be drawn for virtually all forms of social life. The distinction is more than analytic. It demarks a qualitative difference between how we feel, act and think in situations. We have learned that following rules in a formal sense is quite different from following rules for interaction with our friends. For example, to comply with safety rules for operating an automobile, we must take our automobile to an inspection station, have an expert check the brake linings and, perhaps, test the emissions levels for our automobile's exhaust. But how we get our car to the inspection station may well require that we juggle work schedules, arrange for a babysitter, postpone meeting a friend for a drink at the local pub or even take advantage of the locale of the inspection station to "steal" the rest of the afternoon for the pursuit of happiness.

□ Form and content

Conventional social science has identified intimate social interaction in terms of both its form and content (Goffman, 1974). For example, intimate social interaction usually has meanings that are bound or limited to a restricted set of participants. Those meanings are coded; that is, the way one communicates is usually marked by specialized phrases and terms, and in some circumstances, even a dialect or language. Generally, the content of interaction is emotional and thus volatile. In the world of intimate interaction, things are often not as they seem. The more intimate the interaction, the more esoteric the meanings and the less likely that the meanings and rules will generalize to other venues of social life.

Intimate social life, however, is the cradle of society. In our lives with family and friends, we form the core attributes of social self—who we think we are and who we think others think we are—and here we acquire competencies for social life. Charles H. Cooley wrote that the primary group was the essential component of all social life. How we operate an automobile and, most importantly, with whom and under what circumstances, is a part of our system of intimate social life.

For those teenagers on that March day more than twenty years ago in St. Paul, Minnesota, their intimate social life—who they thought they were and what they thought they were doing—was deconstructed by the crash they were responsible for. The crash challenged their definition of what they were doing (having a good time) with the reality of a human death. In a very real sense, the crash can be seen as the alienation that results from mixing the intimate social forms of interaction with the formal rules of operating the car.

We are offering a way to see what actually happens in a crash (cf. Gusfield, 1990). We do not suggest that every crash can be understood this way, for there are many reasons for crashes, such as a driver simply falling asleep or suffering a heart attack or some mechanical failure in the vehicle. Identifying all these "causes" is, of course, important, and we are suggesting that one frequently overlooked "cause" is the nature of the social interaction taking place concurrently with the operation of a vehicle. Moreover, we suggest that a particular kind of interaction, one that is a consequence of the coming together of formal and intimate social life, can be a particularly dangerous component of the complex system we know as driving a car (Wallace, 1965). So important may this coming together be that understanding it could change the way we interpret well-documented associations between certain demographic variables and the likelihood of crashes. In particular, we refer to the increased probability that the young and the old are more likely to be dangerous drivers than those of other ages. Looking to social phenomena as cause allows us to see that it may well be the co-occurring interactions accompanying driving rather than diminished physical skills or immature thinking and judgement that account for the association between age and probability of crashes.

■ Mixed or Confounding Social Forms

Underlying our thesis is the concept of "mixed social form" (Nash & Calonico, 1996, p. 131–35). Mixed social form refers to the way the meanings of interaction are framed or organized according to what people take for granted as appropriate for a given situation. We know of the intimate form—for example, that small numbers of people communicate with each other in specialized ways that tend to carry high emotional content and require considerable attention to perform. We must pay attention to the stories our friends tell or risk challenging the assumption that we do not care about them. In the formal setting, rules are disembodied and the things we do result from our knowing what to do and having done it before. When we have friends in our car, we combine the world of intimacy with the routine of operating an automobile.

The act of operating an automobile can be seen as an enactment of social forms. One form or the other can shape and influence the content of the interaction within it. A form can be a highly rational performance that merges judgement and control of a machine. This act entails obeying signals, reading signs and the actual control of the speed and motion of the vehicle. Of course, the competency of performance depends on age, reflexes and perhaps native intelligence. However, the increased simplicity of driving (power steering, automatic transmissions, controlled-access highways, cruise control, etc.) creates circumstances that minimize the driver's consciousness of the act of driving, thereby creating "room" for other forms. Of course, the increased ease of operating an automobile allows automotive manufacturers to exploit the space created by selling devices to fill. Such devices include navigation, complicated music reproduction and climate-control systems. For young drivers and passengers, who are still practising the enactment of forms and for whom the automobile affords special opportunities for being intimate, spending time with friends and doing that "hanging out" thing (a code for being social in a way that adds specialized character to "who" the young want to be), mixing the rules of driving with the rules for being young can be dangerous.

Ideally, these two forms (formal and intimate) would be sequential—that is, the informal would take place while the formal is inactive and vice versa. However, forms are enacted simultaneously and may confound one another, creating in the act of driving a mixed form that may be alienating by its very character, encouraging such emotions as "road rage." What happens is that formality and informality clash. Attention to one interferes with the other. This juggling of one form over the other requires a great deal of practice. No doubt as one grows more mature and acquires more experience with forms the juggling becomes easier. But another process accounts for the ease of the balancing act among more mature drivers. The mature driver simply does not mix forms as much. He or she is more likely to drive a route, a familiar path from work to home or from home to the store and back, than the younger driver whose driving is "all over" in order to enact informal forms of interactions. So the chance of conflicts, of clashing between "safe" driving and having fun with one's friends, increases. How the conflict works has never been completely depicted in social science literature, but we can offer a rough sketch of it.

On that afternoon in March, the young man and his friends constructed their social reality by acting outside a formal form (in this case, removing themselves from the close, rational control that their school imposed on them). The freedom the automobile afforded them involved more than the opportunity to be together. It allowed them to act like friends, and in doing so, surely unintentionally, to take a human life.

■ Community and Traffic: Doing a Survey

Having outlined the elements of interaction that make the actual driving of a automobile the occasion for mixing or confounding intimate and formal life, we need to depict what more "objective" conditions might give us clues as to when the confounding takes place. In 1997, in Springfield, Missouri, the Center for Social Sciences and Public Policy Research (formally the Center for Social Research) conducted a telephone poll of drivers in the city. The poll was conducted to measure actions, knowledge and attitudes toward local traffic situations and driver behaviours. The questions were developed through focus group meetings of Center researchers with local key informants from organizations with a vested interest in traffic conditions and public safety, as well as with sociology students from Southwest Missouri State University.

The sample was selected from a computer-generated set of random telephone numbers, and the interviews were conducted by trained interviewers under supervision of a professional staff. Steps were followed to ensure that the target 300 interviews would be representative of licensed drivers in Springfield. While most of the findings of this study do not directly inform us about what happens in mixed social forms concurrent with the acts of operating an automobile, they do allow us to profile who is driving, what they typically think about when they drive and who is likely to express the idea that driving is somehow problematic to them. The following summary gives a brief overview of the results:

- About half of Springfield drivers say they get angry or frustrated when driving in congested or backed up traffic.
- Half of Springfield drivers are in favor of Springfield police using high-tech video cameras to issue traffic tickets. Seventy-five percent say they would be willing to pay additional taxes for this capability.
- Almost 90 percent of Springfield drivers believe first-time applicants for a driver's license and persons with multiple traffic citations should be required to take a driver-education course.
- Fifty-eight percent of Springfield drivers say they see someone driving in what they consider to be an unacceptable or unsafe manner every day.
- Almost 80 percent of Springfield drivers say they believe using a cellular phone while driving is a hazard, but only 40 percent say using a cellular phone while driving should be illegal.
- Eighty-seven percent of Springfield drivers are in favour of random road blocks to check for intoxicated drivers. Of those favouring random road blocks, 81 percent felt police should search vehicles when they have reason to believe the driver is using alcohol or drugs.
- Fifty-six percent of Springfield drivers believe the penalties in Missouri for driving while intoxicated are too lenient. Only four percent say they believe the penalties are too stiff.

- Almost half of Springfield drivers say they sometimes honk or shout at a discourteous driver. Fifteen percent say they get angry enough with discourteous drivers to want to assault them. Twelve percent say they occasionally make obscene gestures at other drivers, while eight percent say they sometimes try to cut off or get even with a discourteous driver.

Who said these things? Fifty-one percent of respondents were female. Their age-groups ranged from teens to seniors: 16 percent were between 16 and 25 years of age; 19 percent between 26 and 36; 20 percent between 37 and 45; 20 percent between 46 and 55; 10 percent between 56 and 65; and 15 percent over 65. Their average number of years of education was 14.15, with a standard deviation of 2.1, and their average income per year was $38,000, with a standard deviation of $20,000.

While these data do not directly depict the mixed form, correlation coefficients between conventional variables and answers to questions about driving can uncover patterns that suggest the validity of the way we conceptualize the act of driving. Rank-order analysis using age as the predictor revealed that younger drivers and, in particular, the very young (between 18 and 25 years of age) are more likely than older drivers to say they become angry and frustrated, use obscene gestures on occasion, even use illegal cutoffs (turning into parking lots) to avoid traffic jams, and to express ideas that might indicate aggressive driving habits and lenient attitudes toward traffic laws.

Such findings are hardly surprising. Extant data (*Sourcebook of Criminal Justice Statistics*) reveals, for instance, that when US high-school seniors were surveyed over a twelve-year period (1984 to 1996), the portion involved in at least one crash that resulted in injury or property damage has remained fairly constant at between 17 and 19 percent. This pattern persists despite a reduction in the percentage saying they drove while drinking at least once during the last twelve months. So even with successful results from campaigns to dissuade young drivers from drinking, they are involved in crashes.

Clearly, youthful drivers are at risk for crashes, and their perspective on driving (that is, the meaning driving has for them) reflects their competencies and degree of involvement in peer social life. Data from the survey of Springfield drivers support the hypothesis that youthful drivers tend to be more preoccupied with social activities such as interacting and impressing their peer passengers than the formal activities of navigating to a desired destination in a safe manner.

Tables 5.1, 5.2 and 5.3 show the Spearman's Rank Correlation Coefficients for four conventional variables and various self-reported behaviours and opinions for a random sample of Springfield, Missouri, drivers. Spearman's is a widely

TABLE 5.1

**Relationships between general sociability questions
and predictor variables**

General Sociability Questions	Age	Income	Education	Gender (M=1 F=2)
Require Passengers to Use Seatbelts	0.137*	0.135*	0.103	0.239**
Against Road Blocks	-0.188**	0.052	-0.009	-0.098
Use Cellular Phone	-0.115*	0.339**	0.135*	-0.010
Drive All Over Town	-0.203**	-0.020	0.034	-0.107
Against Ban on Cruising	-0.162*	0.156*	0.088	-0.195**

used measure of the degree of association between variables that can be ranked or placed in categories. A positive correlation indicates that either the older, the higher income, the higher educated or the females, as the case may be, tended to report higher levels of the particular behaviour or opinion. The asterisks indicate how confidently we can assume that the particular relationship must exist among the population of all Springfield drivers, with one asterisk indicating 95 percent confidence and two asterisks 99 percent confidence.

Table 5.1 shows that youthful drivers are less likely to require their passengers to wear seat belts and more likely to use a cellular phone while driving, drive all over town as opposed to a few standard routes, oppose a city-wide ban on "cruising" and oppose road blocks to check for intoxicated drivers. Other significant relationships suggest that more affluent youth, in particular, are even more likely to use a cell phone while driving, whereas lower-income youth may be even less likely to require passengers to use seat belts. The data also suggest a tendency for young male drivers, as opposed to young female drivers, to be less likely to support a ban on cruising or require their passengers to wear their seat belts.

We suggest that this depiction of age as a cause of risky driving and even crashes is only partial. More to the point is that young drivers are more likely to engage in multiple kinds of social interactions while driving and therefore are diverted from following the rules for safe operation of an automobile. As Rothe (1987, 1991, 1994) has demonstrated, social principles govern what happens inside automobiles. To the degree that these are omitted from an

TABLE 5.2

Relationships between aggressive driver questions and predictor variables

Aggressive Driver Variables	Age	Income	Education	Gender (M=1 F=2)
Friend/family killed/hurt in accident	-0.295**	-0.085	-0.016	0.000
Honk/shout at discourteous driver	-0.368**	0.036	0.025	-0.096
Get angry/frustrated in traffic	-0.293**	0.009	-0.059	-0.020
Obscene gestures at discourteous driver	-0.190**	-0.011	-0.050	-0.128*
Cut off/get even with discourteous driver	-0.198**	0.008	-0.014	-0.113
How fast drive when late	-0.291**	0.012	0.007	-0.064
Favour higher speed limits	-0.345**	-0.067	-0.066	-0.072
Against video-camera tickets	-0.220**	0.033	-0.021	-0.069

analysis of safety, misunderstanding and ineffective policy may follow. The problem is exacerbated when that social interaction is heavily based on norms of defiance against the courtesy and the well-ordered road rules dictated by traffic law. Rebellion against these imposed standards is readily exhibited by the proverbial aggressive driver who, when challenged by a similar type, often vents the resulting frustration through a relatively recent phenomenon known as "road rage."

Several survey questions were constructed to measure various indicators of aggressive driving. The correlation coefficients between them and each of the four predictor variables are shown in Table 5.2. The strong and highly significant negative correlation coefficients for age and the aggressive driving variables

TABLE 5.3

Relationships between aggressive driver questions and predictor variables by gender

	Age	
Aggressive Driver Variables	Males	Females
Friend/family killed/ hurt in accident	-0.232**	-0.353**
Honk/shout at discourteous driver	-0.278**	-0.431**
Get angry/frustrated in traffic	-0.233**	-0.349**
Obscene gestures at discourteous driver	-0.156	-0.211**
Cut off/get even with discourteous driver	-0.163*	-0.231**
How fast drive when late	-0.239**	-0.345**
Favour higher speed limits	-0.306**	-0.375**
Against video-camera tickets	-0.228**	-0.202*

indicate that young drivers were much more likely to report exhibiting these opinions and behaviours than older drivers. Almost as striking are the lack of significant relationships with the income, education and gender variables, suggesting little difference in these characteristics between affluent and lower-income drivers or between males and female drivers. These data strongly suggest a culture of defiance against the system dominating the youthful driver's social interaction. Was the passing manoeuvre that resulted in the death of the young woman due to the driver's youthful inexperience in judging safe passing conditions, or is it attributable to an effort to impress his friends with his daring defiance of the formal road rules of prudence and courtesy?

Interestingly, while the negative coefficients in the Gender column of Table 5.2 suggest that aggressive driving is a predominantly male phenomenon, Table 5.3 shows that the correlation coefficients between age and aggressive driving are stronger for females. This finding suggests that females are much more likely to "mellow" with age, exhibiting more rapid declines in aggressive driving behaviour with each passing year than males.

Survey data may sketch the broad profile of the consequences of mixing or confounding social life while operating an automobile. To understand fully the way that intimate social life contributes to risky driving, however, requires a detailed look at the nature of what transpires inside the car. Although that afternoon two decades ago provided an eyewitness account of only one instance of the confounding, it may all too often be prototypical. The tragedy for the young driver involves the conflict between the requirements of friendships and "taking an afternoon off," and safe driving. Policies and practices on the part of government, parents and schools to promote safe driving among youthful drivers need to accommodate the social uses to which young drivers put the automobile.

6

RURAL VERSUS URBAN DRIVING
Social Behaviour and Lifestyle

J. PETER ROTHE

WHY DO SAFETY STRATEGISTS want to compare rural and urban drivers? How do rural and urban drivers differ in social behaviours, community and cultural values, views on risk and temperaments? These questions require researchers to dig beneath standard traffic-safety variables such as violations, collision characteristics, age, gender, causes of crashes and exposure—factors that gloss over people's psycho-social behaviours. To understand rural drivers better, we must unearth and screen these psycho-social behaviours within a rural context.

Rural areas increasingly experience serious crashes. According to Baker et al. (1992, p. 27), Canada's rural areas have 50 percent higher mortality rates than urban ones. Alberta statistics show that 76 percent of fatal crashes occurred in rural areas (Alberta Transportation, 1997), where only 20 percent of the Canadian population lives (Ramp, 1999). Standard epidemeological reasons for the high rural traffic mortality and morbidity rates show that there are fewer trauma centres in rural areas, resulting in delayed access to emergency care, limited follow-up surgical care and fewer EMS professionals trained in advanced life support (Grossman et al., 1997).

Researchers have historically paid little attention to the drivers' social context (Clark, 1976; Rhodes, 1999; Rothe, 1994). But today, researchers investigating road rage are focussing on social scenarios like family hassles, friendships, work demands, road construction and community standards (Gulian et al., 1998; Hennessy, 1998; Hennessy & Wiesenthal, 1997). Hennessy (1999) concluded that the driver's social and cultural life is a strong indicator of driving behaviour. Psychological literature suggests connections exist between individual stress, view of self, and social behaviour (Krech, Crutchfield & Ballachey, 1962). For example, Rosenberg (1986) and Neff and Husaini (1985) reported that stress and feelings of depression and worthlessness often lead to increased alcohol consumption and dangerous driving.

Furthermore, several rural health-based academics have compared rural and urban social behaviours. For example, Forrest (1988) described rural-dwellers as being more independent in spirit, passive in conflict, religious, and ethnocentric in personality than urbanites. Millar and Lulaff (1981) commented that rural-dwellers are more passive and fatalistic than urban-dwellers, while Hansen and McIntire (1984) reported that loneliness is more common in rural areas than in urban ones.

The literature demonstrates a need to investigate driving and social context further. Thus, a qualitative study was undertaken to answer two basic questions: (1) What social characteristics influence temperaments (e.g., moods), relevant attitudes (e.g., values about family or safety), driver behaviours and beliefs about risk and safety (e.g., fatalism and luck)? and (2) How do rural and urban drivers differ in general and specific driving-based temperament in ways that suggests driver action and attitude?

■ Basic Assumptions

Five assumptions support our thoughts. First, "rural" denotes a region charac-terized by a small population that is primarily involved in farming, mining, forestry or fishing (Miller & Luloff, 1981); urban designates large towns or cities. Second, traffic is a social phenomenon that is created, formed and changed in and through people's responses to cultural values, sentiments, moral/political forces and ideals (Gusfield, 1981, 1996; Rothe, 1993). Third, emotion or temperament is constantly played out with families, friends, work-mates, local institutions and organizations. It therefore influences driving behaviour (Rothe, 1990). Fourth, interview data embody events and activities that drivers choose to describe their realities (Cicourel, 1974; Freund & Martin, 1997). Fifth, qualitative research descriptions about driving support the imple-mentation of effective rural-based intervention programs (Rothe, 1994; Ramp, 1999).

■ Methodology

Two researchers travelled throughout Alberta interviewing drivers about rural and urban socio-cultural features. Participating drivers were volunteers aged 23 to 55 years old and lived in Edmonton, Calgary or rural locations. Professionals, retailers, tradesmen, farmers, ranchers, office workers and agricultural college students participated.

Two strategies were used to choose participants. First, every third candidate from a sampling frame provided by a major insurance company's policy-holders was invited to participate in local focus groups. Next, "table-top inter-views" were initiated, in which random patrons in local coffee shops shared their points of view. This procedure provided spontaneous information and greater randomization of participants. The focus-group sessions lasted from twenty (three interviewees) to ninety minutes (twelve interviewees). One hundred and fifty drivers participated, of which eighty-three were rural and sixty-seven were urban. Saturation set in as respondents repeated themselves and comprehensiveness was verified. Distinct patterns of behaviour, attitudes, temperaments and structures of reasoning were noted.

Semi-structured interviews focussed on (1) risk and surrogates of risk (locked houses, vehicles and seat-belt use), (2) personal responsibility, luck and fatalism, (3) temperament and (4) anger-producing traffic scenarios. Although the entire interviews included 22 questions, specific queries relevant to this chapter were as follows:

- What role does luck play in driving? How does it relate to crashes and injuries?
- Do you always lock your house/vehicle when you leave? When do you not lock your house/vehicle? Do you always wear a seat belt? Why or why not?
- How would you describe your everyday temperament? How would you describe your temperament while driving a car?
- What kind of traffic event or kind of driver upsets you the most, if any? How do you typically respond?
- What does the home/workplace mean to you? Please describe.

Data analysis included a series of steps. First, the audio-taped interviews were transcribed and printed. Two researchers analyzed the volumes of data. One researcher reviewed all of the transcripts and extracted broad relevant themes. Theme extraction was guided by the pre-defined questions asked in the inter-views. After the first-order themes were defined, the data were analyzed for articulation of subthemes and refinements of broad themes. A second researcher reviewed the transcriptions and analyzed the data according to second-order themes—themes that are relevant to the study but are more deeply embedded in the discourse.

The second researcher used analytic induction as the sense-making tech-nique. Much like a puzzle, first-order themes were fit into a frame. Second-order themes were used to refine the original pieces and extend the frame. As new concepts, ideas, issues and problems were located and the frequency or distribution of the phenomena was noted, the puzzle took the form of a model that supported evidence not included in the first-order analysis (Lindesmith, 1953; Becker, 1970). Consistent with analytic induction, the data were interpreted according to embedded patterns, significant concepts, beliefs, concerns, values and normative behaviours. The goal was not to overwhelm with detail or undermine with practicality. The analysis was intended to be the brick and mortar for developing the foundation of a socially based theoretical framework on rural-urban driving (Strauss & Corbin, 1994).

■ Feelings About Home Life

Homes are drivers' micro-worlds—launch ports from which they start their daily journeys. Home is—at least in theory—the most important locale of private life, where drivers should find self-fulfilment and satisfaction (Berger & Berger, 1975). But major differences in the images of home were noted between urban and rural drivers. The urban drivers show a mental image of home life constructed on an ethos of hurry, hustle, busyness and "temporary permanence"—a temporary escape, a place to eat and sleep. For example:

- I would describe my lifestyle as varied. I have different interests that keep me from getting bored .... My home is where I have my meal and watch the news, and read a bit, and sleep. That's about it. The rest of the time I do biking, walking—those sorts of things.
- You come home from work and you eat and find something to do. Usually I am looking to go elsewhere. I don't like to stay at home. Just eat and sleep.
- My home is peaceful. I really enjoy being inside it. However, I consider myself quite active; there's not too many evenings in the week that I'm home. Maybe Friday, because I'm exhausted and getting ready for Saturday.

While "temporary permanence" was embraced by some urban drivers, others defined home as a refuge where they feel comfortable, relaxed and in control. For example:

- It is a nice home base from which I leave for the world.
- My house is my castle ... Going home is where I relax, so I want it to have comfortable chairs, comfortable atmosphere you know!
- When I am by myself, I am quite content. I consider my home my refuge where I am in control. I am satisfied, pretty much.

- I can describe my home as being comfortable. I see my home as a home base more than anything. That is where I keep all my materials. It's where I leave from and come back to. That's where my wife is, that's where my family comes to visit. It's quite enjoyable.

For some drivers, a hectic city life requires a peaceful and relaxing home:

- You come home right away. It's chaos out here, you know.
- My home life would be quiet, but the work life would be quite busy, quite active, and a lot of things to do. At times it is stressful, but manageable.
- Work is busy and stressful. Home life is peaceful and relaxing as I can get it.

Others linked hectic homes to busy urban realities. Their answers refer to work and children as key reasons for living in hectic households:

- Very hectic at home! Two parents who work. Two children rushing!
- Hectic home life. Pick up the kids. Drop off the kids ...
- I would put both my home life and my work life as pretty high stress. I have a pretty active family. I have a lot of stress at home and a lot of stress at work.
- I have a very high stress job that eats into my family life. It's a 24-hour-per-day job; and my husband has the same job. And it's very, very stressful, and very, very hectic; and it is never finished.

As the quotations show, for some urban drivers, the relationship between work and home has a negative connotation. Work stress relates to home stress. But children are different. Although they represent a collective factor for hectic home lives, they are more like "loving evils," an essential ingredient for successful family life.

Rural drivers repeatedly defined their homes as happy and stable places. Home represents a refuge, a welcoming location of family interaction and a place where drivers find support, love and social intimacy:

- I come from a very close family. We spend a lot of time together. Everybody is concerned about each other, and that is very good— very good family life.
- Work is something I do during the week. I really enjoy going back home.

- My home, it's great. Very supportive—both my daughter and my husband. My husband has taken on more of my duties at home, and my daughter has learned how to cook. So I only find it a positive thing.
- I have a close and loving relationship with everybody in the family.

Unlike urban drivers, it is customary for rural drivers to experience self-fulfilment and emotional satisfaction at home. It is a significant part of their lifestyle, not a staging area for lifestyle. Homes provide rural participants with a safe haven from the outside world; the following short responses are typical:

- Happy, not much stress. Kids have left home.
- Easygoing, happy.
- Quiet, happy.
- Fairly busy, but happy.

■ Feelings About Work

Drivers' lives are organized according to rhythms of home and work; the latter is ideally defined as a vocation in which drivers find a measure of fulfilment. However, urban participants described work as barely tolerable places where they experience lack of control, alienation and low financial rewards. These features contribute to stress, pressure, apathy and frustration which in turn influence driving (Broome, 1985). The following quotations reflect work and tolerance.

- Yeah, it's ongoing and mega overtime and the whole office is like that. I am just one other fish in the bowl, you know.
- Work is disgusting. Complex usually, 'cause I am fielding a lot of the problems from a lot of people who are not into computers.
- I am not happy with my job. Who would be happy? Yeah, very stressful. It has contributed enough to my sickness. I really feel that way.

Work tends to be "busy," "hectic" and "stressful." Frustrating computer problems! Too much overtime for too little cash! Little time for doing hard work! Bosses who only consider profit! Witness the following comments:

- You make the best of what you got. Our company was bought internationally, and now they are talking about getting us a third computer. Oh, goodie, we get to do this again ... more pressure ...

- I got a really hectic job 'cause I travel a lot. Fly here and there in the car. Really, I am all over the place. It's really hectic.
- My manager pushes and pushes ...

Farmers mused about the crossover between farm as work and family; one blends into the other. Hence, it is difficult to remove farming from family and tradition. Farming is all-embracing; the end goal is to earn sufficient money to continue the tradition for at least one more year. Work stress becomes economic stress because of low market prices offered for farm products. Extensive time needed to milk cows or harvest grain was considered a way of life, not work. One farmer said, "I very much enjoy agriculture. I am very committed to it. It's my life's passion and my work."

For non-farmers, work was described as a life necessity. The earnings allowed them to pay for family events, outings and other lifestyle needs. Work was seldom acknowledged as a vocation or professionally valued activity on its own. It was usually linked to family, lifestyle, home and spousal responsibility.

■ Risk Surrogates

Risk-taking has strong cultural and social bonds (Wildavsky, 1982; Rothe, 1994). Drivers usually decide to avoid risk on the basis of social behaviour (Rothe, 1994). How drivers account for risks and safety within different contexts reflects how drivers partake in risk-avoidance and safety activities. Three common risk-avoidance actions are locking houses, securing vehicles and wearing seat belts.

People's efforts to lock their houses and cars serve as surrogates for risk-taking (Cooper, 1992). Safety- and health-related institutions promote crime-prevention measures like locking doors through awareness campaigns, popular literature and personal communication. Yet people act according to social factors like trust, community and neighbourliness.

As city residents, urban drivers experience a context of violence, anonymity, uncertain policing and distrust. Homes are generally locked, regardless of whether drivers visit their neighbours, go shopping or take extended trips. Their vehicles are locked for similar reasons: it has become a habit:

Of course I lock my car ... I always do. It's just one of the things I do without really thinking about ... Just do it. Why take a chance?

Some urban drivers fail to lock houses or vehicles, using a prominent reason like, "Older cars have low value; no one wants to steal them, so they can remain unlocked. New cars have high value; thieves want to steal them, so they must be locked." Additional noteworthy comments went along this line:

- My piece of trash ... If somebody hauls it away, it is not a big deal. And in the summertime, what are they going to steal? My jack?
- Away from my immediate home area, I lock the doors. Before, I didn't because I had an old vehicle, so if somebody did steal it, that would be OK.
- I have two old beaters! If they want to take them, goodbye. Now I have another vehicle, so maybe I will start thinking different about it. It is more expensive, worth more.

Another argument for not securing vehicles is that locked cars mean little to professional thieves intent on breaking in, and collateral damage like smashed windows or vandalized doors is more expensive than the cost of stolen items and is inconvenient to repair. The old adage "locked doors keep out honest people" captures such thinking. The following responses are non-equivocal:

- [Lock my car?] Not very often! Only at shopping centers, or so. Not at home! I probably should. I mean any car could be open in 2 to 3 minutes. Even if it is locked! If someone wants to break into your car, if you lock it, it doesn't help.
- If someone wanted to break into my car, he could just smash the window. Now I have to pay for a smashed window. By leaving the door open I avoid that cost.
- No [I don't lock the doors], and I leave the window open too. Yeah, take whatever you want but don't break the windows.

A number of urban drivers live in cities, but they often drive and stay in the country. They lock their vehicles in the city but not in rural areas:

- Not in small towns, but in larger areas or cities. I don't want my truck stolen.
- I lock the truck most of the time if I am in town or in the city, but if I go out to my parent's farm, no, never.
- Probably about 98 to 99 percent of the time in the city. If you are visiting a small town where everybody knows everybody, I leave it [my truck] unlocked. But definitely not in the city!

As urban drivers see it, there is less need to lock vehicles in the country because they are more familiar with and trust rural people. They lock doors in urban settings because they are unfamiliar with and distrustful of urban citizens.

Rural drivers differed from their urban counterparts. They are less likely to lock their houses or cars, have less fear of violence and are more trusting of their neighbours:

- I never lock the house ... I never bother with it. What for?
- Very seldom! There's no need in the country. People trust each other.
- Who has the time? Neighbours look out for each other, and they have dogs.

One farmer highlighted the issue when he said that his house is always unlocked so that people who "drive in the ditch in the winter, get lost or get into trouble on the road" can find refuge.

Rural drivers heading to the cities to work, shop or visit treat locked cars similarly to their urban counterparts. They are more likely to lock their vehicles in the city than the country:

- Not always! Not around here! There's no need. You know the people here.
- Not all the time! What for! There's no need. Nobody's gonna take it here. But the city's a different thing ... Always, always lock cars.
- I do in the city. When I'm home on the farm I don't, because everybody knows everybody.

Seat belts can be seen as an extension of locked houses and cars (Cooper, 1992). Seat belts demonstrate a continuity of risk based on lifestyle and perception of safety.

□ *Seat belts*
Urban drivers are generally aware that wearing a seat belt reduces the risk of mortality. Media blitzes, radio and newspaper articles tell them so. However, many urbanites buckle up for another major reason: legal repercussions. They want to avoid receiving traffic citations, large fines and demerit points for failing to wear seat belts: "Oh, yes! Seventy-five-dollar ticket! Otherwise I wouldn't." For others, seat-belt wearing has become a habit, except for short trips: "Usually but not always, like if I was running over to the store I probably wouldn't wear it."

Wearing seat belts should not be considered a natural part of the rural drivers' travel habits. Interviewees were reluctant to believe that seat belts reduce death and serious injury. Their skepticism was based on second-hand information shared by family members or friends. The social grapevine is a dynamic feature of rural life. Family, friends and colleagues share local news, information and gossip. Stories are told about drivers and passengers who escaped serious consequences in crashes because they did not wear their seat belts:

- My wife and kids wear it all the time. I never do. Never have—never will. Why? Because my brother saved his life four different times because he never had one on! We talked about it for a long time.
- I had a buddy who told me about an accident a few years ago. If he was locked in, strapped in, he wouldn't be here today. I take that back. If I am downtown, and I see a cop car come, I will throw my seat belt over.

For many, wearing seat belts is a discriminating rather than habitual act. Rural drivers may wear seat belts when travelling on the highway but not wear them while driving in town. Witness:

- Long drives, I wear it. In town, I don't.
- Usually I do; on occasion, at work. When driving around ... no I don't, and occasionally going up town.

Few rural drivers can be considered seat-belt wearers. Restraints are removed for reasons like "backing up a car," "making trips on gravel or country roads," "feeling comfortable in trucks" and "desiring to be independent and free."

■ Developing a Consistency Rule

A noteworthy consistency rule evolved from the data. Locked houses and cars (surrogates of risk) relate to seat-belt wearing. Urban drivers who regularly lock their houses and cars may be more likely to wear seat belts. Witness the following exchange:

Interviewer: Do you lock your doors whenever you leave your house?
A: Yes, they are always locked.
Int: Even when you are going to see a neighbour?
A: Yes, of course.
Int.: Do you lock your car whenever you leave?
A: Always.
Int: Do you wear your seat belt?
A: All the time!

Conversely, drivers who do not lock houses or cars may not be as likely to wear occupant restraints:

Interviewer: Do you lock your house or apartment whenever you leave?

B: No.

Int: Under what circumstances wouldn't you?

B: Well, if I am just around the neighbourhood or if I am nearby the house, I wouldn't lock it. Same with the car! I would leave the car in the driveway or in the front of the house unlocked because we are usually going in and out. And I have not put my seat belt on coming back from the video store, which is ten blocks away.

Int: So, short distances.

B: Short distances? I won't do it, even if the kids are in the car. I don't want to get into bad habits, and I think it's more convenience and speed.

Int: How so?

B: Well, rationally you know, I would be getting out [of the car] in a second anyway ...

Int.: Do you wear a seat belt?

B: Sometimes, mostly never. I don't think they really help.

■ Personal Responsibility or Luck

Although researchers manifestly deny luck, rarely is it excluded from people's expressions of daily life. Although luck cannot be proved, both rural and urban drivers routinely invoked it as justification for their driving. Luck has simplicity; it helps explain unexplainable experiences and it demonstrates basic outlooks or philosophies of life. It is used to explain involvement or avoidance of collisions, close calls and escape of death or injury. It has coherence, stability and meaningfulness.

Luck plays a role in avoiding motor-vehicle collisions:

- Yeah, sometimes I have been pretty lucky not to have been in an accident.
- There have been many times that I've been lucky. Lucky, as somebody not hitting me, because they end up hitting the curb and move out of position.
- Yeah, I would have to say there is some luck. You never know how it is going to happen, or what is going to be at the end. I would have to say that there is a bit of luck.
- A tough question! Sometimes it [luck] has all to do with it. That's all I'm going to say.
- A lot! Cause, well, it is only a matter of a split second, and that can't be placed on your reflexes. Part of it has got to be some luck involved.

Luck gained prominence when drivers explained their collision experiences. It was featured whenever drivers had difficulty defining the factors of a crash. A rule evolved from the data: good luck helps avoid crashes while bad luck helps create them! There was agreement that it is bad luck when other drivers cause crashes or when drivers are confronted by severe environmental conditions like sleet, rain or snow storms. Drivers can find themselves in the wrong place at the wrong time, a situation for which drivers hesitate taking responsibility. Here are some personal announcements:

- There are irresponsible drivers out there. I mean it could be luck if you happen to be the one closest to that irresponsible person. Somebody is responsible, but you're out of luck if you are there and can't help it.
- Luck is important. My wife and I were driving in separate cars. She was in one lane next to me, but a little further back, and I was further ahead in another lane. We were stopped at a red light ... and a drunk driver came and smashed behind her ... and totalled her car. It had nothing to do with my wife. She was in the wrong lane at the wrong time.
- The only time that luck has a role in anything is when you are rendered totally helpless. Like turning around the bend in a mountain valley and hitting a fog bank! Then it's truly luck ....
- I would say there is luck, depending on conditions. If you are on a steep icy hill, and you're far away back from somebody, if he starts sliding down the hill, and you start sliding down after him and hit him. Just luck!

Rural and urban drivers agreed that they adhere to safe driving practices like carefully watching other drivers, paying attention to roadway exigencies and driving carefully. Still, they noted that luck contributes to their collision-free driving histories:

- I try and pay attention. Probably experience, and a whole bunch of luck.
- Pure, absolutely, unadulterated luck which I try to create myself. I do defensive driving, constantly second-guessing what is happening on the road. It sounds terrible, but I don't trust anybody behind the wheel.
- I would say part of it is luck. There are some accidents that you cause, and there are some that are thrust upon you. I try to be careful, and on the occasions that I haven't, I've been lucky.
- I think it's a combination of defensive driving and good luck. I can't nail it down to anything specific. I have always been pretty careful.

■ Fate or Divine Intervention

Fate, divine intervention or destiny was an object of explanation used more often by rural than urban drivers. They offered alternative thoughts to help explain the unexplainable, by proposing that fate contributes to the creation of traffic crashes. Fate or destiny is beyond the driver's control, so drivers share little or no responsibility for their actions. Noteworthy phrases in the data included "when your number is up, it's up" and "if it's meant to be ...." Because the drivers cannot control traffic issues, they become victims or beneficiaries:

- I was in a collision. Someone rear-ended me. And the fact that I haven't been in any more ... I think angels are protecting me.
- Luck hasn't anything to do with it. If your number is called, it's called.
- A part of me seriously believes that when it is your time, it is your time. If you are in the wrong place at the wrong time, you were supposed to be there.
- It is luck and also when it is your time to go, then you are going to go because I see a lot of things happen and I have no idea how those people made it ....

Deterministic accounts suggested that geographical location, other drivers and culture are major contributors to collisions. Because they are considered to be basic and real, drivers make decisions accordingly:

- You're used to driving in the city. So you're are used to driving with 100,000 vehicles out there. You get into a small town or farm area, you are the only vehicle for miles. You don't look then. Yet farmers are pulling off their field, out onto the road. Quite frequently, they don't check.
- I grew up in a rural community. You can go to a small town and they park their car in front of the drugstore. They got what they need and get in their car, and just back up. They don't look! They are ready to go and they just leave. I seen it happen where I come down a main street in a small town that I grew up and it's like—whoa! You better have your foot on the clutch and brake all the way down the main street or you'll be toast. They just pull out.

Urban drivers repeatedly blamed other drivers' behaviours or personal characteristics for their collisions. One such behaviour is other drivers' momentary
inattention:

- If we drive down the road and started counting the number of people
  we see on the cell phone ... shame on all those people. They always
  seem to hurt someone down the line.
- There are a lot of people smoking, and they drop cigarettes, or whatever. Sometimes, they are drinking coffee and spill on themselves. I
  mean lots of people are doing things like that. They cause accidents.

■ Everyday Versus Driving Temperament

Hennessy (1999) concluded that driver temperament contributes substantially
to driving behaviour. He singled out such observable actions as honking horns,
yelling profanities at other drivers, weaving or passing on the shoulder, lashing
out vengefully, creating momentary inattention and distracting drivers. To
provide an accurate portrait of driving and life temperament, a series of mental
states and subjective experiences are described.

The data in Table 6.1 make it clear that a proportion of urban and rural
drivers consider themselves to be easygoing but they change once they enter
their vehicle. Easygoing people can become agitated, impatient and aggressive
drivers.

Major traffic features that upset these drivers include senior drivers at intersections, rush hour or traffic congestion, tailgaters and running red lights.
Even-tempered urban drivers' responses to such features are essentially passive:
"I try to get by them if I have to. I will stop for them." Easygoing rural drivers
who experience irritating traffic situations tend to produce measured, low-key
responses. They talk to themselves, shake their heads and "let things be."
There is a consistency between their general and driving temperament:

- I don't get agitated. I just say "well, we have to take it in stride and
  relax."
- You can't do much; you just have to follow them ...

In Table 6.2 we see that some drivers defined their temperament as moderate
except for circumstances that force them into a different frame of mind. This
dualism leaves a large grey zone filled with drivers who change temperaments as
they experience different life scenarios. They are the normal or moderate
majority whose rationality includes a fitting temperament for a fitting life event.

TABLE 6.1

Driver temperament: From easygoing to aggressive (samples)

General temperament	*Driving temperament*
Urban drivers	
I'm reasonably laid back.	Every now and again I get a bit agitated and impatient. I have to rein myself in.
Easygoing.	Not quite road rage, but close. You can't afford to hit people ...
I would like to say I'm even tempered.	I have road rage, where I get frustrated at drivers who aren't thoughtful or considerate. I don't react as calmly as I should.
Fairly calm.	More aggressive, just with my language, not with my actions ....
Rural drivers	
I don't get mad; I am very even tempered—always friendly and happy.	I don't take it personal when people do stuff. I know they shouldn't be doing that and I don't let it bother me.
Friendly and easygoing!	I try to keep easygoing, but it's hard.
Easygoing. But I can blow up pretty fast.	I do get frustrated when I drive. Not so much up here because there are four lanes, but you get down where I am from and there are two lanes, and you get what I call the weekend drivers; I get frustrated.
I am fairly even tempered. I will get annoyed with other drivers but I won't act on it.	I tell myself "don't react." Some drivers who are driving too close, or cut you off, or merge on top of you! I find that frustrating, but I don't let myself get angry.

TABLE 6.2
Driver temperament: From moderate to irritable (samples)

General temperament	*Driving temperament*
Urban drivers	
I'm okay. Depends on things that happen. I'm up and down.	I get mad when drivers screw me around. I try to stay cool, but at times you just can't.
Easygoing, but no pushover.	I'm fine as long as some guy doesn't push my button. Sometimes, though, you feel like lashing out at some of the Calgary drivers.
I don't think I'm one thing or another. I'm just me.	It all depends on what's happening. More times than not I let drivers know how I feel.
I guess the best way to describe myself is even tempered … with a bottom line.	Generally I'm careful and give a measured response to some idiot. I let him know how I feel, but what's the point of taking it overboard and somebody gets hurt.
Rural drivers	
I find that, generally, I am a pretty reasonable guy.	I'm okay except when some guy passes me and then slows right down. That pisses me off.
Good days and bad days.	If I am mad getting into the car, then it probably is going to reflect in my driving, but basically, give me music—that is all I need. Country and Western!
I would say really easygoing. It takes a lot to push me over the top, but when I do it's not pleasant.	I gesture if some guy is not signalling. I would speed up and not let him by, box him in, that kind of thing.

Moderate rural drivers were found more likely than urban ones to become aggressive when they confront irritable traffic circumstances or drivers. Some consider it reasonable to tailgate or follow offending drivers so that they can later confront them. They have major problems with impaired drivers, tailgaters, drivers who fail to signal intentions and drivers who cut off other vehicles. Typical rural drivers' responses include chasing offending drivers, purposefully reducing speed to frustrate other drivers, honking the horn and experiencing rising aggravation:

- I followed guys home because I wanted to give them a piece of my mind.
- I honk my horn if somebody really ticks me off.
- If they have pulled out in front of me where I had to swerve, I'll chase them.
- I usually give them the bird, lay on the horn; sometimes turn around and chase them, pass them, be erratic. If I'm mad I'll tailgate them.

Traffic congestion, buses and culturally specific law-breaking drivers upset moderate urban drivers. Their typical responses include aggressively passing non-violating drivers, forcing entry into another lane and becoming extremely aggravated:

- I keep my distance until I've had enough crawling. Then I roar by them.
- Keep away from them. Pass them and go like hell so I can the hell get out of their sight.
- It's okay at first, but then I get sick of it. My fuse gets shorter and eventually I get really pissed off.

As shown in Table 6.3, some urban drivers considered their general temperament to be uptight, angry or stressed; no rural drivers defined themselves in these terms. At worst, participating rural drivers discussed having a moderate disposition that changes when they encounter life hassles. Already irritable, some urban drivers become even more frustrated when they encounter traffic events like being cut off by other drivers or when other motorists don't allow them into their lanes. Responses can be extreme:

- Punch out their headlights and tail lights, using my walking stick. Hey, I'm big.
- You just lose it sometimes. You would probably cut off the other driver. You get your chance and you take it.
- Short of getting out of the car and smacking someone.
- When someone cuts you off I roll down the window and call him an asshole.

TABLE 6.3
Driver temperament: From moderate to irritable (samples)

General temperament	Driving temperament
Urban drivers	
Hot.	Very hot!
Kind of on the edge, very short tempered.	Fairly angry, quick off the mark.
I'm generally uptight and depressed.	Look out people, get out of my way.
Constantly stressed from all the crap in the city.	Short fused and pushy ... real pushy.

Urban drivers who described their general temperament as frustrated allow irritations to become exaggerated in traffic. They become short fused and increasingly agitated behind the wheel, taking measures intended to insult, hurt, harm or destroy.

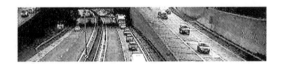

URBAN AND RURAL DRIVERS defined everyday reality differently. Key differences serve as a starting point for attending to rural traffic safety issues. Five propositions help construct the rural driver's reality.

PROPOSITION 1: For rural drivers, home or family life is composed of meanings and actions that primarily reflect comfort. Standard concepts excavated from the data are relaxation, warmth and togetherness. For urban drivers, home life denotes hectic everyday events like attending to children, staging leisure events outside the home, and valued but brief stays to relax. For many urban drivers, home life is a form of "temporary permanence."

PROPOSITION 2: Rural drivers define work in terms of involvement and sociality. For example, farmers consider work a way of life that interrelates with family. There is no dualism. Workers tend to see work as an extension of family activities. Urban drivers describe home life as efficient utilisation of time. They are more likely to define work life as stressful, time controlled and busy.

PROPOSITION 3: Rural drivers normally do not extend their work and home lives to driving, whereas urban drivers tend to drive according to work stress, pressure and haste.

PROPOSITION 4: Rural drivers' versions of securing homes, locking cars and protecting their bodies by wearing seat belts included trust of neighbours, belief in family values and reliance on friends helping friends. They are less likely to lock their houses and vehicles and more likely to drive unbelted than are their urban counterparts. A consistency rule can be invoked: drivers who lock their homes also tend to lock their vehicles and wear their seat belts.

PROPOSITION 5: Rural drivers are more likely to have easygoing or moderate temperaments. They are likely to give measured responses to traffic situations. Urban drivers are more likely to define their temperament as angry, irritable or stressed because of their work and home lives. They are more likely to become increasingly aggressive when they confront traffic problems.

The common-sense formulation and application of social, psychological and cultural behavioural patterns help construct the social reality of rural driving. They help construct the rural driving world; one where the large number of crashes are linked to driving behaviour, which in turn reflects social and cultural patterns of living. The latter require attention and scrutiny for proposing prevention or intervention traffic safety strategies.

7

DRIVING IDENTITIES
OVER THE LIFESPAN

Codes for the Road

MIKE BOYES &

PHIL LITKE

CONSIDERABLE RESEARCH, policy and legislation development, enforcement and engineering energy have been expended in an effort to improve the level of safety in the human activity of driving. While much has been done to change driving for the better, there is consistent concern that much more can and must be done to reduce the toll of the road in human lives and misery. To a greater or lesser extent, most traffic-safety initiatives focus upon individual drivers as the proper unit of analysis. After all, driving is seen as a solo activity within western culture. Road-safety professionals consistently express how difficult it is to change individual driving behaviour for the better. Individual drivers do not seem to listen to road-safety messages and do not seem inclined to shift their driving behaviour in positive directions. Young novice drivers (and especially, young male novice drivers) are still at significantly higher levels of risk on the road than other drivers. Elderly drivers are still at increased risk for collisions and for not self-selecting themselves from the road at the appropriate time. Middle-aged drivers, while identifying road safety as a concern, do not seem seriously inclined to make it a behavioural priority. What are we to do about this state of affairs in road safety?

What we propose is a shift in how we as researchers and practitioners interested in road safety think about and approach the task of driving, our understanding of the individual driver and our understanding of the ways in which we might influence the behaviour of individual drivers. To accomplish this shift we propose a significant change in the theory of driving and drivers used to direct our intervention efforts. To accomplish this change we suggest that we reconsider several theoretic approaches that have been proven in the past but have not as yet been fully or effectively applied to understanding drivers and driving behaviour. Specifically, we will consider driver identities and the range of psychological *and* social forces argued by identity theorists like Erikson (1968) to impact on the formation and maintenance of personal identity.

Beyond looking at this existing model, we will argue that consideration of a theory of moral conduct codes, which can be shown to follow from this view of personal identity, may provide new options for the development of effective interventions aimed at shifting driver behaviour in more positive directions. This theoretical approach overlaps the boundaries of both psychology and sociology and views personal identity as something that is negotiated between individuals and the groups to which they belong (or to which they desire to belong) and not as something intrinsic to the individual. Such an approach enables us to view driving behaviour as an ongoing social enterprise.

Within North American culture, drivers are viewed as purely autonomous beings, solely responsible for their goals and directions while driving. They embody the North American ideal of individual choice, individual responsibility and personal (identity) determination. While there is only one driver per vehicle (excluding, of course, the back-seat variety), the individual driver is a component of a larger system that includes other drivers on the road, pedestrians and, ultimately, society as a whole. A safe journey requires cooperation at all levels. While there are various laws and conventions aimed at promoting traffic safety, the effectiveness of these too depend on the cooperation of all drivers and, again, society as a whole. Such cooperative effort is evident in the mundane workings of traffic law.

Highway 401 is one of Ontario's major traffic arteries. The posted speed limit on this and all other highways in Ontario is 100 kph. But normal traffic flows at between 110 and 115 kph: i.e., the road users, including the police, have negotiated an actual speed limit 15 kph above the posted limit (Keegan, 1997). This "soft limit" was tested by school teacher Gordon Thompson, who protested the low posted speed limit by exceeding the posted speed limit by an ever-increasing amount until he was ticketed. Thompson further tested these negotiations when he and a friend clogged traffic by driving the same stretch of highway in tandem at the posted speed limit. Once again Thompson's action was counter to the established norm and threatened the social negotiation process, and again Thompson was ticketed (Keegan, 1997).

Whenever another driver's behaviour draws our attention on the road, we comfortably attribute that behaviour to the driver's personality, personal skill level (or lack thereof) or state of mind—that is, we view people's driving as a reflection of who they are (Bierness & Simpson, 1988). For young drivers, obtaining their drivers' license affords them an important level of autonomy and even "a living room on wheels" (Rothe, 1993). For middle-aged drivers, driving is, at its simplest, an ongoing reminder of one's autonomous status in the world; but how we drive and what we drive is also a public statement. All driving behaviour is interpreted and understood in the social context of other drivers on the road. As with one's choice of career, political stance and religious preference, driving behaviours and choices may be understood as identity issues.

Erikson (1963, 1968) has made it clear that while identity is most centrally a concern of young adults, who are consumed with its vicissitudes, identity issues are at play at all points in the lifespan. Adolescents eagerly anticipate the rite of passage that allows them to ascend to the rank of driver. The elderly must contemplate the decision to hang up their keys and cease being drivers. As we will discuss below, the only way to understand the impact of driving cessation among the elderly is to see it as a profound loss of identity.

Road-related identity issues can also be seen to be at work in the lives of young, pre-driving children. Specifically, the roots of such central driving issues as safety, risk-taking, peer influence and concern for fellow drivers are planted in early childhood. We will argue that the potential effectiveness of parent-focussed traffic-safety programs for pre-school and early school-aged children may be rooted in the impact such interventions have on the driving identities of children and youth.

Erickson's overall model of development is described as psychosocial, in that it is intended to track both the psychological and social forces that shape individual growth and development across the lifespan. Further, Erickson (1968) identifies eight stages or ages at which these psychological and social forces come together in a series of distinct defining moments. In infancy, for example, the issue is basic trust versus mistrust. That is, in the process of forging and then relying upon some kind of attachment relationship with its primary caregivers, the infant comes to a basic realization (based upon the nature of the care it receives) of whether it is a care-worthy individual and whether relationships and those with whom one enters into them with can be trusted. How this early phase of psychosocial existence works out has life-long implications. Both the child and his or her primary caregivers (the social context) play a role in determining this outcome.

The crisis of identity, for Erikson, works the same way. At its most poignant in the late-adolescent and early young-adult years, the identity-formation crisis involves psychological drives to identify and establish a coherent sense of personal identity. These psychological issues must be worked out in a series of social contexts that both push for identity commitments to be made and limit the number of options from which the youth can legitimately select identity components. In other words, identity formation involves both psychological issues of preference and choice *and* social support and validation of potentially available identity options. To consider one component of identity formation without the other would be to miss the fundamentally interactive nature of the formation and maintenance of identity. While the transactional nature of driving identity is fairly clear when we consider concerns about peer-group influences on young drivers, it is important to remember that identity issues are at play across the lifespan.

It is necessary at this point to introduce a further aspect of the concept of identity. The tension between psychological identity desires and social identity affordances carries with it certain moral implications. Specifically, once an identity has been taken up (that is, psychologically selected and socially validated), it brings with it certain role obligations and duties that an individual must live up to in order to claim that identity. Rom Harre (1984) refers to these duties and obligations as honour codes. An *honour code* is a moral code that details which behaviours are to be exhibited in which situations to maintain one's status as an honourable member of a particular identity group. The code of Bushido, for example, detailed precisely what behaviour was expected from a Samurai warrior if he was to maintain his honour; regimental codes of honour within the military operate in a similar fashion.

If a young male driver is to maintain his status as a fast driver with quick reflexes, he *must* take a risky alternative when faced with several ways to complete a particular driving task; otherwise, his identity may be compromised. Likewise, to maintain their professional identity and status, driving instructors must consistently make safe driving choices. In either case, to fail to make the "appropriate" driving behaviour choice is to risk losing one's driving identity. Honour codes provide a novel and powerful way of understanding the relationship between driver identities and driver behaviours. Further, they offer a new approach to the task of developing driving-safety interventions that are appropriately targeted at both the psychological and the social supporting components of driver identities and behaviours. For example, reminding adults who speed through park zones of their parental code responsibilities may positively influence their driving behaviour.

In what remains of this paper we will sketch out how the related concepts of driving identity and honour codes may help in designing traffic-safety initiatives for children, novice drivers, middle-aged drivers, and elderly drivers.

■ Road Safety for Young Children

Young children do very little conscious identity work. For Erikson (1963), the main psychosocial concerns of this age group centre first on initiative, or doing things for themselves, and then on industry, or the application of initiative to building basic skills and competencies. These activities set the foundation for later identity development. Because there is not a lot of detailed inflection on matters of identity at this young age, much of what may serve later as the foundation for identity formation is simply taken for granted. For example, the material resources children routinely have available to them will set expectations for the levels of resources (allowance, computer access, transportation access) they will incorporate into their identity expectations in adolescence.

Parents and teachers have an opportunity to influence a number of basic safety behaviours in children. For example, legal and social movements that promote zero tolerance for improper infant and child automobile-restraint devices have produced a cohort of children who take for granted that the fastening of some sort of restraining device is pre-requisite to vehicle movement. That is, it is part of the honour code for travelling in a car. Child traffic-safety programs like the Canadian Tire Kidestrian program work by taking parents through exercises to help them guide their children in establishing basic traffic-safety behaviour codes.

Thia (1996) examined the increase in traffic-safety knowledge of school-age children as a function of their parents' specific instruction in the Kidestrian program. The study found that parents who had received the Kidestrian package were more likely to have worked through the program with their children, and the children demonstrated higher levels of pedestrian safety knowledge on follow-up assessments. This finding demonstrates that the optimal place to intervene with traffic safety for children is with their parents rather than with the children directly.

Whether this sort of intervention carries implications for the levels of risk tolerance these children exhibit later as they begin to drive for themselves remains to be seen. It does suggest that we might benefit by tracing the roots of other safe-driving identities back to the competency-building years of early and middle childhood. For example, it may be possible to raise the level of intolerance for risky behaviours at an earlier age so that children's peer groups as they are reach driving age will be less tolerant of behaviours that place others at risk.

■ Young Novice Drivers: Forming Driver Identities

The formation of safe driving attitudes and behaviours is a central purpose of driver-education programs (Lonero & Clinton, 1997). The risk-related behaviours of young male drivers in particular are well documented. What is not currently well understood, however, is the range of driving identities that young drivers perceive as being available to them and the social forces that act to move them in the direction of one identity over another. Remembering that identity is both a psychological and a social issue opens up the possibility that effective driver-safety interventions could be focussed upon the social and peer groups young drivers use as identity reference points. For example, recognizing that risk-taking is a central part of many young male novice drivers' identity helps us see the honour codes of this reference group that support and promote risky behaviour.

Driving behaviour may be more effectively influenced by challenging the norms of such population sub-groups directly, by challenging the norms of other peer groups or by developing ways to show young drivers the actual extent of the risks they take. (This may help them to see that much less extreme behaviour may still meet the code requirements of their identity reference group.) Alternatively, we could work to create separation between driving and identity, that is, work to promote the notion that driving is just driving and need not be considered to be a central part of one's identity. This is much easier said than done in current North American culture but has been effectively accomplished in Europe where pedestrian and cyclist identities are valued on par with those of drivers (Gunnarsson, 1998). In such places less emphasis is placed on the view that driving represents a fundamentally valuable individual activity.

■ Middle-Aged Drivers: Maintaining Identity and Code Expectations

Identity is of less obvious concern during adulthood when people are mainly getting on with the business of living, rather than forging, their identities; however, identities are not set in stone beyond adolescence. The stereotyped middle-aged male buying a red sports car can be viewed as an attempt to "re-do" the identity formation process, that is, to start over. Other, more mature identity issues can be seen when we recall that *both* the formation *and* the maintenance of identity are as much social issues as psychological issues. Identity reference groups are still very much at work, although they may be less easily identified, as they may not consist entirely of one's direct peer group. For example, being sufficiently well off that one can afford both a fast, expensive car and the photo-radar tickets that can go along with it suggests a particular identity and an attendant driving code. In such cases the optimal course for intervention may not be to focus upon the individual but rather to attempt to shift the social support for the particular driving identity.

The significant success of the Mothers Against Drunk Driving (MADD) movement in the 1980s can be attributed to their effectiveness in shifting the level of acceptability of drinking and driving in the larger social community (Reinarman, 1988). MADD's success may have been at least partly due to its not having tried to influence the behaviour of individual drivers directly; instead, MADD focussed on significantly lowering the level of tacit social acceptance of driving while drunk. In effect, MADD affirmed the immorality or honour code-violating status of drunk driving without having to change any laws.

Public-service advertisements aimed at middle-aged drivers are also effective to the extent that they can raise the moral-code aspects of driving. The Australian Traffic Accident Commission (TAC) advertisements are particularly effective in this sense (Dow, 1998). By presenting individual drivers in an accessible manner, showing them going through the day-to-day activities of their lives (including unsafe driving practices) and showing the socio-moral consequences of their bad choices, the TAC commercials provide powerful incentives for adult drivers to rethink components of their driving identities. By depicting normal people doing "normal" things while driving and by showing the moral consequences of those actions in ways that directly affect the identities of the drivers themselves, the TAC commercials cut to the moral core of routine but problematic behaviour and seem, as a consequence, to play a powerful role in both social and individual change (Litke, 1999).

Thus, the ideal avenue for driving-safety interventions among adult drivers is socially directed toward re-establishing the identity and moral codes and highlighting the driving-pattern changes necessary if one is to live up to other codes and identity requirements.

■ Driving Cessation Among Elderly Drivers: Integrity Versus Despair

The issue of identity re-emerges, for Erikson (1968), in the latter years of life. At this point, however, the task is not to form or maintain a sense of identity but rather to reflect on the life one has followed and begin to consider whether the identity choices one made were right. Referring to it as the stage of integrity versus despair, Erikson argues that the elderly review their identity projects in light of the effects they have had upon themselves and others. To the extent that they view their choices as incomplete, they experience despair about the purpose of their lives. However, to the extent that they can see their contributions, they can begin to withdraw with a sense of self-accomplishment or integrity.

For many elderly drivers, the automobile represents an ideally convenient form of transportation. While they may have more free time in retirement, that free time does not necessarily translate into more flexible transportation options (University of Michigan Transportation Research Institute, 1995; Marottoli et al., 1997). Public transportation systems tend to be built to maximally convenience the working population, with fewer options available in non-rush periods. The elderly may feel they need to continue driving for pragmatic reasons. However, the decision to cease driving involves far more than pragmatic concerns. Decommissioning oneself as a driver or, even worse (from the individual's point of view), having one's license or insurance removed translates to a loss of personal autonomy and can have a powerful impact upon older drivers' identities. This impact will be felt more severely to the extent that the decision was made for, rather than being made by, the elderly driver (Bahro, Silber, Box & Sunderland, 1995; Eisenhandler, 1990; Marottoli et al., 1997; Persson, 1993).

Beyond recognizing how central driving may be to personal identity for elderly drivers, Erikson's model also suggests a means by which older drivers may be assisted in coming to terms with the necessity that they cease driving. Rather than simply helping them to let go of or shift away from a sense of identity that includes themselves as drivers, it may be possible, as Bahro et al. (1995) demonstrated, to involve the elderly driver in the process directly. Faced with an Alzheimer's patient who refused to see the need to be off the road, Bahro et al. avoided a potentially nasty power struggle for the driver's keys by enlisting the driver himself as a collaborator in their research to develop a better understanding of how to help drivers stop driving. This shift enabled the elderly driver to move beyond driving with integrity, having provided a valuable contribution to the area rather than simply despairing at his failure to maintain an aspect of his identity.

Another possible re-framing of the issue of driving cessation could include enlisting the aid of elderly members of the community in developing a seniors' transportation plan that does not significantly restrict their mobility if they do not drive.

■ Conclusions and Speculations

If we accept even for a moment that on-road driving behaviours result from and contribute to honour codes and formations of identity constitutively, then we may begin to hypothesize about the relative lack of success of past interventions. These interventions aimed at unsafe individual drivers or specific driving behaviours. We imagine it is highly unlikely that an individual would consciously create an identity as an unsafe driver. Ironically, however, problem behaviours were identified as part of a safe-driver honour code or to present an image of a safe driver (for example, the quick reflexes of a fast-driving teenager).

The model outlined here suggests that driving is an inherently social—and therefore negotiated—activity. While not denying conscious action in driving, this model posits a conscientious component to the complex act of driving. Interventions at the social level may have some success where interventions at an individual level have not. To that end, we propose supplementing traditional traffic-safety initiatives with interventions aimed directly at shifting drivers' honour codes, much in the manner adopted by the Traffic Accident Commission in Australia.

8

RISKY VEHICLES, RISKY AGENTS

*Mobility and the Politics of Space,
Movement and Consciousness*

PETER E.S. FREUND &

GEORGE T. MARTIN

AUTOCENTRIC TRANSPORT SYSTEMS now domi-
nate everyday human mobility in the developed world and are expanding
rapidly in the developing world. An autocentric system is characterized by a
high dependence on the auto for daily transport; alternative modes of mobility
are neglected and underutilized.[1] The United States has the most autocentric
transport system in the world; there, 86.4 percent of all person-trips per
household in 1995 were by auto (Hu & Young, 1999, p. 14).

Growing automobility is not restricted to the US; it is also true of Western
Europe and Canada. For example, "it is clear that in the past 40 years the car has
risen from being a marginal form of transport, to being the predominant mode,
accounting for more than 70 percent of all mechanized trips undertaken by
London residents" (Pharoah & Apel, 1995, p. 47). While the level of autocentricity is highest in the established market economies, the greatest growth is
taking place in the formerly centrally planned economies of Eastern Europe
and in the developing world. As the auto is becoming the world's dominant
mode of daily transport, it is also becoming a leading cause of death and injury.
The world toll from motor-vehicle accidents in 1990 was estimated at about 1
million deaths and 40 million injuries (Murray & Lopez, 1996, p. 468).

Autocentric transport requires a particular organization of space—for
example, a built environment of roadways, parking and support facilities. This
auto infrastructure commands a relatively large amount of land that is not

easily shared by other transport modalities. As a result, auto traffic tends to dominate all transport space, and the other means of mobility (walking, bicycling) are subordinated to its demands. Indeed, increasingly in countries like the US, the social organization not only of transport space but also of all public social space tends to be organized around the automobile (Freund & Martin, 1993). Thus, autocentric transport systems are defined not only as transport systems in which the automobile dominates mobility, but also as systems whose infrastructures dominate social space.

While it is not difficult to speak of rail systems as systems, the systemic nature of mass motorization is not so readily visible. This is partly due to the split between the individualized, privately owned vehicles that are used and the public infrastructure on which they depend. Trains are fixed to rail—the vehicle is wedded to its private platform. Autos do not have a fixed path—the private vehicle and its public platform are separable.[2] Yet mass motorization can be viewed as a system. It requires a vast network of roads, as well as storage, fuelling and repair facilities—a now-embedded material infrastructure. Additionally, there is a less visible embedded social infrastructure. Various organizations, including police departments and departments of highway and transport, manage this system at considerable cost to taxpayers.

In countries like Canada and the US, where autocentric systems are most developed, "harder" forms of automobility (such as sport-utility vehicles [SUV]) are becoming increasingly dominant. Most significantly, autocentric systems in the US and Canada are more and more coming to be characterized by hyper-automobility. We can date the period of hyper-automobility in the US from the years of the late 1970s and early 1980s, coincident with and a vital component in the beginning of a radical restructuring of economies. Between 1970 and 1980, annual growth rates in auto fleets outpaced increases in auto use by a factor of 1.2; since 1980 the relationship has been inverted. Between 1980 and 1995, annual increases in use outpaced increases in fleets by a factor of 1.9. In the US, between 1977 and 1995, the number of vehicles per household increased by a modest 12 percent, while the daily vehicle trips per household increased by 61 percent and the daily vehicle miles increased by 65 percent. The average occupancy for all car trips declined from 1.9 to 1.6 persons. Thus, hyper-automobility represents a shift from the extensive development of auto transport, in which more people have to own cars, to its intensive development, in which people have to use cars more and for more individual trips. Key to this transition has been the creation of a socio-material infrastructure that mandates increased automobility.

The hegemony of the automobile in space has consequences for health and safety. Thus, Hanson (1995, p. 23) concludes,

[t]he growing distance between activity sites along with the over-whelming automobile orientation of American society makes travel on foot or by bicycle difficult and often dangerous. One might argue, there-fore, that part of the urban transportation problem is the threat to health posed by the monopoly that motorized vehicles seem to have in urban travel. Air pollution, traffic accidents (some 40,000 traffic deaths per year in the US), and lack of exercise are all health problems that stem from the current configuration of urban transportation.

Two properties of this monopoly (particularly in the US) concern us here. First, hard means of mobility ("risky vehicles") dominate in traffic space and create an attendant ecology of vulnerability. In such an ecology, soft means of mobility are vulnerable and disadvantaged in their use of public space. Second, in the new, "harder" hyper-automobility, larger and heavier vehicles dominate traffic space, saturating public spaces. Such a system makes very stressful demands on the consciousness of those who participate in traffic (in any capacity—even as pedestrians). These demands are for constant "sobriety." (This term is used in the broadest sense, meaning general psychomotor competence.) Such demands for constant and universal sobriety conflict with the ubiquity of factors which can disrupt psychomotor competence and are a feature of everyday life, making most agents potentially "risky" traffic participants. After briefly looking at some data on accidents,[3] we explore these properties in greater detail.

■ Fatalities and Injuries

Death by auto is the most dramatic of its negative effects on health. There were an estimated 999,000 traffic deaths in the world in 1990. This statistic repre-sented two percent of all deaths and was the ninth leading cause of death. While this may seem to be a low share of deaths, the absolute number is high. Indeed, more people died from traffic accidents than from any one of the following causes of death: sexually transmitted diseases; HIV; malaria; breast and prostrate cancers; cirrhosis of the liver; violence; war; or self-inflicted injuries. While road deaths are a problem that afflicts whole populations, there are especially vulnerable demographic groups. Road accidents are the leading cause of death, for instance, for males aged 15 to 44.

With regard to injuries, a composite epidemiological measure to assess the impact of disease and accidents is the Disability-Adjusted Life Year (Murray & Lopez, 1996). It reflects time lost to premature mortality and time lived with disability. Traffic accidents were the ninth leading cause of DALYs in the world in 1990, accounting for 2.5 percent of the total. Again, men aged 15 to 44 were particularly vulnerable; traffic accidents were the leading cause of DALYs for this group. Motor-vehicle accidents are responsible for a wide range of injuries, but especially those of the spine and head. In the US, they are the largest single trauma-induced cause of paraplegia and quadriplegia, as well as being a major cause of epilepsy and head injury (Claybrook, 1984).

Considerably more deaths occur from auto accidents than from any other injury-producing event in the US. In 1992, 47.2 percent of all accidental deaths resulted from motor-vehicle crashes; the next largest source, 14.6 percent, was falls. Similar data exist in countries such as the UK (Adams, 1995). Indeed, the World Health Organization in 1996 estimated that heart disease, depression and auto accidents will overtake infectious diseases as the leading causes of death and disability by the year 2020. It will mark the first time that non-infectious causes will kill more people than germs do. Deaths from traffic accidents will increase as poorer nations become more autocentric in their transport systems at the same time that the proportion of young adults in their populations (those at most risk) grows larger. By 2020, the worldwide death toll from traffic accidents is expected to rise from the current level of about 1 million to about 2.3 million.

It is important to note that a goodly proportion of motor-vehicle fatalities are not occupants of autos. Pedestrians and cyclists accounted for 19.3 percent of all traffic fatalities in the US and 13 Western European nations in 1992. Outside of Western Europe and North America, pedestrians and cyclists fare even more poorly. In 11 nations of Eastern Europe, they accounted for 41.8 percent of all traffic fatalities in 1992, a figure comparable to those experienced in the developing world. The greater vulnerability of pedestrians and cyclists in Eastern Europe and the developing nations can in part be attributed to their poor segregation from motorized traffic and to low levels of traffic control. However, even in developed autocentric systems, where softer means of mobility are segregated from harder ones, a spillover of harder means into adjacent spaces meant for softer means may occur. In New York City in 1997, for example, "five percent of pedestrian and cyclist deaths occurred on sidewalks or other off-road areas where it is illegal to drive an automobile" (Komanoff, 1999, p. 37).

In the developed world, auto safety has improved considerably. For example, in the US, between 1950 and 1997, the motor-vehicle death rate per 100,000 population declined from 23.0 to 16.1 and per 100 million vehicle miles, from 7.6 to 1.6. However, these decreases in fatality rates have to be placed within a larger context. The absolute number of deaths remains high— 41,967 in the US in 1997, compared to 34,763 in 1950—because increased safety has been counterbalanced by increased auto use. There is also some evidence that increased safety causes increased risk-taking. Nonetheless, safer vehicles, improved roads, quicker medical interventions, more effectively monitored and socialized drivers, and better traffic-control systems have contributed to safety—especially for those in automobiles. One of the questions raised here concerns the structural limits of such interventions to improving auto safety. Despite all the safety improvements, auto travel still carries considerable risk.

Additionally, the aggregated and decontextualized nature of the quantitative data used in epidemiological analyses of accidents provides a broad and refracted view of macro social patterns. Such data give little insight into the micro social processes of traffic and the sociocultural conditions in which risky behaviour and accidents occur. Thus, epidemiological studies may show general patterns but do not explain the meaning of those patterns and their connections to micro-social situations. The qualitative data needed for more detailed micro-analyses of the sources of risk in traffic simply do not yet exist (Davis, 1993).

■ Risky Vehicles: The Ecology of Vulnerability

Autocentric transport is dominated by "hard" means of mobility; that is, by large and heavy vehicles capable of moving at high speed. Safety discourses emphasize vehicle occupants over pedestrians, and hard vehicles afford greater protection for their occupants. However, harder vehicles also have a greater impact on other, smaller and lighter vehicles: e.g., compact cars, bicycles, and pedestrian bodies. Additionally, while auto-safety regulations and more crash-worthy cars have helped to decrease fatality rates for auto occupants, they may have had some negative effects on pedestrians and bicyclists because of offsetting behaviour by auto drivers (Crandall et al., 1986). Risk compensation theorists (e.g., Adams, 1995; Davis, 1993) have argued that increased crashworthiness may produce a sense of greater security, which, in turn, leads drivers to engage in riskier behaviour.

Three interacting components (or agents) of the ecology of traffic may be identified for analytic purposes: the spatio-temporal relationships among vehicles or platforms, drivers and other vehicle occupants, and non-occupants. Adams (1995, p. 30) provides an example of a hypothetical traffic encounter:

> Throughout the world hundreds of millions of motor vehicles mix with billions of people. A pedestrian crossing a busy road tries to make eye contact with an approaching motorist. Will he slow down? The motorist tries to divine the intentions of the pedestrian. Will he give way? Shall I? Shan't I? Will he? Won't he? As the distance between them closes, signals implicit and explicit pass between them at the speed of light. Risk perceived is risk acted upon. It changes in the twinkling of an eye as the eye lights upon it.

The agents here are a driver of a car and a pedestrian whose "vehicle" is his or her body. Compared to the driver's car, the pedestrian's body is a safer means of mobility overall, but it is much more vulnerable in any interaction with a car:

> On the road, and in life generally, risky interaction frequently takes place on terms of gross inequality. The damage that a heavy lorry can inflict on a cyclist or pedestrian is great; the physical damage that they might inflict on the lorry is small (Adams, 1995, p. 20).

In apportioning blame for accidents, users of either soft or hard means of mobility are treated as equally culpable, when it is those using harder means who have a potentially destructive weapon at their disposal (Komanoff, 1999, p. 17). Some US courts have ruled that the automobile is a lethal weapon (Novaco, 1991) and "motor vehicles and guns are vehicles of mechanical energy in epidemiological parlance" (Robertson, 1992, p. 10). The implications for a transport system in which the right to use such a weapon is almost universally granted to adults has not been explored in safety literature. The heavy and potentially high speed vehicles that predominate in autocentric traffic render soft vehicles (including human bodies) vulnerable. While as the cliché would have it that "guns don't kill people, people using guns do," it is also the case that a person using a machine gun can cause much more carnage than one using an air gun. In a recent case, a woman whose car had been hit by a SUV sued the company making the SUV, claiming that such vehicles were a threat to cars (Reed, 1998).

Hard means of mobility are potentially more dangerous in that they have a stronger impact on whatever they hit. Obviously a heavy object travelling at high speed packs quite a punch and is likely to be more fatal or injurious in crashes with smaller objects. Thus, the risks that vehicles pose for other vehicles (including walking bodies) in transport space depends not only on their individual weight and speed but also on the overall mix of vehicle weights and speeds. When a car collides with a SUV, the driver of the car is thirteen times more likely to be killed than the driver of the SUV (Bradsher, 1997b).

Speed is the premier cultural icon of modern societies and is a valourized feature of autos. Speed symbolizes manliness, progress and dynamism; slowness, however, signifies age, weakness, backwardness, sickness, unproductiveness and femininity. The thrill of speed is a combination of fear and pleasure, and of control versus abandon. The US National Safety Council estimates that the risk of fatality roughly doubles for each 10 miles per hour of added speed over 50 mph (Wald, 1996). When the US instituted the 55-mph speed limit in response to the oil crisis in the 1970s, road fatalities declined by about one-third. In Britain, a Royal Commission (1994) concluded that lower speed could lower the number and severity of accidents. Data from Germany support the idea that lower speed limits decrease fatalities. In one study in Buxtenhude, although the number of accidents did not decrease, the number of fatalities and serious injuries did (Hickmann & Kaser, 1988). A Hamburg study demonstrated that the probabilities of pedestrian injury and death increase with vehicle speed (Siegfried, 1991). Denmark had a similar experience: lowered speed limits resulted in fewer road fatalities (Gallagher et al., 1989). That lower speed in heavy vehicles can reduce fatality and possibly the seriousness of injury is not surprising. Ironically, fatality rates are lower where there is traffic congestion (although the injury rates are higher) because vehicle speed is slower (Adams, 1993).

Crashworthiness is not simply a matter of sheer weight and speed but is affected by "crush space"—that is, the amount of material capable of absorbing impact before it reaches a vehicle's occupant. While heavier vehicles may afford their occupants greater protection, they pose a larger threat to lighter vehicles and pedestrians (US General Accounting Office, 1992; Royal Commission, 1994).[4] What is most significant here is that the relationship between weight and fatality rate is related to systemic properties of traffic such as the overall weight-speed range and distribution. Thus, downsizing cars is not necessarily more dangerous if the weight of the whole auto fleet decreases. While it is not always speed per se that is risky—Rothe (1994) has suggested that it is deviation from the mean speed that is a problem—speed remains a problem for slower and more vulnerable traffic participants.

The emphasis on the crashworthiness of cars glosses over the fact that the individual car is part of a traffic matrix in which vehicles mix with varying degrees of protection. This way of thinking, Adams (1995, p. 154) pointed out, is analogous to the logic of an arms race, which would argue that roads will be safe when all softer means of mobility are banished and all that are left are tanks. Indeed, "SUV purchases are being made as 'defensive buys'" (Andersen, 1998, p. 23). Such a Hobbesian traffic condition has obvious social drawbacks, including the fact that it seriously disadvantages traffic participants who are walking, cycling or using relatively light autos.

Autocentric transport systems favour hard means of mobility, the controls over which rest in the hands of many individuals who are potentially vulnerable to psychomotor impairment. The dominance of hard vehicles in traffic increases the likelihood that softer vehicles that mix into traffic will be more vulnerable. If one includes pedestrian bodies and bicycles as vehicles in this mix, then the power asymmetry in traffic becomes quite pronounced. In both the US and the UK, walking is a more dangerous way to travel (standardized for miles travelled) than moving by bicycle, car, rail, bus or air. Pedestrians are more likely to be killed in traffic than are car occupants by very large factors—by a factor of 16 in the UK, 14 in the US (The Guardian, 1997; Surface Transportation Policy Project, 1998).

Autos embody cultural meanings of speed, power, and invulnerability, and these meanings are considerations in auto design. There is a lot of culturally rooted resistance in the US to downsizing and slowing autos. An editor of one car magazine complained that the obsession with energy efficiency would "put all of us who love cars into devices that looked and ran like enclosed riding lawnmowers" (Wald, 1990). These psycho-aesthetic desires for size and power coincide with the fact that such vehicles are more profitable. As Commoner (1990) argued, style and profit considerations, more than function or social need, combine to shape the design of cars with the result that they are greater than necessary in size and power ("minicars make miniprofits").

Auto manufacturers have again turned to building faster, larger, more powerful vehicles, especially light trucks. Given the historically low price of gasoline in the US and the desire to tap the market for size and speed, crash-worthiness and power, the predominance of hard means of mobility in traffic has increased. The proportion of light trucks in the US fleet increased from 22 percent to 35 percent between 1990 and 1995. Now, about one-half of all new fleet sales are light trucks. Predictably, traffic deaths from crashes involving a car and a light truck passed the number of deaths involving two cars in 1992—and in crashes between light trucks and cars, 80 percent of the deaths are car occupants (Bradsher, 1997a).

The psycho-aesthetic appeal of the automobile combines the sense of being in a safe, armoured, womb-like environment (one's private space within a public arena) with enormous power at the touch of a pedal (Lupton, 1999; Freund & Martin, 1993). SUVs amplify this experience.[5] The perceived security of being in a SUV thus may contribute to "risk compensation."

■ Risky Agents: The Politics of Consciousness
The application of technology to the routines of daily life involves intensive and extensive use of complex and potentially dangerous inventions. As individuals are socialized into a "technological society," historically unprecedented levels of psychomotor and technical capabilities and skills are developed in the mass of the population. Driving at high speeds, manoeuvring through traffic and even managing movement as a pedestrian through transport space become a part of everyday routines and taken-for-granted abilities. Yet the pervasive and intensive dependence on being able to use or relate to such technologies can be a source of stress and can disenfranchise or put at risk those unwilling or unable to meet such demands. However routine participation in technologized

socio-material environments is for many people, there are others who are excluded.

Given the nearly universal access to traffic, high levels of auto dependence, the dominance in traffic of hard means of mobility and the highly individualized nature of automobility, accidents then are inevitable. As one observer noted,

> When each individual is driving their own two-ton machine, our safety is dependent upon the mental state of all the other individuals behind the wheel. Competition for road-space and the need for momentary decisions makes constant vigilance essential. The reorganization of communities around the auto means we have to drive at all different times of the day, no matter what our state of mind might be right then: fatigued from the day's work, angry at the boss's remarks, upset over breaking up with one's lover, tipsy after a few beers at one's favorite tavern or spaced-out from a couple joints. Momentary lapses by individual drivers are inevitable. (Wetzel, 1990, p. 18)

There are structural limits to universalizing high social standards of self-regulation. These systemic limits constitute the boundaries of accident prevention techniques, which focus on individual behaviour.

Modern social systems make it mandatory for most people to participate in road traffic every day. A significant proportion of this population cannot be expected to be "careful" and "alert" every day. Every morning some proportion of the road users must be under stress because of some personal tragedy or problems at work or home. In addition there would be those who drank too much the previous night or who are on medication. Children, teenagers and the elderly also cannot be expected to be ideal road users. Persons suffering from psychiatric disorders cannot be expected to behave perfectly on the road. If one adds up the total number of all these groups on the road, it may amount to almost half the population. There is a theoretical limit to the influence of accident "prevention" measures focussed on modifying behaviour of road users by "education" (Mohan, 1997, p. 139). Thus, a significant latent reason for traffic accidents is the autocentric transport system itself, a system that demands an unrealistically high and constant level of human functioning.

As more and more space is appropriated by the car, as more drivers travel and travel alone, the demand for an instrumental, diligent, wide-awake state of being increases. This demand leaves less psychosocial space and time for other states of mind, including playfulness, and for altered states of consciousness such as daydreaming. The imposition of a particular kind of subjectivity while driving, walking or cycling in traffic represents one of the subtler forms of social control that accompanies autocentric transport. It is in this sense that we can speak of a politics of consciousness. As Kay (1997, p. 107) observes, "on the road we forfeit the otherwise forgivable right to muse, to fantasize, to fight—to live"; the result is "a constricting test of concentration."

The constant vigilance and self-control that driving and moving in driving space require are not the natural condition of subjectivity. The rather narrow band of consciousness—and its constancy—demanded by successful movement in auto-dominated space poses problems for humans. For example, in a transport system as homogenized as autocentric transport, what alternatives to driving are there for those who choose to get high or tipsy and then must get home? What happens to those who are impaired and should not be driving, but who, given that the car is the only vehicle affording them access, must drive? In 1994, 88 percent of the US population 16 years old and older was licensed to drive. It is not surprising that some considerable percentage of them have the potential for psychomotorical impairment at any given moment. In an auto-dependent society such as the US, the granting of licenses is based on permissive criteria, including allowing people who are illiterate to get licenses, and there is a great reluctance to revoke licenses because livelihoods depend on being able to drive. There are, in other words, always a certain number of people driving who should not be.[6]

To lose one's licence in most parts of the US is to become dependent on others, to be forced to use often inadequate and culturally devalued transport modes such as mass transit (in Los Angeles, buses have been called by some "loser cruisers"). Just as gaining one's license has become a rite of passage, the loss of one's license is not merely the loss of the freedom to move autonomously but also a loss of status. Among older people, a valid driver's licence is the ultimate status symbol. Driving means vitality, independence and the American way of life. In nursing homes in Florida, residents display their driver's licences like trophies on their bureaus. To give up your licence because of illness or disability is a painful rite of regression (Rimer, 1998, p. 78).

The modes by which we transport ourselves are not unrelated to how dangerous various altered states of consciousness (e.g., being drunk) may be. The issue of whether or not people should get high (on substances or activities) or daydream is one issue. How safely we can do this in the context of a particular mode of transport is another issue. In the debates about drunk driving few have defended people's rights to get drunk or have criticized the lack of transport alternatives. That drunk driving is dangerous and that drivers who get high are more likely to cause accidents are self-evident facts. What is not apparent is the taken-for-grantedness of the need for a more general sobriety in a technological society. Increasing reliance on the car makes sobriety, wide-awakeness and optimal bodily functioning unquestioned norms demanded of anyone who wishes to have full freedom of movement.

The image of the "killer drunk" is a convenient one, for it allows society to demonize particular individuals and hence to sequester the problem. Yet most drunk drivers in the US lack prior convictions and are themselves accident victims (Ross, 1993). Drunk-driving fatalities have decreased in the US since the 1980s because of shifts in attitudes and because of improved enforcement of laws. Yet drunk driving is still a significant problem and will remain so if the focus remains on individuals and neglects a system of transport that requires some people to drive a potentially lethal weapon and requires others (cyclists and pedestrians) to navigate through dangerous zones. As indicated earlier, there is a tendency to hold users of softer means of mobility equally culpable with harder ones for impaired driving. Despite New York City Department of Transportation campaigns for educating and managing "drunken walkers," a study showed that in 1997, the driver of the automobile was "largely or strictly" at fault in 74 percent of cyclist and pedestrian fatalities (Komanoff, 1999).

Drugs (some of them prescription drugs) may contribute to impairments and thus to risky behaviour. There is, however, little discussion of this in the safety literature—despite the fact that, according to one estimate, approximately 1 million drivers in the UK take prescription drugs that can contribute to psychomotor impairments (Davis, 1993, p. 190). One British study implicated prescribed tranquilizers in a significant proportion of auto crashes (Barbone et al., 1998). It is reasonable to speculate that such numbers will increase as the population becomes greyer and as the general use of pharmaceuticals continues to increase.

While alcohol and various sources of chemically caused psychomotor incompetence certainly merit attention, other sources of distraction and interference with the appropriate road traffic subjectivity are probably more common. What can be called "normal distraction" (as opposed to chemically induced distraction) is an important factor in auto accidents. The rapidly growing use of mobile phones by drivers is an example of the accretion of mundane distraction. The National Highway Traffic Safety Administration ranks inattentive driving, which includes talking or eating while driving, as the fourth most common in its list of eleven reasons for fatal crashes in the US. Sleepiness was the eighth most frequent reason for fatal crashes. Additionally, Rothe (1987, pp. 116–17) has observed that normal emotional arousal contributes to car crashes:

Almost all the young drivers felt comfortable on the day of the drive. Yet, significant variables could be highlighted which may indicate some form of temporary emotional instability. To illustrate, aroused emotions arising from sporting or work activities, aggressions resulting from romance problems, tensions because of car and weather conditions, resentments because of negative circumstances like having sprained an ankle, and thoughts about mental escape caused by poor work days may have influenced the driving act. Further, attention to passengers, the radio and/or cassette player, upcoming events and surroundings possibly contributed to the crashes.

What is significant here is that to participate even as a pedestrian in an auto-centric system one cannot be distracted by emotions or thoughts during one's travel time. Daydreaming and the intrusion of personal troubles must be held at bay in an auto-oriented subjectivity. Thus, the sources of impaired driving, cycling or walking are myriad.[7]

There are other socio-economically structured causes of traffic accidents. Economic pressures contribute, especially among truck drivers (Rothe, 1991). Truck drivers frequently operate under time pressure and have a relatively high rate of drug consumption, particularly of stimulants. Because many drivers are self-employed, economic considerations can lead them to drive long hours with unsafe equipment and overly large loads. Additionally, truck loads and size have increased over time, contributing to the seriousness of accidents. Driver fatigue may contribute to as many as 40 percent of all trucking accidents in the US (Brody, 1994; Karr, 1995). In one study, long-haul truck drivers were observed moment by moment using video recordings and electroencephalo-grams for one week. The study concluded that most drivers did not get enough sleep and a minority lapsed into sleep-like states while driving (Mitler et al., 1997). In discussing the impact of economic pressures on truck drivers, Perrow (1984, p. 180) argued

> the work truckers do puts even irresponsible drivers in a situation where irresponsibility will have graver consequences than it does for most of us. Again it is the system that must be analyzed not the individual.

In addition to altered consciousness and common distraction there is the factor of human error. Studies show that drivers routinely commit significant numbers of errors (Rothe, 1994, p. 27). The possibility of technological failure only adds to the problem. Furthermore, in interaction with other agents in traffic, individual errors may be compounded as they converge to produce incidents that are uncontrollable. Such compounding of error is dramatically illustrated in multi-car pileups involving tens, even hundreds of vehicles caused by, for example, the sudden fogging of a major roadway.

In order to further improve traffic safety in highly developed autocentric systems, we need systemic changes to reduce autocentricity. Those changes may ameliorate the contradictions between the demand for constant sobriety and psychomotor fitness and the inevitability of human and mechanical errors.

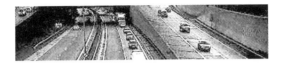

HEAVIER AND LARGER VEHICLES increasingly predominate in autocentric traffic space and render softer and smaller vehicles more vulnerable. Any intervention to improve safety is limited, as Davis (1993, p. 10) points out, by a system which puts many fallible human beings in charge of many vehicles "with an exceptionally high potential for harming others." High levels of dependence on the auto for access, as well as its importance as a means of self-expression and its potential as a dangerous weapon, impose a requirement for sobriety and safe behaviour on all those who would move in traffic. Given the myriad factors that can disrupt sobriety or encourage risky behaviour, it is highly probable that some participants cannot or will not behave safely. Following Foucault (1979), one might argue that potentially unruly (and never totally manageable) mind-bodies limit the power of the necessarily self-imposed discipline of modern traffic systems which govern behaviour and make safe participation in intensely and pervasively motorized traffic systems possible.

Traffic-safety discourses are defined by two themes: technological improvements in vehicles and their platforms, such as safety belts, air bags and limited-access roads; and modification of the behaviour of individual traffic participants, such as the social control of drunk drivers (Gabe, 1996). However, the social problem of roadway injuries and deaths needs to be understood in a broader context, a context that includes the systemic nature of transport and its accidents. A full appreciation of transport systems will include an understanding of the social organization of space. Social space is materially embodied and "the profound impact of the material world remains something which may experts risk find difficult to incorporate into their 'value frameworks'" (Williams et al., 1995, p. 120). In fact, there is an identifiable social ecology of vulnerability produced by societally normative and materially embedded autocentric transport systems.

Altering the accident toll significantly would mean changing "the event space within which accidents occur" (Prior, 1995, p. 140). It is not so much that the present safety orthodoxy is wrong but that its focus on technical and individual interventions leaves collective and structural factors unaddressed. This orthodoxy illustrates the fact that discourses about accidents take place in "politicized environments which involve partly the need to assign blame or credit" (Sagan, 1993, p. 42). Roadway safety is currently dominated by an expert technical and engineering paradigm that keys on vehicle safety and roadway safety while it neglects, or only secondarily considers, the safety of pedestrians and cyclists. Thus, for example, a current focus is the danger of rollover for SUVs, a problem only for occupants of SUVs. This is a rather narrow focus considering the safety problems that SUVs pose for others in traffic (i.e., blocking the horizon). Even among drivers, it is mainstream drivers—able-bodied healthy adults—who form the focus, neglecting the elderly and the impaired.

The political nature of auto-hegemonic space is often obscured by technocratic discourses about traffic. When traffic engineers, transport planners and other experts promote improved traffic flow, they generally mean motorized traffic flow in which other modalities may be viewed as obstructions. When they talk about safety, they may mean keeping pedestrians and "softer" transport modalities from interfering with motorized traffic flow. Improved flow increases speed (thus allegedly saving time) and thus the fastest transport modalities are given priority in public space. Safety and flow are impeded when there is a mix of modalities and conflict between them. Conflicts between modes of transport are resolved by having slower ones yield to faster ones and by giving autos priority in the use of the road (a public space) over walkers, bikers and others; the increase of harder autos in traffic further disadvantages them.

At its root, much of the roadway-safety issue centres on a competition for the most desirable socio-material space of daily mobility—the built environments created to provide people with channels for access to sites where they work, shop and live. In autocentric transport systems, the decision has already been made—and embedded, materially and socially—to favour those who move in private autos. So plans to relieve transport congestion focus on technical improvement to cars and on the more efficient management of car traffic (i.e., "smart" cars and roads), rather than on creating or retrofitting transport spaces to include viable channels for cyclists or pedestrians.

The social organization of movement in space raises issues of distributive justice and degrees of political empowerment. Political rights and the ability to exercise them in traffic centre around safe access, as well as the quality and rhythm of access, including the ability to enjoy movement and the space one is moving through. A recent case in the US dramatically illustrates this issue. A black teenager was hit and killed by a truck while trying to cross a busy seven-lane highway to reach the shopping centre where she worked. The intersection at which she crossed from a bus stop to the mall had no pedestrian signals or crosswalk. The owners of the mall were accused of using the highway for racial exclusion because they had banned city buses from discharging passengers in the mall (Chen, 1999). This incident illustrates how the social organization of traffic space (which is, after all, public space) can work to exclude certain groups and even to put them at considerable risk.

In recent years there has been a resurgence of what one might call "anti-auto" movements. Local opposition to road construction, collective struggles over who can safely use transport space and campaigns for better mass transit are examples of these movements. Of course it is not "the auto" but autocentric transport systems and their dominance that is the problem. In many cities, cycling and pedestrian activists contest the organization of space-time in transport and campaign for the rights of access of other means of movement. In the UK, groups such as Reclaim the Streets have repeatedly "liberated" auto-dominated streets for a day, making them auto-free and transforming them into safe places for play, entertainment and other activities. The contested terrain of these movements is autocentric space, time and motion.

At issue is the need for more multi-modal, inter-modal transport space and less auto-hegemonic space ruled by "risky" vehicles. As people are pressured and encouraged to use autos, the likelihood of risky behaviour increases. A viable multi-modal and inter-modal system would offer a wider range of transport possibilities and temporal rhythms of movement. Such a system would be more inclusive and would have more spaces that older people, people with disabilities, people without cars (including children)—a wider spectrum of mind-bodies—could safely use, move through and enjoy.

NOTES

Unless otherwise indicated, data sources were the following: American Automobile Manufacturers Association, Motor Vehicles Facts & Figures, 1997 (Detroit); United Nations, Human Development Report, 1996 (New York); United Nations, Statistics of Road Traffic Accidents, 1994 (New York); US Department of Commerce, Statistical Abstract of the United States, 1998 (Washington); US Department of Transportation, Traffic Safety Facts, 1992 (Washington); US Department of Transportation, 1995 American Travel Survey (Washington); US Department of Transportation, 1995 Nationwide Personal Transportation Survey (Washington); World Health Organization, The Global Burden of Disease, 1996 (Geneva).

1   There are, of course, three motorized vehicles in addition to the auto—the bus, truck and motorcycle. However, we speak of autocentric transport because of the sheer numerical domination by the auto. Autos represent about three-fourths of all vehicle registrations and about seven-tenths of all vehicle miles of travel in the US and in the world at large. With regard to accidents, 95 percent of the 11 million motor vehicles involved in crashes in 1992 in the US were

autos. Additionally, the rapidly growing use of SUVs (which are light trucks) is blurring the boundary between autos and trucks.

2   Historically, railroads were built on new, separate, and private right-of-way, while the auto usurped the traditional public right-of-way used by others (i.e., walkers).

3   It should be noted that the term *accident* implies a surprise or chance occurrence. The term is gradually being replaced in epidemiological research by more precise terms such as unintentional injury (Baker et al., 1992). Accident also focusses on the agent utilizing an injury-producing object rather than on the social and material contexts in which injury occurs. Thus, the very definition of events as accidents (as opposed to, perhaps, socially produced but preventable incidents) has policy implications. However, we use the term accident here since it is more generally familiar.

4   While auto manufacturers have downplayed the risks that heavier vehicles pose for other traffic participants, they have used that risk to resist US regulations to make cars more fuel efficient. They have argued that more fuel-efficient cars will be lighter and hence at greater risk in encounters with heavier vehicles in traffic (Bradsher, 1997b).

5   According to one report, SUV drivers become less attentive than other car drivers while driving, drive more aggressively and are less likely to wear seat belts (Rutenberg, 1999).

6   An extreme example of official tolerance towards licensing can be seen in the case of a Houston, Texas, woman who needed three tries to pass her written exam. During her road test she stepped on the gas rather than the brake, killing two children. Yet she was to be allowed to take the road test again (International Herald Tribune, 1996).

7   What is called "road rage" is a case in point. The National Highway Traffic Safety Administration estimates that about one-half of the deaths on US roads are partly or totally the result of some driver losing emotion control. Moreover, "violent aggressive driving" on roads seems to be increasing—by 7 percent a year—while such causes of death as drunken driving are decreasing. One reason given for the increase of road rage is growing traffic congestion (The Economist, 1997). Others link the increase to growing sprawl (Surface Transportation Policy Project, 1999).

SECTION TWO
INSTITUTIONAL SUB-SYSTEMS

INSTITUTIONS TYPICALLY REFER to complex, large, formal, legitimate organizations that are designed to organize people toward fairly explicit goals and to direct individuals' activities. Government, courts, media and the school are examples of institutions whose rules govern the activities of their members. They represent a clear and hierarchical structure.

The underpinnings of society reside in the institutions to which we grant the authority to represent our interests and to assume agency at a scale that individuals cannot. This section examines how traffic safety is affected by the day-to-day interactions of institutions and individuals, and the resulting social organization.

A persuasive justification of government is that people would not cooperate to realize their interests and needs without it. Hobbes' *Leviathan* justified the state as an expression of social order, peace, security and defense. As Hobbes said, it is rational to institute a powerful government to ensure that all citizens keep the peace. His writings paved the way for today's popular slogan "For the common good." In recent years, the common-good argument has led to follow-up questions. Who defines and promotes the common good? Is the common good interest-free? Who benefits most from the common good? Should the common good be a higher virtue than individual fulfillment or do the two interrelate?

In a Hobbesian sense, the common good includes the roadway. All roadway users seek to maximize their gain. Let us assume for a minute that the roadway itself is a great "common." What control is required to avoid a tragedy of the common? How much control is required before drivers collectively threaten the safety of themselves and other roadway users?

■ The Economic Sub-System
The pursuit of cooperation at the expense of the individual is a significant stratum of activity that gives shape to community traffic safety. A broader area of the familiar is self-interest displayed by different parties on the roadway. Most pronounced is economic self-interest, which varies from individual drivers assessing the worth of their cars, valuing their insurance premiums and attending

to auto repairs, to auto manufacturers seeking profits, civic governments seeking cost effective transportation, lobby groups yearning for special money-making privileges, and transportation-based corporations operating for profit.

Economics can be addressed through macro- or micro-perspectives. Charles and Lester Lave (1990) shed substantial light on the macro-level of economics and traffic safety. However, micro-components of economics have not to date been substantially addressed. For example, little initiative has been assigned to establish the role dispatching plays in traffic safety. The transportation industry relies on it. Truckers operate their vehicles according to it. Yet it has escaped scrutiny. A similar account can be given for workers who commute. Their economic worth to a corporation or business depends on their being injury free and in a state of well being. Downtime is expensive for employers.

■ The Legal Sub-System

A complex institution primarily concerned with enforcing compliance on the road is the law. It includes primarily the police, judges and attorneys. They enforce the traffic laws and investigate the causes of crashes. They apply the rules to help standardize behavior or help modify risky or deviant behavior. Unfortunately, the job of upholding the law and punishing guilty drivers is ambiguous: officially sanctioned actions and duties fall prey to informal norms and codes. For example, police monitoring a stretch of highway with a 100-kph limit require personal tolerance and detachment discretion. Who will be targeted for a speeding citation? Will the person driving 101 be as guilty as one travelling 110, 120 or 150? Do all drivers deserve the same punishment? Is an impaired driver recklessly driving over the centre line and hitting another vehicle as guilty as a fatigued driver waiting too long at an intersection and getting hit from behind while standing still? What is a fatigued driver? These are but a few questions that remind us that the laws are constructed by some authorities to control activities, create greater safety and make it easier to apprehend and label risky drivers at the side of the road or in a court room. Because of the importance of the legal system, energies are now spent on closer scrutiny of the police and courts. These strategies present alternate perspectives on the law.

■ The Media Sub-System

The media have become the institutional authority of social communication. They contribute to the function or dysfunction of the roadway system. Media creations appropriate and transform a vast range of symbols and ideas that directly impact on traffic safety. The media have a vitality that could play either a destructive or constructive role for a better understanding of the interrelating sub-systems that operate in the roadway system.

■ The Education Sub-System

Closely related to the ubiquity of the media is the school. Traffic safety has been taught in public schools for a long time. The primary instructional methods have been presentations, lectures and simplistic activities like matching words, doing quizzes and colouring pictures. These activities have been largely non-reflective. The police may visit on a special day, bringing the Seat Belt Convincer to the school to demonstrate the effectiveness of seat belts. Children participate in the program and go home to tell their parents about it, after which time little is ever heard about the demonstration again.

Recently, practical action research has re-energized schooling. In action research, students and educators relate theory to everyday practice, teaching themselves and others about important social issues within their confines of operation. When students engage in this forum, they become increasing reflective about how issues like traffic safety affect their communities. They learn to solve puzzles collaboratively as they grapple with their lived realities.

9

*Understanding and Interpreting
the Political Basis of Traffic Safety*

DAVID MACGREGOR

*In our wounds we celebrated the traffic-slain dead,
the deaths and injuries of those we had seen dying
by the roadside and the imaginary wounds
and postures of the millions yet to die.*

—J.G. BALLARD, CRASH

■ The Dialectics of Mobility

ON SEPTEMBER 3, 1999, near Windsor, Ontario, on the 401 Highway that connects an endless stream of traffic with the American border, a thick early-morning fog swiftly blanketed unwary motorists. Some would later say the heavy mist fell like a sheet around their windshields (Crawford, 2000). Transport trucks and automobiles careened across the highway. Blinded drivers hit the brakes and steered to avoid obscured vehicles. On both sides of the road, ghostly cars and trucks piled into one another, as though in a giant, deadly game of bumper cars. Twisted wrecks oozed gasoline. Stunned passengers debated in the gloom whether to stay put or risk fleeing into the maelstrom.

Leonard Shognosh sat terrified in the passenger seat of his battered van; beside him, his wife Elaine Shognosh gripped the steering wheel. Leonard's mother, Eleanor Shognosh, a tribal healer in the Anishinabae band at nearby Walpole Island, huddled in the back seat. She and Elaine urged a run from the van, as the vehicle was pummeled again and again by wailing phantasmic automobiles. Leonard counselled it was too dangerous to leave; they might easily be squashed in the mounting nightmare outside. "They've already been hit three or four times, spinning around so that the van faces the wrong way on the west-bound lane, which is how, materializing out of the fog, Ms. Shognosh can suddenly see the tractor trailer, barreling straight at her windshield" (Anderssen, 2000).

There may no better illustration of G.W.F. Hegel's dialectic of freedom than the state of traffic safety in advanced industrial nations at the beginning of the twenty-first century. Freedom involves, among other things, opportunity for movement: speedy, secure and rewarding circulation within the human community. As Hegel argued, freedom comes at great cost. The sacrifice of life to mobility must surely rank as a world-historic tragedy. In no other human endeavour, except modern warfare, have so many lives been wasted and so much treasure needlessly expended.

In the US alone, three million people have died in traffic accidents since the birth of the automobile; many millions have been seriously injured; countless lives have been shortened by toxic emissions from cars and auto-related industries. Sacrificial offerings to the deity of locomotion have no respect for childhood innocence. Traffic accidents are the leading cause of death for US children from five to fourteen years of age. An average of 7 US children 0 to 14 were killed and 866 injured each day in motor-vehicle crashes in 1998 (US Department of Transportation, 1999, p. 1). The World Health Organization reports that 120,000 died in traffic accidents in the European region in 1995; 2.5 million were injured (World Health Organization, 1998, p. 1): "Pedestrians and cyclists stand out as a particularly vulnerable group. In the United Kingdom, they make up 45 percent of all road deaths. In Hungary, the proportion is even higher, being over 50%, though it is substantially lower in most Western European countries (17 percent in France, 20 percent in Germany and around 30 percent in Denmark and the Netherlands)." Norwegian researchers determined that "pedestrians and cyclists have fatality risks of seven and five times the risk faced by car drivers" (Elvik, Kolbenstvedt & Stangeby, 1999, p. 2).

Hierarchy propels the dialectic of motion. "There are signs on the US side of highways near the US–Mexican border which portray women and children running across the highway in the same way that other areas have signs warning that deer and cows may be crossing" (Kopinak, 2000). Animal life perhaps suffers most from worship of speed. "Millions of vertebrates—birds, reptiles, mammals, and amphibians—are killed every year by vehicles traveling on America's roads. For example, roadkill has helped reduce the population of a federally endangered cat—the ocelot—to about 80 animals" (US Federal Highway Administration, 2000). Fish habitats are obliterated or poisoned by the automobile. Traffic in British Columbia and the American Pacific Northwest, for example, has helped to devastate the wild salmon population.

The declining rate of traffic fatalities in many rich countries may herald an era requiring no daily allotment of human blood, bone and tissue to the mobility god. Indeed, in 1997 the Swedish Parliament embraced a goal of "Vision Zero" for traffic casualties in the next decade (Carlsson, 1998). For the rest of the world, however, a sunny epoch of safe roadways lies in the far distance; we must traverse an ocean of gore before reaching the promised land.[1]

The dialectic of motion is nowhere more evident than in Canada, a land of vast distances, multiple time zones and the longest national highway in the world, where remarkable progress goes hand in hand with depressing reversals. Transportation policy in this country focusses on individual behaviour as the chief cause of accidents and a major factor in environmental pollution. Consequently, government is mostly blind to the larger picture of societal neglect, industrial malfeasance, and political irresponsibility that lies behind unacceptable death and injury rates, and dangerous air quality in major cities.

Overwhelming attention to individual behaviour and disregard for other factors in traffic safety are consonant with the dominant ideology of neoliberalism, which guarantees sway of the free market, regardless of public need.[2] The market system itself mostly serves as a screen for the "new imperialism," "a non-territorial empire with its imperial capital in Washington, D.C." (Panitch, 2000, p. 18), as recently clarified by protests against trade policy in Seattle in 1999 and Washington in 2000. For reasons discussed below, Canada may represent an extreme instance of neoliberal influence on traffic planning.[3] This paper employs an analysis of the Federal Government's "Road Safety Vision 2001" (Transport Canada, 1998b) to elucidate the neoliberal foundations of Canadian auto-safety policy.[4] It also presents an alternative traffic-safety agenda, drawn in part from Sweden's radical Vision Zero program, "founded on a long term goal that nobody should be killed or injured in the road system" (Carlsson, 1998, p. 1). Initially, however, I want to survey the politics of traffic safety more generally.

■ Traffic and Neoliberalism

The contrast between Canadian and Swedish approaches to traffic safety may hinge on an important philosophical difference between the two countries. With Canadian neoliberalism, the market colours almost every facet of society.[5] In the Swedish model, however, commodity relations are influenced to a greater extent by government. A United Nations Children's Education Fund study on child poverty in wealthy nations illustrates the consequences of these two approaches. Sweden has the lowest rate of child poverty in the world, with 2.6 percent of children living in relative poverty. The Canadian child-poverty rate places it among the worst for advanced industrial nations, with 15.5 percent of children considered to be poor. Sweden's record is the result of universal government programs aimed at supporting family life. Canada's unsatisfactory performance is mostly due to lack of public support for families, especially those headed by a single parent (Phelps, 2000).

Arguably, the factors at work in traffic accidents are more complex than those for child poverty. The part played by the state in reducing crashes remains unclear. Nevertheless, Swedish roads are among the safest in the world; Canada's motor-vehicle fatality rate is about a third higher than Sweden's (Transport Canada, 1998b, p. 5). The contrast between Sweden's Vision Zero program and Canada's plan for traffic safety, discussed later in this chapter, may stem from Canadian discomfort with an interventionist role for government.

The philosophical dissimilarity between Canada and Sweden reflects a lengthy debate. At the dawn of the industrial era, Hegel drew a distinction between civil society and the state, where civil society comprises the self-regulating market and non-governmental organizations.[6] Hegel recognized the value of market relations for human autonomy, but he also pointed to terrible danger in giving precedence to relations of buying and selling over community needs. The market rests on a misguided idea of freedom as identical with freedom of choice: "I am free when I am left alone, not interfered with and able to choose as I please." This false idea ignores historical movements that control the choices people make. "Real freedom," in Hegelian terms, "begins with the realization that instead of allowing these forces to control us, we can take control of them" (Singer, 1995, p. 339). The North American option in favour of private automobiles over mass transit, for example, arises from badly loaded dice. "History has shown us how the government's bankrolling of car costs and car-based land use has made the automobile look economical and become essential. Our subsidies, not ourselves, have ruled" (Holtz Kay, 1997, p. 345).

Concrete freedom, Hegel suggested, arises from participation in a democratic state armed with resources to curb destructive behaviour in civil society (MacGregor, 1998). Market relations, Hegel wrote (1967, pp. 147, 276), would inevitably bring the interests of producers and consumers into conflict, and require "a control which stands above both and is consciously undertaken." The requirement that government exercise its authority over the market "depends on the fact that, by being publicly exposed for sale, goods in absolutely daily demand are offered not so much to an individual as such but rather to a universal purchaser, the public; and thus both the defence of the public's right not to be defrauded, and also the management of goods inspection, may lie, as a common concern, with a public authority." Instead of democratic leverage over the market, as Hegel recommended, we have government dancing to the tune of auto giants and other large corporations. Later in this paper, I will discuss new forms of state intervention required to protect the public from the perils of the automobile.

Despite the inroads of neoliberalism, most citizens agree with the Hegelian view that the market should be subordinated to the needs of the larger community. In the US, for example, a "1999 Louis Harris poll reflects the largest support yet for a strong federal presence in safety matters including highway and auto safety. A record 93 percent of respondents said that it is 'important' for the federal government to be concerned about uniform safety standards. This continues the trend of increasing support for federal activity to ensure uniform safety standards" (Advocates for Highway and Auto Safety, 1999, p. 38).

Free-market hazards are ubiquitous in the auto age. Benign tolerance is the rule, for example, when it comes to driving while chatting on cellular phones or fitting lethal "brush bars" to the front ends of sport-utility vehicles (SUVs).[7] Market shifts heavily promoted by the auto industry have compromised important advances in vehicle design. After a twenty-year fight, minivans now mostly adhere to passenger-car safety standards. Not so SUVs, which currently dominate luxury-vehicle markets and pose a disproportionate hazard to other road users and to air quality. "As an example, the chances of death for small-car occupants when their vehicles are struck in the side by a large pickup truck or a SUV are more than 20 times greater than when the collision is with another small car" (Advocates for Highway and Auto Safety, 1999, p. 63). Half of new vehicles sold in the US are now light trucks or vans, so that US (and to a lesser extent, Canadian) roads now contain two separate fleets of vehicles. These two fleets are fundamentally incompatible in multiple-vehicle crashes. One fleet is made up of comparatively light, vulnerable passenger cars that are relatively stable in both weight and mass. The second fleet consists of substantially heavier, crash-aggressive light trucks and vans (TVS) whose market share has surged during the 1990s. The average disparity in mass between these two fleets is now close to 1,000 pounds (Advocates for Highway and Auto Safety, 1999, p. 189).

Neoliberal approaches to traffic safety are accompanied by hot-button political strategies that target "scapegoats and villainous minorities" as the cause of societal ills (Laird, 1998, p. 155). These strategies erode civil liberties and criminalize certain forms of social behaviour while having a questionable effect on traffic safety. Moral crusades against drunk drivers and squeegee kids (homeless individuals who earn an income by cleaning windshields at city stoplights) have helped to blunt the impetus for safer, pollution-free automobiles and highways that gathered momentum in the 1960s and 1970s. In Ontario, for example, the Mike Harris Tories devised a clever "anti-pollution" strategy aimed at drivers of older vehicles. Under Ontario's Drive Clean program—which relies on stereotypes of belching rust buckets—cars more than three years old are tested biannually for exhaust emissions. The lax standard catches only the most egregious pollution cases—about fifteen percent of vehicles tested. The program thus avoids confronting both the auto industry and high-income voters who populate the Tory heartland.

Neoliberalism promotes road freedom for the privileged and comfortable, and in some ways, it merely continues a hoary auto-age tradition. "It is almost axiomatic by now," observe Freund and Martin, "that transport policy neglects the interests of the poor, the aged, women, children, and the physically and mentally impaired" (1993, p. 129). But in its mistaken quest for individual freedom, neoliberalism has reversed proven safety measures.[8] "In 1995 the US Congress, flushed with the victory of less-government slogans, raised the speed limit [on freeways], increasing the risk for more accidents" (Holtz Kay, 1997, p. 106). The Harris Tories achieved office in the same year by promising to scrap a highly effective photo-radar program on provincial highways; Ontario initially blocked municipal efforts to install red-light cameras at intersections because they were judged to interfere with driver privacy.[9]

Neoliberal policy harmonizes with the *Zeitgeist* of speed and personal indulgence. Red-light running is common practice in Toronto and other large Canadian urban centres. In the US, speeders take advantage of lax police enforcement and view speed limits as suggestions. A report in the *New York Times* (Zielbauer, 1999) provides a revealing perspective on speeding and aggressive driving: "'There's no debate that speeds now are higher than they have ever been in the history of this nation,' said Richard Retting, a senior transportation engineer with the nonprofit Insurance Institute for Highway Safety. 'There seems to be no stopping that trend.'" The increased presence of light trucks poses new problems:

> Other drivers, especially those steering burly sport utility vehicles with mammoth engines, seem ill-equipped to handle all that power, said Sgt. Paul Vance of the Connecticut State Police. These days, his troopers see more drivers than ever fly by them at 80 and 90 m.p.h., he said. Once caught, more of those drivers now simply blame their vehicles. 'They'll say, "The car just got away from me,"' he said.

Following Alberta's lead (Harrison & Laxer, 1995), Ontario downloaded authority for road maintenance onto municipalities and ended subsidies for public transport. Tory policies have encouraged urban sprawl, especially in the Greater Toronto Area. Unlike that in other countries, Toronto's transit system operates without government assistance. Public transit in Canada's biggest city is crumbling even as pollution, much of it from auto emissions, reaches record high levels. Privatization and deregulation, both of which—whatever the ideological justifications mounted for them—are really innovative forms of government patronage for industry and the wealthy, threaten what remains of a nationally integrated transportation network. In the critical Great Lakes corridor, the North American Free Trade Agreement (NAFTA) has turned Canadian freeways over to north–south freight truckers. Like a stop-action film, the Windsor crash, which involved 87 vehicles and took 8 lives, provided grim evidence for the takeover of public highways by the trucking industry. About a third of the vehicles involved in the Highway 401 crash were tractor trailers (Anderssen, 2000); a tanker-truck fire may have accounted for most of the deaths, as trapped auto passengers were immolated in the flames.

Ontario's "Common Sense" Revolution presents a special case of neoliberalism's impact on public services, including traffic regulation. Bent on eliminating "red tape" and convinced of the nullity of government supervision, the Harris Tories slashed the budget of the Ministry of Environment by 42 percent and laid off a third of front-line staff, including technicians and inspectors (Diemer, 2000). Industries were set free to regulate themselves, and vital programs, such as the Drinking Water Surveillance system, were dropped. The Walkerton *E. coli* disaster, which began in May 2000 and left 2,000 people ill and as many as 18 dead from drinking municipal tap water, was likely a direct result. Data on the impact of Ontario's deregulation policies on traffic have not yet been assembled. The government admitted in June 2000, when one Ontario Provincial Police officer was killed and two other officers were badly injured in a truck crash on the 401, that it had still not hired sufficient road and truck inspectors to maintain the province's highways.

Neoliberalism treats public funding for mass transit as a "subsidy" rather than an investment. Transit riders supposedly benefit from government largess while trucks and autos are cost-free. Yet US estimates suggest the public confronts a tab of $3,000 to $5,000 (or even more) for each automobile; Canadians likely bear a similar cost. "Things we rarely consider bear a dollar sign: from parking facilities to police protection, from land consumed in sprawl to registry operations, environmental damage to uncompensated accidents ... 'Driving's not just a free lunch,' says one activist. 'It's a free lunch you're getting paid to eat'" (Holtz Kay, 1997, pp. 120, 357). While drivers benefit from the free lunch, the trucking industry benefits even more. Trucks, for instance, cause an estimated twenty times more damage to roadways than automobiles do.

American neoliberalism inflicted tremendous damage on the movement for traffic safety, especially under President Reagan, who blocked the airbag rule for many years and seriously weakened the National Highway Traffic Safety Administration (NHTSA) (Luger, 2000). The NHTSA has rebounded in recent years, however, and traffic safety is once again on the political radar, and the US never neglected its infrastructure to the same extent as Canada and other countries entranced by neoliberal doctrines (Galbraith, Conceicao & Ferreira, 1999). American roads, for example, are in much better condition than those in Canada. With one-tenth the US population, the Canadian road deficit is equivalent to that of the US; both countries require an injection of about $17 billion to bring their respective road systems up to standard.

An energetic $7-billion transportation plan for Vancouver features a large investment in public transit, although it has met resistance because it will be partly financed by levies on owners of private automobiles. The federal government recently announced enhanced funding for Via Rail after decades of neglect, as well as $600 million over 6 years for highway infrastructure. In addition, Ottawa established stiffer pollution rules this year, although these remain voluntary. The 2000 Report of the Federal Commissioner of the Environment and Sustainable Development noted that the federal government has made no progress on curbing pollution—more than half of which is generated by transportation—for the past ten years.

Transport-related industries are central to the Canadian economy; moreover, these industries are linked by NAFTA to the world's leading industrial power, the US. The American economy sucks up twenty percent of Canadian industrial production—much of it related to transport—a proportion similar to the dependence of less-developed nations on the industrialized world. Foreign capital controls much of Canada's resources and enjoys majority ownership of shares in many Canadian firms. Consequently, traffic-safety initiatives must navigate terrain cornered by wealthy outsiders with an attentive ear in government. Writes Madelaine Drohan (2000), "It would take a brave politician to challenge the biggest employer in town for the broader public interest." The huge auto-industry complex in southwestern Ontario, which exports much of its output to the US, enjoys tremendous political clout. Oil extraction, dominated by US firms, plays a major part in Alberta. Similarly, refining looms large in Ontario, Quebec and New Brunswick. In the US, by contrast, big oil and the auto makers must contend with other powerful players and thus may be more vulnerable to public pressure.

Unlike the US, Canada never developed a well-organized movement to demand regulation of the auto industry. Heward Graftney, a Conservative MP, fought to raise awareness of the issue among Canadians in the 1960s, but no Canadian Ralph Nader ever emerged, and robust European sensitivity to the issue of traffic safety finds only a modest equivalent in Canada.[10] Award-winning Canadian designs for safe, non-polluting autos never reach the production stage (Nader, Milleron & Conacher, 1993). Most Canadian auto-safety regulations are piggyback versions of original US legislation. The economics of large-scale production on the North American continent mean that Canadian consumers benefit from US auto rules, such as the revolutionary airbag requirement (which Canadian transport engineers initially opposed because they feared airbags would reduce seat-belt use). Canadians are typically more willing to alter individual behaviour than to tackle industry giants on auto-safety issues. Accordingly, once the US government legislated seat belts in passenger cars in the early 1970s, after a vicious battle with automakers, Canadians joined world leaders in seat-belt use thanks to strongly enforced provincial laws that required motorists and passengers to buckle up. Canada also took a primary role in the use of child-restraint systems.

These developments partly account for the spectacular decline in Canadian traffic deaths, which began in 1973. Despite a huge increase in traffic volume, the death rate has shrunk by half over the past quarter century. (Canada's excellent universal health system also probably played an important role, since rapid medical response significantly reduces road deaths and severity of injuries [Nathens, Jurkovich, Cummings, Rivara & Maier, 2000].) Indeed, "Sports injuries have overtaken automobile accidents as the leading cause of disabilities and deaths in the age group of 15 to 24" (Christie, 2000). However, aside from universal medicare, the individual is the focus of legislative efforts on auto safety. Ottawa sat on the sidelines during the struggle for the seat-belt standard; automakers were never compelled to offer child safety seats. An exception to this rule is the Canadian government's requirement for daytime running lights, which has no counterpart in the US.

In some instances, where the government has acted in the public interest, transnational trade agreements (of which neoliberal Canada is a big booster) have thwarted these efforts. A key example is the case of MMT, a gasoline additive with adverse health effects that was banned by Ottawa. The product's maker, Ethyl Corporation, took the Canadian government to court claiming unfair restriction of free trade. Ethyl won a claim of $13 million for court fees and lost profits, and won the right to supply its toxic product to gasoline retailers. The MMT case aside, government failure to act is more general. As discussed earlier, Ontario cut the Ministry of Environment by almost 50 percent since 1995. The province allows sulphur levels in gasoline higher than any other jurisdiction in Canada or the US. Promising federal environmental initiatives have either misfired or stalled.

■ Sweden's Vision Zero and Canada's Road Safety Visions 2001

They call the stretch of the 401 Highway between Chatham and Windsor "Carnage Alley" (Anderssen, 2000). Built in the early 1960s, the artery was never meant for the swelling volume of north–south commercial traffic that accompanied the 1989 Free Trade Agreement between Canada and the United States and the 1995 NAFTA that brought Mexico in as a third partner. Mike Harris' Tories, and the federal Liberals shrank from the daunting cost of upgrading the 400 series of highways that criss-cross Ontario; cosmetic changes to the 401 around Windsor did little to stem the tide of blood. Probably alone among North American superhighways, the 401 still features soft rather than paved shoulders, a factor cited by some for the road's rising death toll.

Three hours after the Windsor accident, Nelson Shognosh (2000) approached his sister-in-law and brother's burnt-out van. Most who succumbed in the smoke and fog, including Nelson's mother Eleanor, did not die immediately. A fourteen-year-old girl pleaded for her life while rescuers stood helpless, separated from her by burning trucks and automobiles. Flames caught Eleanor Shognosh, who lay pinned under the seats of the van. "Elaine Shognosh climbed out of the shattered back window and dashed across the highway, to where farmers had already gathered with pickup trucks to assist the wounded." She saw the fires starting and she was afraid to go back: "'I thought they were both dead.' She found her husband later, bloody but alive" (Anderssen, 2000).

Like his mother before him, Nelson Shognosh is a traditional healer and teacher; aboriginal communities across the continent know him affectionately as Sugar Bear (George, 2000). Alerted by the Ontario Provincial Police, Tom Doxtator reached Nelson Shognosh soon after the crash.[11] Officers let Sugar Bear through the yellow tape into what they labelled "the hot zone," where 27 vehicles and 6 people were crushed and incinerated (Crawford, 2000). First Nations peoples recognize the living must help the spirit of the suddenly departed along in their journey. "Nothing stops," says Nelson Shognosh (2000); the lost spirits enter another phase of life, "and death is part of it." Sugar Bear stood in the hot zone to reassure his departed mother and the other lost souls. "What was it like in those last few seconds? Those dying must have felt so alone. We are there to help the dead to enter the spirit world." No priests or ministers reached the wreck. Only Sugar Bear could comfort the dead. "The firefighters and police were glad to see me," observed Nelson Shognosh. "Someone had to be there to acknowledge the lives that were lost."

In 1997, 3,000 people died on Canadian roads and 200,000 suffered injuries. In the same year, Sweden recorded 540 road deaths; 4,000 were seriously injured. The Canadian fatality toll has steadily receded since the early 1970s, while Sweden recorded about 540 deaths in 1996, 1997, and 1998 respectively, after a long period of falling casualty figures. Both countries agree that these statistics are intolerable and unnecessary, but their solutions differ markedly. Frustrated by lack of progress in lessening road fatalities, Sweden has set policy targets for reduction of traffic deaths and injuries (Carlsson, 1998). The Vision Zero program recognizes that it is not realistic to eliminate accidents in a road system that "is very complicated and essentially uncontrolled." Rather, the program aims to eliminate serious injury and death that may result from accidents. By the year 2007, for example, fatalities are to be reduced to 250 per year. Unlike Sweden and other countries such as the UK, Canada sets no reduction goals. Nor does Ottawa's Traffic Safety Vision 2001 program underline the difference between accidents and the human consequence of accidents, as does Vision Zero. Instead, Vision 2001 suggests that "most accidents can be avoided with common-sense solutions," which include shunning alcohol and excessive speed, and wearing seat belts.

The crucial distinction between an accident and its effects on the occupants of a vehicle was initially proposed by the traffic safety pioneer, William Haddon, the first director of the US NHTSA. Haddon also devised the traffic-safety matrix, which includes "vehicle design and equipment, driver behaviour or, more generally, human factors, and the highway environment" (Advocates for Highway and Auto Safety, 1999, p. xxv). Accepting the inevitability of accidents and the limited malleability of human behaviour, Haddon emphasized improving the crash worthiness of automobiles and redesigning the highway environment. As Lawrence Ross (1992, p. 7) points out, even such lamentable behaviour as drinking and driving would be of scant concern if no deaths and injuries resulted from it: "From the traffic safety viewpoint, drunk driving might be tolerable if its links to errors and crashes, and subsequently to injuries and deaths, could be severed."

Canadian authorities suggest that the relative safety of Sweden's roads compared to Canada's may result from Sweden's strict laws on drinking and driving. The legal limit for a driver's blood alcohol level (BAC), for instance, is 0.02 in Sweden compared to 0.08 for Canada. Vision 2001 calls for "more active enforcement with increasing fines and harsher treatment of repeat offenders to spread the no-tolerance message on this irresponsible driving behaviour." However, Sweden's success in fighting drunk driving relies only partly on criminal law. Contends Ross (1992, p. xiv), "More central to this achievement is recognition of the causes of drunk driving in social institutions, leading to countermeasures based in alcohol policy—reducing drinking—and transportation policy—reducing driving." The Transport Canada Vision statement mentions neither of these countermeasures. Significantly, Sweden's Vision Zero places driver behaviour, including drunk driving, in the background.[12] "The road transport system must be designed so that people's mistakes do not have disastrous consequences" (Carlsson, 1998, p. 3).

Pronouncements against drunk driving, as in Canada's Vision 2001, are more about public performance than saving lives. Anti-drunk-driving campaigns, remarks Joseph Gusfield (1992, p. x), constitute "a statement about who the good guys and the bad guys are ... [Their] ritualistic character is a way of asserting the moral values and ethical choices that are present as the dominant norms ...." Gusfield warns against confusing "the ritualistic nature of public acts with expediential ones ... Saving lives and saving souls may not be the same game." There is no question that drinking and driving poses considerable risk and imposes extravagant societal costs. Nevertheless, anti-drunk-driving campaigners exaggerate the contribution of drunk driving to traffic accidents. No more than 25 percent of fatal collisions in the US are alcohol-related (Ross, 1992, pp. 37, 47). Moreover, the role of alcohol in many of these accidents remains unknown. "A driver who was operating his vehicle flawlessly and who could pass a field sobriety test would still be guilty of drunk driving if a breath test showed his BAC to be 0.10 [0.08 in Canada] or greater." Driving while under the influence of alcohol is much less hazardous than many legal activities, such as operating a motorcycle. "Comparison of the number of alcohol-related fatalities with the estimated number of miles driven by drivers with BACs over 0.10 percent shows that there is less than one fatality for every six hundred thousand impaired miles driven."[13]

Along with reducing drinking and driving, Vision 2001 recommends increasing seat-belt use and deterring speeders. Seat-belt use is already at 90 percent in Canada, an enviable figure that leaves limited room for improvement (the report calls for 95 percent seat-belt use). Speeding is at least as risky as drunk driving. "Because higher speeds reduce the time available to react to emergencies and increase the amount of damage suffered in crashes, it seems reasonable to regard speeding as a dangerous law violation, other things being equal" (Ross, 1992, p. 48). US studies show that with favourable road conditions, the vast majority of drivers "will engage in this violation." Moreover, effective deterrence of speeders requires enormous investment in law enforcement. Neither factor is emphasized in Vision 2001.

"If we can have modern roads and vehicles surely we can also modernize individual attitudes to road safety" intones Vision 2001 (Transport Canada, 1998b). For Canadian traffic-safety policy-makers, road construction, road maintenance and vehicle safety are secondary to altering individual behaviour. "All levels of government are uniting to put more focus on the safety aspects of roads in their jurisdictions," says the report—in plain defiance of considerable evidence to the contrary. "The vehicles on today's roads are much safer than they were a quarter century ago. They perform better in crashes and they are increasingly equipped with safety devices to avoid crashes in the first place."

This rosy statement ignores the preponderance of SUVs on Canadian roads, and the fact that these vehicles may not conform to automobile-safety standards. Nor does it address the urgent need to improve on existing safety regulations, such as (to name only three) "vehicle stability (rollover prevention), vehicle crash compatibility, and pedestrian safety (vehicle-pedestrian impact)" (Advocates for Highway and Auto Safety, 1999, p. 189).

There is one encouraging departure from the focus on the individual in Vision 2001 (Transport Canada, 1998b). The report rightly calls for improving national data-collection on traffic safety in Canada: "A national task force is ... at work to improve data quality and compatibility and to encourage cross jurisdictional sharing of information." The report recommends linkages with insurance claims, hospital records, and driver and vehicle registration. Compared to other nations, Canadian traffic-safety data is hardly stellar. We hope the report's commitment to enhanced communication "will be reflected in an improved National Collision Data Base."

Sweden's Vision Zero reflects a homogeneous political culture that differs sharply from Canada's. The Swedes are motivated by a "passion for equality" (Bergqvist & Findlay, 2000, p. 119) that has no parallel in the Canadian context, in which considerable energy is expended in reconciling various communities within the nation and class inequality is tolerated. "The importance of diversity" in Canada, writes Linda Briskin (2000, p. 22) in a study of women's organizing in the two countries, "cannot be over-estimated—racial and ethnic diversity, regional diversity, language diversity, all of which are framed within the context of debates about Quebec as a distinct society and about the right of First Nation peoples to self-government." The Swedish "passion for equality" encourages traffic-safety strategies that embrace the needs of all road users: the young and the old, rich and poor, motorcyclists, pedestrians, bicyclists and motorists alike. Canadian traffic-safety policy, more in tune with "the ideology of automobility" (Freund & Martin, 1997), privileges the rights of motorists over other road users. In Sweden, the small and relatively homogenous population and the unitary character of the state encourage national initiatives that enjoy real chance for success.

For Swedes, the ability of the human body to withstand collision forces sets "the limitation of the maximum speeds in the [road] system." High speeds may be permitted only where they can be technologically controlled and pose no physical danger. Vision Zero directs that "vulnerable road users (pedestrians, bicyclists, elderly people, etc.) will determine the safety demands of the system." The Swedish program is informed by studies that show that even if all traffic laws were strictly followed by every road user, only 50 percent of deaths and 30 percent of injuries would be avoided. "This shows that the road transport system really is very unsafe and it is too easy just to blame the road users. The system designers have to take a much greater responsibility [for] the safety of the system."

Transport Canada mentions proudly that BAC tests are performed on more than 80 percent of fatally injured drivers (Transport Canada, 1998a). Some may be less comforted that resources of busy emergency rooms and pathology labs are strained in this way. Rather than focus on driver guilt, Vision Zero recommends investigating accidents with a view to determining "'What could have been done to prevent the fatality or injury?' and this knowledge has to be used to improve the system" (Carlsson, 1998, p. 4). Vision Zero recommends reducing speeds across the system, especially in areas where motor vehicles, pedestrians and other road users compete for available space.

The Swedish focus on speed may appear to place attention once again on individual driver behaviour. Vision Zero planners recognize, however, that speed must be treated within a structural context. In other words, "speeders" are not the focus of traffic-safety efforts, but rather average speeds within the system. When the US reduced highway speed limits in response to the fuel crisis of the 1970s, for example, overall death rates fell dramatically. Death rates increased with legislated higher limits in the mid 1980s (Freund & Martin, 1993, p. 39).

Neither Vision Zero nor Canada's Vision 2001 mention the dreadful loss of animal life to the traffic system. The obliteration of companion animals and wildlife is more often mocked as "roadkill" than considered as a serious issue— even where collisions with large wild animals such as bear, deer and moose also threatened human lives. This is beginning to change. In Banff, Alberta, for example, Parks Canada built a series of underpasses and overpasses to facilitate passage by deer, antelope and grizzlies. We must find ways to discourage dandelions—a bear delicacy—from growing by the highway. The US Transportation Equity Act for the 21st Century provides funding support "for wildlife crossings on both new and existing roads." American initiatives embrace turtle crossings in California, deer culverts in Washington state, bear underpasses in Florida and salamander tunnels in Massachusetts. In the Netherlands, where 20 percent of the badger population was killed annually by cars, highways now feature fences and badger-tunnels, which have helped double the badger population in some areas (US Federal Highway Administration, 2000).

■ Prospects for Traffic Safety
Programs to severely reduce injuries and fatalities in the road system necessarily aggravate the jealous god of mobility. Heavy constraints must be placed on speed, traffic flow and individual choice; and societal resources need to be

redirected away from autos to public transport. Instead of laying down more roads, the prevailing network must be improved. Research suggests, for instance, that a investment by Sweden of $10 to 15 billion in improving infra-structure safety "can reduce the number of fatalities by 80–90 percent" (Carlsson, 1998, p. 5). These measures require an extraordinary degree of state intervention into social and economic communities within civil society. Powerful political interests must be confronted, including the auto-safety establishment (which concentrates too heavily on individual behaviour), road builders and automobile makers. The success of Vision Zero will depend largely on the ability of policy-makers to overcome these obstacles. Exporting the Swedish program to other countries, such as Canada, will be extremely difficult, for it goes directly against the neoliberal celebration of an unregulated market.

In 1993, when almost 700 Swedes were killed annually in auto accidents, the government announced a national road-safety program with a goal of 400 road deaths by the year 2000. That target may be unattainable, given that progress in reducing road deaths has stagnated. Similarly, Vision Zero may be overly ambitious. Writing about women's organizing, Bergqvist and Findlay (2000, p. 141) observe that Sweden's "passion for equality" led government to underestimate civil society's opposition to change: "Regardless of the fact that Sweden has demonstrated a greater commitment to women's equality than Canada, resistance to the introduction of initiatives that threaten the tradi-tional balance of power between women and men in public life continues." Both countries are leaders in furthering women's participation, but Sweden's more centralized system of government, stronger political will and greater openness to democracy forged a larger role for women in the state and civil society.

Factors that created an outstanding record for women's equality in Sweden may also work in favour of Vision Zero. Swedish authorities are working closely with traffic-safety NGOs, which have adopted Vision Zero "as the 'leading star' of [their] work for improved safety" (Carlsson, 1998, p. 5). Even automobile associations, which have traditionally fought speed restrictions, are coming onside. In contrast to Swedish centralized planning, any compre-hensive program for traffic safety in Canada must negotiate the sensitive zone of federal–provincial responsibility. Canada's greater diversity also presents obstacles to a truly radical traffic-safety initiative.

In some ways, however, Canada has forged ahead. Motorcycle helmets have been mandatory across the nation for many years. Ontario legislated bicycle helmets for children in 1996 (ten years after California passed similar legisla-tion)—a critically important measure the Swedes have not yet adopted. Seat-belt use is roughly equal in both countries. Toronto leads North America in bicycle use. Perhaps most important, the Canadian traffic-calming movement

(Transport Association of Canada, 1999), which aims to reduce speed and increase pedestrian and cyclist safety in urban areas, has gained considerable strength. The neoliberal thrust foundered at the municipal level, where citizens are anxious to control the automobile and state intervention (in the guise of municipal authority) is widely favoured. Traffic calming involves physical additions to city streets, such as speed bumps or sidewalk extensions, and changes in traffic flow, including one-way street systems (Engwicht, 1993). Canadian traffic engineers recently produced traffic-calming guidelines for application across the nation.

Like Canada, Sweden harbours strong transport interests. Swedish automaker Volvo is a pioneer in vehicle safety. The firm recognized early that "safety sells"—something that US automakers did not fully appreciate until the 1990s. Nevertheless, even this manufacturer does not come close to the safety standards suggested by the authors of "Stuck In Neutral" (Advocates for Highway and Auto Safety, 1999), a comprehensive report on auto safety in the US. For example, the report recommends on-board crash recorders for passenger vehicles that would enable emergency response and crash notification systems. It also calls for changes in vehicle design to avoid and reduce pedestrian injury. A large part of the problem with pedestrian crash safety is that many serious injuries and deaths occur at relatively low vehicle-impact speeds. Despite the low speed, such a crash can often result in death because people are killed from head trauma when the upper torso and head strike stiff, unyielding portions of the vehicle front end, including fender tops and windshield cowls, that inflict terrible injuries. Making basic changes to the aggressive quality of passenger-vehicle front ends could save scores of lives and prevent hundreds of serious injuries (Advocates for Highway and Auto Safety, 1999, p. 80).

Unlike Sweden, neoliberal Canada faces the problem of a deregulated trucking industry; transport traffic, along with trailer size and unwieldiness, is increasing exponentially. Profit-making in this highly competitive industry places tremendous demands on drivers' mental and physical health. Trucks have few of the safety features built into passenger cars, and their handling characteristics are inappropriate for highways designed primarily to accommodate smaller vehicles. The mix of truck and auto traffic on Canadian roads is a recipe for disaster—as shown in the Windsor crash. "Nationally, deaths in big truck collisions are 17 percent of all road traffic deaths and five per cent of all traffic injuries" (CRASH, 1999). Blissfully unaware of the danger, the Canadian government is quietly negotiating to allow multiple trailer-truck trains under NAFTA. Ottawa already delegated responsibility for truck safety to the provinces, making trucking the only commercial freight mode not regulated at the federal level. Some provinces do a good job; others, such as Alberta and Ontario, maintain slipshod regulatory regimes.

When Sugar Bear stepped across the yellow tape into the hot zone, smoke still rose from tangled hulks. Nelson Shognosh had been working only about 400 metres from the scene where his mother died after a tractor trailer crushed the Shognosh van. Eleanor Shognosh was one of about 500 Canadians who died in large truck collisions in 1999.[14] According to Sweden's Vision Zero, the world's traffic network can be constructed so that tragedies like that suffered by the Shognosh family need never happen again.

During an open-line radio show from Owen Sound, Ontario, which concerned a rash of local traffic deaths just before the first holiday weekend of the Canadian cottage season, I awkwardly mentioned the visionary Swedish project. The radio host politely acknowledged my remark but wanted quickly to move on to more important matters, such as how to educate errant drivers. Yet the genuinely effective task may be to challenge what Ross (1992, p. 168) calls the "dominant paradigm," which "focuses on a blameworthy driver," and look instead to making the roads safe for every user: " We have to look on road safety in the same way as we look upon safety in our work environment, in air transport or in rail transport. In those fields every fatality or serious injury is regarded as a failure which should not happen again. If we succeed [with Vision Zero] we can, as real professionals, proudly say we have created a mature road transport system" (Carlsson, 1998, p. 6).

NOTES

1   "About 1 million traffic deaths and about 40 million traffic injuries occurred in 1990 worldwide
    ... The World Health Organization projects that deaths from traffic accidents will rise by 2020 to
    about 2.3 million, more than doubling the toll for 1990. Deaths will increase as developing
    nations adopt auto-centered transport systems, at the same times as the proportion of young
    adults in their populations (those most at risk) grows" (Freund & McGuire, 1999, p. 59).
2   Peter Rothe's *Beyond Traffic Safety* (1994) offers a useful corrective to standard views of traffic
    safety. He argues that driving should be seen as a social relationship that takes place within a
    complex, multi-level framework. Reducing the driving experience to individual behaviour has
    mostly negative effects for our understanding of traffic safety.
3   Canada's Liberal government is proud of its commitment to neoliberalism. At the Berlin
    Summit on Modern Governance in the 21st Century, for instance, Canadian representatives
    insisted that other world leaders "recognize Canada as a pioneer in adopting social democracy to
    global economic competition" (*Globe and Mail*, 1 June 2000, p. 4).
4   For the balance of this paper, Transport Canada's "Road Safety Vision 2001" will be referred to
    as " Vision 2001."
5   The Canadian medicare system forms an exception to this generalization. Canadians are justly
    proud of the role played by government in providing health care. Canadian neoliberals and their
    powerful allies in the United States have targeted Canada's universal program for privatization
    with some success in the past few years. The outcome of this ideological battle remains in
    doubt. Barbara Cameron and Lena Gonäs (1999, pp. 52–60)offer a useful comparison between
    Canada's and Sweden's support for universal state programs.

6   Civil society has recently become an important term in political discourse, though "there is little agreement on its precise meaning" (Anheier, 2000). Usually it refers to various citizen groups and non-governmental organizations (NGOs) that stand outside the established power networks of the state and the market. By contrast, Hegel saw the market and economic organizations such as corporations and unions as interdependent parts of civil society. The Russian experience after 1991, during which citizen-led opposition to the Soviet state was swallowed up by market forces, indicates that Hegel's original concept, which stresses the interdependence of the state and non-market aspects of civil society, may still retain its validity.

7   Betsy Wade (1999) reports that the US government anticipates there will be 80 million American cellphone users by the end of 2000. In March 1999, the little town of Brooklyn, Ohio, put an ordinance into effect against "use of a cellphone held in the hand while the car is in motion." Similar legislation is proposed for the city of Chicago. A recent study in Toronto found that cellphone users are four times as likely as non-users to be involved in a collision, regardless of whether the cellphone is hand held or hands free. An National Highway Traffic Safety Administration study also found that cellphone use increases risk of a crash: " Tim Hurd, a spokesman for the agency, said that as a general rule, 'distraction causes fatalities.'" Nevertheless, cellphones may also increase safety on the highways. "Charles F. Richmond, a troubleshooter for the Connecticut Department of Transportation, speaks for many when he says, " The cellphone has saved more lives than the ambulances. Outside North America, cellular phones are regulated more strictly. Thirteen countries, including the UK, Australia and Italy, have banned their use while driving.

8   Rothe (1994) rightly criticizes traffic-safety programs that focus on speed and electronic detection; but his objections are leveled within a framework that emphasizes all levels of traffic management. The neoliberal abandonment of traffic regulation does not constitute responsible traffic policy.

9   A Norwegian study found that stationary speed enforcement (traffic radar) brings a reduction in traffic fatalities of up to 14 percent (Carlsson, 1997b, p. 7).

10   This may be changing. A burgeoning traffic calming movement in this country, discussed below, may bring Canadian awareness of traffic issues to European levels.

11   Tom Doxtator is Aboriginal Resource Instructor at the Chatham campus of St. Clair College.

12   "Increased control of drunken driving is barely cost-effective in Norway and Sweden," notes Gunnar Carlsson (Carlsson, 1997a, p. 1), "but is probably more cost-effective in many other European countries."

13   About 40 percent of fatally injured Canadian drivers in 1996 had been drinking or were impaired (Transport Canada, 1998a). Fatally injured drunk drivers generally are involved in single-vehicle crashes; the stereotypical drunk driver who collides with a sober motorist or pedestrian features far less in accident statistics. Traffic deaths often result from shock that accompanies trauma and severe bleeding. Persons with significant BACs are more susceptible to shock, and more likely, therefore, to succumb to crash injuries. The role played by increased susceptibility to shock in those with high BACs needs further study.

14   A coroner's inquest on the Windsor collision that took the life of Eleanor Shognosh and seven others called for the return of photo radar (abolished by the Harris Tories in 1995) and an increased police presence on the 401 Highway to deter speeders. It also called for design changes to improve safety on the fatal stretch of road, including roadside fog alerts to warn drivers (Harries, 2000).

10

DISPATCHERS AND DRIVERS

*On-the-Road Economics
and Manufactured Risk*

J. PETER ROTHE

AS ONE TERMINAL MANAGER PUT IT, "The relationship between dispatchers and truckers is similar to that of the pope and the bishops. Only the truckers don't have to kiss the ring." Sit back for a moment and reflect on the concept of dispatch and its relevance to traffic safety. The highways are packed with vehicles of all sizes: bicycles, motorcycles, cars, transport trucks. Although we see them daily, we seldom think about the number of vehicles that are dispatched and what that means for traffic safety. At the micro level, dispatched vehicles are operated by a group of employees, who were sent by agents to deliver a service. But at a macro level, dispatched vehicles represent corporate needs, management–labour relations, blue-collar workers toiling for pay, company profits, breaches of laws and regulations, and the construction of high-risk traffic scenarios. We are uncertain how many vehicles are dispatched at any time, but when we think about the number of semi-trailer trucks, dump trucks, vans and half-ton trucks, emergency vehicles, couriers, taxis, buses and service vehicles that enter our vision, we can easily become overwhelmed. Much of the traffic is time-sensitive, profit-oriented, efficiency-controlled and dispatch-monitored.

Dispatching is a form of labour control on the highways. Drivers define the roadways on the directives of corporate dispatchers and the wishes of industry executives (Ericson, 1984). They are told where to travel, when to arrive, how important the trip is and what earnings will result from it. In most cases, drivers meet the dispatchers' expectations because the dispatchers have the power to define the situation and interpret the need for action. Dispatchers control the drivers' itineraries. They systematically rely on driver compliance during all stages of the trip; truckers are expected to obey. Unfortunately for dispatchers, drivers are not robots. They act and react differently to life circumstances. They defend their abilities and respect their craft. They show emotion. In short, they are exemplar pragmatists. Over and over again, well-meaning older truckers suggested that "You've got to do what's right for you or you'll never last." It is both the dispatchers' demands on truckers and the truckers' responses to dispatch commands that require attention for analysis of traffic safety.

■ Dispatchers

They're my boss. That's the way I look at it. If I don't want to do something they can make me by ultimately pulling rank and saying just shut up and do it. —TRUCKER

It's sort of like having about five contingency plans in the back of your mind all of the time. —TRUCKER

Dispatchers collectively represent the perennial go-betweens: between truckers and shippers, truckers and management, company and customer. They fulfill corporate functions like contracting loads and back hauls, assigning loads to drivers, defining trip expectations or logistics to the truckers, negotiating the cost of loads with shippers and, in some cases, managing company personnel. While concentrating on the freight company's profit margin, dispatchers vary widely in their adherence to matters of road safety policies, driving violations, load sizes and commerce laws. They are in charge. According to Stackhouse (1991), they may force operators to drive longer and faster than regulations permit or may support the driver, acknowledge the importance of road safety and emphasize degrees of reliability. But regardless of dispatcher tactics, their efforts are directly correlated with the profit and expenditure that are essential to maintaining their respective trucking companies.

A dispatcher working for a carrier operating eighteen trucks accepted expediency over safety. He reported,

Look, the most I get out of an over-the-road trucker is maybe ten years. Then he's gone. He'll be married and want to drive local. So for ten years I'm gonna be on his ass to get out of him everything we need. Safety? Shit! That's his own business, not mine.

Dispatchers bridge management and drivers. They possess substantial formal and informal power over truckers and responsibility for the company's financial welfare. Informal power can be seen in the dispatchers' control over truckers without use of policy-driven and guidebook-approved procedures. It is practised behind the scenes, in the backrooms. Measures of informal power are part of the everyday landscape, expected by drivers and considered legitimate by management. Much like a school teacher giving treats to students who have done well and silent treatment to those who have disobeyed, dispatchers assign rewards for drivers who obey and take disciplinary measures against those who refuse dispatcher commands. Informal strategies of discipline are resources available to dispatchers, no matter how perfect, unsafe or illegal a command may be. For example, they can assign the loads, equipment and driving times according to which drivers they prefer to use (Rothe, 1991). If a driver refuses to take a load because of fatigue, or if he invokes the hours-of-service policy, the dispatcher can, and in many cases will, take action against that driver. Retaliation is commonly understood as a significant feature in the world of trucking. By the same token, a driver with back pain may be offered an easy trip as long as he demonstrates an eagerness to work.

Traffic-safety professionals recognize that driver error due to fatigue is a significant consideration in commercial-vehicle crashes (Hoffman, 1989). When a driver is unwilling to make a return run without adequate sleep, the dispatcher can accept the driver's decision and search for another candidate, or, more likely, threaten the tired driver with disciplinary measures like loss of future loads and back hauls, or assignment of low-profit loads. For example, a Vancouver trucker legally refused to take a new load because he already fulfilled his legal number of consecutive driving hours. The trucker's move displeased the dispatcher, who consequently assigned the trucker a Vancouver-to-Nanaimo-run, a full-day trip consisting of a four-hour ferry ride. The damaging element of the assignment was that truckers have no opportunity to earn mileage-based pay parked on a ferry (Rothe, 1994).

Interviews with dispatchers illustrate that they readily support safety in principle. Yet it is not uncommon to witness dispatchers encouraging truckers to compromise traffic laws and safety regulations. That encouragement may take the form of an explicit request or implicit wink-wink, let's-get-it-done. As I have indicated previously (Rothe, 1991, 1994), dispatchers are quick to withdraw from the scene if the trucker receives a traffic ticket or is caught driving unsafely by the company safety supervisor. The rationale often used by dispatchers is featured in the following statement made by a dispatcher:

> I tell the guys what they have to do, within what time. I mean we all know, you know, the push is on. But still the guy gets caught, it's his ass

that's in a sling. He's got to be smart enough not to get caught. I don't sit in the cab with him. Not getting caught is his responsibility and not mine—and he knows it. We all know it.

Truckers can take legal action against dispatchers who demand that drivers operate illegally or unsafely. However, they may experience ramifications beyond the formal complaints. At worst, they may be forced out of the job (Rothe, 1994). At best, they will be hounded by a dispatcher. As one dispatcher said of a complaining driver, "I'll be on him [the trucker] like butter on toast until he gets the message ..." The severity of threats against truckers has lessened over the last couple of years. With the shortage of long-haul drivers, and with companies competing against one another to scoop up worthwhile drivers for their expanding fleets, drivers have become more vocal in their opposition to dispatcher demands. Some companies have responded with a kinder, gentler approach to dispatching. Nevertheless, the fact remains that dispatchers have control of drivers and many exercise this control in haphazard and coercive ways.

Some trucking companies give dispatchers the authority to discipline truckers who oppose their demands—or to reward truckers who fulfill questionable demands. Formal disciplinary procedures are invoked on the basis of power vested in the dispatch role as defined by policy or company guidelines. Common practices include suspension, entry into personnel file, outright dismissal, loss of pay and loss of year-end bonus. Larger freight companies assign the head dispatcher or operations manager the right to implement disciplinary procedures. This person usually makes decisions in concert with the dispatcher, trucker and safety supervisor. Many smaller carriers, operating up to twenty trucks are owned, managed and dispatched by the same person. Hence a trucker can be, and often is, fired on the spot for not fulfilling the owner/dispatcher's wishes. These individuals usually pay little attention to labour standards or legalities.

Agar (1986), Bradley (1979), Rothe (1991) and Stockington (1991), among others, have described how truckers are expected to drive overweight, operate poorly maintained equipment, drive over the legal speed limit, overdrive the legal number of consecutive driving hours, purposefully mis-weigh scales and drive in North American locations without proper papers. Of special significance is speeding. According to statistics collected by the Ontario Provincial Police and the M.T.C., 60 percent of all truck-driver convictions under the Highway Traffic Act are for speeding. It is one of the most frequent causes of truck collisions (Ontario Ministry of Transportation and Communications, 1983). This situation is no surprise if we consider Rothe's (1994) research that described how many dispatchers were willing to pressure truckers to complete a trip within a certain time frame—one that demands speeding.

Although dispatchers hold substantial formal and informal power over the truckers, they are seldom held accountable for the actions that influence driver behaviour on the roadways. They are part of the silent backdrop and are seldom included as contributing factors to truck-and-trailer accidents or truckers' traffic violations. Truckers hesitate risking their livelihoods by implicating dispatchers (Rothe, 1994). Whenever the police attempt to investigate a dispatcher's role in a crash, officers are quickly stonewalled with a code of silence invoked by dispatchers and truckers. Why risk disciplinary actions or the loss of a job?

■ The Economic Influence

If we don't show profit, we'll be out of work.

—DISPATCHER

Transport companies exist to make money. To succeed, management depends on the dispatchers not only to accept corporate values but to invoke them in daily transactions, making them a collective, vital piece in the freight delivery puzzle. The best dispatchers are those who make the greatest profit. They are like middle managers who carry the health of their companies on their shoulders. Pleasing drivers, shippers, managers, other dispatchers and dockhands, and constantly attending to timelines, equipment and government regulators makes dispatching a high-stress job.

Above all other duties, dispatchers expedite freight. To accomplish this successfully, they engage in "sharp practices that compromise safety regulations, cartage policies and traffic laws" (Reckless, 1967). Thus, many of dispatcher activities are a mild version of white-collar crime (Reckless, 1967; Sutherland, 1941). Dispatchers readily manipulate drivers to violate important regulations, something of which most road users are unaware. Drivers are at the bottom of the freight industry pecking order. They respond to dispatchers in order to avoid punishment or gain perks. Because trucking is a highly competitive world, drivers know that if they refuse loads on the basis of legality or safety, many other drivers will accept the trips. Truckers, like dispatchers, are in the transportation game to make money; they don't make a living by sitting idle.

☐ *Dispatcher–Truck driver competition*

Discussions about truckers and dispatchers must take into account the fact that dispatchers are middle management or supervisory staff while truckers are line staff. Each adheres to a different set of ground rules, ideals, basic assumptions about business and frames of reference about role definition. The basic thread linking the two is that both strive to maximize incomes. Ideally, the advantages gained by dispatchers translate into gains for the trucker. Unfortunately, this win–win situation is rare because the differences between the two groups predominate. Instead, there is ongoing antagonism between the two, which influences truckers' on-the-road manoeuvres. If the antagonisms turn to hostility, truckers may be compelled to seek other jobs, or dispatchers may feel compelled to invoke disciplinary measures.

Fleet managers often accept the competition, antagonism and even hostility between truckers and dispatchers. However, fleets that are best able to handle exploitation, quarrels and upsurges of emotion between dispatcher and trucker have the best chance in the marketplace. They collaborate on safety and emphasize professional, respectful communication. Loads will not likely be assigned on dispatchers' whims but offered according to agreed-on operating criteria. These companies encourage their dispatchers to understand and appreciate truckers, and vice versa, and hold their dispatchers accountable for safety. There is less competition between drivers and dispatchers, leading to less aggravated driving.

■ Breaking Laws as Routine Practice

No sense trading four quarters for a dollar.

—DISPATCHER

A common belief among truckers and dispatchers is that laws and regulations are elastic: they can be stretched according to business circumstances, immediate needs and the company's expressed ideology of safety. When these features are applied to the roadway, they become compromises in the number of hours truckers drive, their speeds on the highway and the weight of their loads. When interviewed, dispatchers and truckers agreed that compromised safety regulations and traffic laws were common in trucking. One driver in the coffee room said sarcastically, "Oh no, I've never heard of that ever happening anywhere [laughing] ... Or two logbooks, I never heard of that before either ... [more laughing]." Truckers and dispatchers confirmed that the breach of laws and safety policies extends beyond truckers. As one trucker surmised, things are done on the basis of "circumstances behind the scene." Witness the following abbreviated statements:

- I don't think anybody can say that you're never asked [to break laws].
- The laws do get bent quite often.
- Everybody runs illegal.
- If we're swamped with loads, it's amazing how the laws can kinda fall back in the back of the corner for a while.
- In a rush, the laws get overlooked; so does safety, for that matter.

Truckers and dispatchers speak a silent language of implied intentions; dispatchers envision laws and regulations as negotiable for achieving maximum profit, while truckers seldom go out willfully to break traffic laws. Their breaches are manifest in the broader context of the market economy. Hard-to-meet demands are passed along from shipper to dispatcher and trucker, and a simple and practical rule abides: "take the load, lose it." Just-in-time deliveries must get to their destinations at an increasingly fast pace, within a context of restricted consecutive driving laws and logbooks that monitor driving hours.

☐ *Logbooks and hours of service*

It is common knowledge that long-distance truckers cheat on their logbooks; indeed, it is part of the truck-driving mythology. Although many drivers adhere to the legal stipulations, many others do not. They cheat on logbooks so that they can drive more hours than they are legally allowed. For many, it is a common-sense version of driving. As one driver said, "I haven't met somebody yet that runs a legal logbook." Others proposed that cheating on logbooks is "done all the time" or "no big deal."

In tight markets truckers have to "cut corners to make it." In particular, owner-operators have difficulty "making ends meet" within the legal framework. They must drive enough hours per month to pay for their equipment and travel expenses. Their take-home pay consists of money left over after the bills have been paid. As one owner-operator commented,

> If you ran legal, ten hours a day in the States, or thirteen up here, you wouldn't be making any money ... Everybody bends the rules ... but it all ... they work it out to a point ... It's pretty close to being legal ... Even the D.O.T. knows it happens.

Another stated cryptically, "You do what you gotta do."

Freight companies, who actively promote cheating, must share responsibility for altered logbooks. A driver who conceded that he cheats on his logbooks explained:

> You have to, or else you'll never make a dollar. You have to know how to run your logbook the way it can be run, the legal way ... With [one] company, you had to call in every morning with your log hours from the previous day and they put it on the computer and if it didn't look right to them, they'd screw around with the computer to make it look right.

For some companies, the review of the driver's logbook is little more than a façade. They ask the drivers to submit their books but then do little to analyze them accurately. Records are changed, inclusions are altered, and some logbooks are mysteriously lost. A few drivers like it. It gives them a blank cheque to alter the logistics of the drive. The trucking companies benefit. They can keep the driver on the road for a longer period of time. Their only concern is getting caught in a government safety audit.

Truckers employ several techniques for cheating on logbooks. They are commonly referred to as back-filling, keeping two books and having butterfly logs. Regardless of which breach a trucker uses, it must "look good for the government." Back-filling involves truckers driving for a lengthy period of time. After four to six hours, the truckers stop and fill in the logbook according to what they consider believable. It is a technique designed to make up time. Other drivers run with two or more logbooks, where each book has different hours of operation. If the authorities demand that a driver produce his logbook, he can choose one that corresponds to the circumstances with which he is faced. Witness the following trucker response:

> At [one transport company], some guys run two logbooks ... Well, you just pretty well, y'know, you just lie a lot and fill out two logbooks, one that says that you're there and the other book will say that you're sleeping while you're driving, the opposite heh! So you ... if you get caught at nighttime well you show them that one, and that one ... If you're driving in the daytime, show 'em the other one.

Other drivers still believe in butterfly logs. The meaning is simple. When asked to turn over his logbook, he throws it away or hides it. He tells the police officer he has lost it. The rationale for doing so is that the penalty for a lost logbook is less severe than the penalty for a logbook that has been tampered with.

Some drivers related tampering with logbooks to using illicit drugs. A fixed logbook strongly indicates that the trucker is exceeding the legal limit of driving hours. To do so, he has to stay alert, and drugs help him do that. Long trips within tight times—such as, for example, excursions from Toronto to Vancouver or from Florida to Toronto—may prompt drivers to take amphetamines (bennies). When a middle-aged driver who usually makes extended trips was asked if he ever used drugs, the driver produced a large grin and said,

> They [the dispatchers] wanted me there that day already and I was still 800 miles away or whatever, and I called in and the dispatcher said well, can you bring it in? I said I don't know, I'm tired. Well if you can bring it in, bring it right in, we'd really appreciate it if you could just bring it right in. And so I brought it right in and it was ... aah ... about a 36-hour drive non-stop to get there. And that's about as much bending the rules as I've ever done.

So did he pop bennies while driving? "Kind of, hahaha," he said.

Dispatchers and truckers repeatedly suggested that experienced truckers are better at breaching the laws than new ones. As truckers gain experience, they become better versed in how hours-of-service laws can be broken to produce more profitable trucking careers. New truckers are more likely to obey the law. Thus, they are not good candidates for making trips that demand a breach of the legal limits of driving. Witness a dispatcher's perspective:

> You see, you have to know who to ask [to break the legal hours of driving law]. Obviously it's not the new guys. They'd get caught. They don't know any better. But they learn. Then when they're more experienced they'll do it because it means extra money for them.

A senior dispatcher expanded on the issue of youth and inexperience:

> Truckers don't log every minute of the day. They have to get the load delivered. When guys come from California with bananas, no, some other fruit, they adjust their logbooks while loading. They should book on-duty while loading. Instead they book time in sleeper to make sure they abide by the seventy hours per eight days rules ... I don't deal with daily hours much. A lot of drivers are old enough and mature enough to make it work for them ... Our newer drivers don't. They're out there in nowhere land and out of hours. What do I do? I get them home. What else am I going to do? When new drivers come in, they need to talk to other drivers to know what they can get away with.

Although dispatchers support bending the hours-of-service regulations, they prefer to stay silent. They won't discuss drivers who compromise logbook regulations with their company management or safety supervisors. Although they make implicit or explicit requests of drivers, the informal company code says drivers are responsible for themselves. It is part of doing business. Thus, dispatchers are unlikely to support drivers caught by company safety supervisors or legal authorities. At the same time, dispatchers are unlikely to tip off safety personnel about truckers who fix their logs.

According to some dispatchers, it is not the expected arrival time of a trip that is the problem but rather the driver's inability or unwillingness to cut corners. One of the dispatchers emphasized that a Florida-to-Toronto trip should only take two full days. He suggested that a truck load early Friday and be ready to deliver Monday—about 40 hours later. He broke it down to ten hours on duty, eight hours time off, and another ten hours on duty. In the words of the dispatcher,

This is how long it should take a trucker to get to the border. Another eight hours may be needed to cross the border and come up. This means that the trucker should cut corners like gassing up and eating during his time off.

Dispatchers tend to interpret truckers' driving times according to the needs of the carrier. For example, a driver was in Toronto during rush hour. He called the dispatcher to inform him that he was out of driving hours. He drove more than 60 hours during his 7 days of service. It was a hectic time for the freight company. There were no other drivers available who could travel to Toronto, relieve the driver and deliver the goods to the warehouse. The driver was reluctant to do it, but the dispatcher was insistent. Needless to say, the driver ceded to the wishes of the dispatcher and brought the load home illegally on Friday afternoon.

☐ *On weight*
When logbooks are completed, they are submitted to the transport company's log box for examination by the safety supervisor. The policy at one carrier stated that it is the company's responsibility if its employees accept a poorly completed logbook. However, it is the truckers' responsibility if they enter weigh scales and get apprehended by law enforcers for carrying improper logbooks. Enforcement officers and weigh scale operators often check drivers for driving hours and weight.

It is common knowledge that fatigue has a direct impact on safety. An overweight load resembles a moderate risk at best. One driver for a regional carrier said,

Overload? Yeah, I had that. I haven't had it on the highway. I had it in town. It doesn't really bother me because the loads, as far as I'm concerned, if you drive carefully enough with that load, it's not much overweight. I'm not talking about twenty or thirty thousand. I'm only talking about ten or fifteen thousand, where you go from A to B which is not too far.

Depending on the commodities, trip routes and destinations, truckers may expect to drive over the legally allowable truck weight. Some dispatchers encourage drivers to drive around weigh scales or to enter them with higher weight than allowed. The truckers receive special incentives for doing the latter. As one driver described, "They might say sometimes well, you guys know your way around the scales. Just come home or whatever!" Dispatchers often become aware of overloaded trailers after the fact. It all begins with the shipper giving the dispatcher a load weight over the telephone. The dispatcher quotes a price on the basis of the weight and distance. Upon arrival, a load that is heavier than quoted becomes a major issue for the trucker and shipper. If overloaded, the trucker may phone the dispatcher and ask for guidance. Most of the time that guidance goes along the lines of "do the best you can, but make it easy for our company"—meaning, try to take it.

Dispatchers are usually willing to close their eyes if the load is for a preferred customer. Truckers take the brunt of responsibility. In the final analysis they are supposed "to know what their load is. It's part of their job." The vice-president of operations for one transport company explained his company's policy. The driver takes responsibility for loads that are under gross weight but over axle weight. If the load exceeds the gross weight, the driver is expected to contact the dispatcher, who may "cut the load" or switch to a lighter tractor. Some company executives explained that drivers do not like reporting weight predicaments to dispatchers. Cutting loads takes valuable time and changing to lighter tractors usually means another driver comes with a lighter truck to pick up the load. As a result, the original driver no longer has a profitable trip. A company executive commented that if truckers complained about weight, their dispatchers would likely answer like this:

> Fine, we'll put a light tractor on it. We won't cut the load, just put a different tractor and trailer on it. Guys don't like that. They know that the size of the load will go out and that someone will be hauling it. A trip to Texas is a good one. So they'll take the chance and haul the load, despite the fact that they are running a heavier truck ... Owner-operators have heavier trucks and therefore carry less weight. If they don't take the chance, others will.

Owner-operators are left in a bind. They do not appreciate the additional stress an overload puts on their equipment; furthermore, they are responsible for all fines. Being caught at a weigh scale means paying a fine, losing time or having to pay for another trucker to take some of the excess load. At the same time, owner-operators do not want to lose a good haul and have dispatchers consider them "whiners." Most of the time, they accept the overweight load.

Drivers are often powerless to take action against overloading. The trailer is sealed or the driver is placed in a position in which the dock workers threaten him to unload and reload, a situation that takes valuable time. Time becomes the commodity shippers and dispatchers use to position drivers into pulling overweight loads. Several drivers indicated that breweries, whether located in Canada or the US, are known for their attempts to overload trailers. And running overweight is not just a casual compromise of the regulations. It can be a stressful experience. A trucker en route to Cornwall, Ontario stated that he was not only overloaded, but his freight was damaged because of the poor loading. He said,

I'm really upset with the company ... I'm supposed to be in Cornwall by
11. I've got two loads in front of the trailer that have to be dropped off
first. We're overloading ... The load is being damaged ... I'm too stressed
to do this and they wonder why people are killed on the road.

□ *Time pressure and speeding*

A popular trucker dictum is, "the sooner you get there, the better it is." Although
refrigerated-truck drivers are hit the hardest, all truckers and dispatchers feel
the pressure to keep daily schedules. Just-in-time deliveries demand it. A safety
supervisor gave an example of time pressure and driver behaviour represented
in Figure 10.1.

A company driver unloaded at point A, after which he was destined to unload
at point B. He jumped the curb and ripped the overhead wires to save time. His
safety supervisor stated, "It's ridiculous. And you know what was to blame?
Time pressure. He wanted to save time so he went over the curb, and made a
bunch of destruction." When money and profits lead to time pressure, drivers
often feel the need to speed up to reach their destinations. If the time limit is
broken, drivers lose a significant amount of money for being late. Witness:

> But that's where the thing comes in and the shippers dictate the arrival
> time. They say it's gotta be delivered 7 o'clock or 6 o'clock in the
> morning at the market, you know and stuff like that. And aah, that goes
> the same from California, from Texas from everywhere, but the times are
> different, but the rest is the same. Like I've had one yesterday I had a ...
> the same company where I used to work, they called me in to help them
> out because the other guy that took my place already quit. So I went back
> there yesterday and there was a claim there for $800, no $1200 claim for
> late delivery, and you know what they say, aah, decline in market value.
> That's what they call it. Decline in market value. If you would've brought
> it in at 6 o'clock in the morning to the market, that's, I mean the market
> starts at around 5 o'clock in the morning. That's when the buyers are all
> there and everybody's starting to buy. At 5 o'clock in the morning. So
> the truck is supposed to be there early, 5 o'clock, 4 o'clock, 5 o'clock in
> the morning. If you get there later, well of course the prices are starting
> to drop because now everybody's bought their stuff. But it doesn't
> change the fact that it's illegal what they're doing.

Experienced truckers are aware that the commonly voiced theme, "decline in
market value," is a major reason they are fined for late arrival at the auction.
Lateness may be invoked for truckers arriving less than two hours behind
schedule for trips consisting of thousands of miles. Owner-operators are most

FIGURE 10.1

Time pressure and driver behaviour

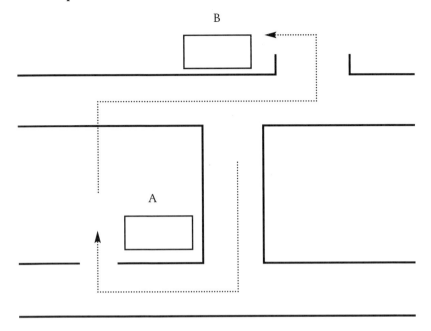

prone to being fined. One dispatcher addresses the owner-operator scenario and suggests that he

> tells the guy you gotta be at such and such a place at such and such a time. So he goes hammer down, he says, well hammer down, make tracks. So the driver goes like crazy. He gets a speeding ticket. Who pays the speeding ticket? The driver ... Now he's overweight you know, he picks up a load from a company that calls the dispatch and he says you know I'm three thousand pounds overweight. What am I supposed to do? "Well, run around the scales," the dispatcher tells him. Run around the scales, which is illegal.

As in the case with overweight loads, time pressures are institutionally bound. They are part of doing business—big business. According to several truck company executives and dispatchers, unloading appointments also create pressure on drivers. Shortly after a shipper faxes an order to the freight company, the dispatcher establishes a delivery appointment at the destined warehouse. Drivers are expected to honour the arrival time. Some shippers are flexible about time as long as dispatchers or drivers notify them about delays ahead of time. Others demand that drivers arrive at predetermined times. Dock workers are ready to unload and dock space is at a premium. For some industries, such as auto-parts manufacturers, manufacturing materials need to arrive on time so that the plant can keep working.

The nature of some businesses suggests that it is not imperative to have trucks arrive at precise times. It is a matter of principle, and shippers have normalized it as typical business. The reasoning goes something like this. Establish arrival times, withhold money from the bill from truckers who are two or more hours late, and get your goods cheaper than market transport value. In some cases, shippers get their loads hauled for free on the basis of a negotiated contract.

☐ *Safeguards against speeding*
Many fleets use trucks with governors set at 100 kph. Thus, truckers travelling around 95 to 98 kph should not consider passing and stay in the right hand lane. They should not be found in the left-hand lane. According to one safety supervisor,

> If you're going between 95 to 98 k's per hour I shouldn't try to pass you … Our drivers all know what trucks can do and can't do.

To help assure safety, the safety supervisor sits on the side of the roads and uses a hand-held radar to measure the speed of his company's trucks. The safety supervisor then sends every driver a copy of the roadway observation assessment. If the observation is negative, he sends a letter that says the trucker is "a professional and shouldn't do it." If the observation is favourable, he sends "a note telling him why his actions are good for the trucking image."

■ On Dispatchers Affecting Driving
There is little doubt that dispatchers influence truckers' on-the-road behaviours. As corporate representatives, dispatchers have power. Drivers fear that dispatchers could take action against them, which may lead to economic hardship. This concern can play havoc on the road. Because truckers fear losing their jobs, they may speed and drive aggressively in order to fulfill unloading times. Late arrivals may lead to fines or tongue lashings that include threats of dismissal.

☐ *Morning start up*
A common rule in trucking is that drivers look forward to a good early-morning send-off. They want to begin their trips on a cheerful note. If they get upset with a dispatcher because he uses unreasonable tactics like assignment of

bad loads, bad-mouthing or demanding achievements that are impossible for truckers to attain without breaking laws, truckers become emotional. These emotions often manifest themselves on the roadway through truckers' attention span, aggression or fatigue level. Here is one powerful quotation:

> Sure there's been times I put the boot to the pedal, thinking, you bastard [dispatcher].

A senior driver reasoned slowly and meticulously on how the dispatcher can and does affect his driving. He described:

> Yup, because sometimes you get a load up there and you start at 5:30 in the morning and you got a hand-balmer load coming in and the guy below you will start at 6 o'clock and he's got a gravy load, just take it somewhere and drop it and switch the trailer. You're pretty much in a bad mood. That screws up your driving. But you get over it. Every once in a while they put you in a bad mood. That's no different than your wife waits in the morning time to tell you she's not going to be home at 2 in the morning because she's got a seminar to go to. It's a human thing that happens. Not anything uncommon about it.

Angry drivers are dangerous drivers. Rather than concentrate on the road, especially under rush-hour driving conditions, drivers are preoccupied with feelings of resentment. A senior executive for one industrial carrier said,

> We do our damnedest not to have him go out mad ... We can imagine what he'll be like when he gets to four hundred, five hundred miles.

While sitting alone in the cab, a driver has the opportunity to stew and replay his feelings over and over again. Tension builds as time passes. A point is finally reached where the driver may become bitter and drive dangerously. One driver explained in detail how a dispatcher affected his driving:

> Well, I went from being a person who was down-to-earth, happy and thought a lot to a person that became kinda bitter. And this, like you're going down the road you're thinking of this. Your mind is not totally on driving. I, I know it, I know for a fact I went through it. It's just like having a sickness in the family. That's there, and does play a role, it's a bad thing. You got harmony with a dispatcher, you got a lot going. You're going down that road pretty easy, free and easy. I found myself thinking a lot differently. Like my mind was on what I was going to do about this

problem, instead of sitting there and having my mind on what I was doing about my driving, like I was, my mind was wandering off my driving, because I found myself starting to miss turns. I'd be thinking about this so much, I'd miss a road, because my mind was on something else.

The driver was so upset with the dispatching situation that he eventually quit.

Dispatchers may frustrate truckers so much that the drivers agonize over it at home. Their experiences stay with them for a long time, manifesting themselves in a lower attention span and higher levels of aggression. The extra pressure can inhibit the drivers' sleep, disrupting their sleep patterns, which may affect the drivers' performance on the highway. A dispatcher's early morning actions may create a chain of events, the last link of which is driving.

A single example should suffice. Early one morning, a dispatcher informed a driver that a load was waiting for him in Montreal, a distance of 200 miles. He was supposed to be there in three hours. The driver countered that the dispatcher knew he had to travel at least 75 mph to get to the destination on time. The driver accommodated the dispatcher and, in the process, broadsided a car. Although the vehicle was heavily damaged, there were no major injuries. After the accident the driver went back to the yard and "nearly killed the dispatcher." It was a fight, which led to him quitting driving for a year. He is back on the road today. But he emphasized to the manager, " You make me mad again, I'll quit and never come back." The dispatcher was fired. But to the trucker's dismay, the manager hired a new dispatcher, a former driver. The new man "wasn't any better. He betrayed drivers."

Other drastic events can happen. For example, one company executive spoke about one of his drivers travelling from Montreal to Cleveland. At a truck stop, about 100 miles from Cleveland, the driver called the dispatcher, who in turn blasted the driver for arriving late. The driver's response? He quit on the spot. As he left, the driver locked the rig and hurled the keys in the nearest snow bank. A company official travelled to Ohio and retrieved the vehicle. The keys were never found. The official acknowledged,

Of course it was the dispatcher's fault. You don't dump on a driver when he's out of town. What the hell did he expect? Smiles and roses? If you're gonna give the guy shit, at least wait till he's in your park.

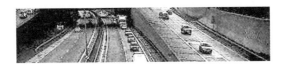

Truckers know that the invisible hand of the dispatcher is always on their shoulder, steering them in a certain direction, influencing their driving behaviour. They play an important role in trucking, and their influence needs to be investigated on a grand scale if traffic safety is expanded into the economic domain. Without a doubt, dispatchers influence safety and risk-taking on the roadways. However, like the truckers, other people pull their strings—the shippers—and future research should also focus on that group.

The descriptions offered in this chapter resulted from research completed with truck carriers in good standing. One must wonder what smaller, less-committed fleets are like—fleets that have a reputation of cutting corners and refusing researchers on their premises?

11

**VOLUNTEER CITIZEN ACTIVISM
AND COURT MONITORING**

JOANNE JARVIS

*Never doubt that a small group of thoughtful, committed citizens
can change the world. Indeed, it's the only thing that ever has.*

—MARGARET MEAD

IN THE COURTROOMS OF THE NATION, ultimate
legal decisions about drivers who breach traffic laws are made. Thus, the courtroom is a key area for creating change. One strategy for highlighting questionable court events is court monitoring. Court monitoring represents a strong
example of the effectiveness and power that an ordinary group of citizens, with
shared beliefs and concerns, can have on the criminal-justice system. Conducted
by volunteer citizen activists, court monitoring can have an impact on the
disposition of criminal cases involving impaired driving, thus assisting in the
improvement of traffic safety in area of drinking and driving.

This chapter explores why Mothers Against Drunk Driving (MADD) performs
court monitoring and looks at the effect court monitoring has on the adjudication of impaired driving cases. Research indicates that court monitoring can be
effective in increasing the likelihood of convictions, decreasing the likelihood
of dismissals and, in cases of repeat offenders, increasing the length of jail
sentences. In addition, I will briefly outline components of an effective court-
monitoring program.

■ Why Monitor the Courts?

Founded in 1980 by Candy Lightner of California, MADD is a massive volunteer movement of victims, their families and concerned citizens. MADD began in response to the carnage impaired driving was causing on the roads and the destructive path it left in the lives of so many people. Victims and concerned citizens were alarmed at the leniency with which drunk drivers were treated by the criminal justice system and the extent to which technical defenses could be used to free them. Today, both MADD Canada and MADD U.S. have thousands of devoted volunteers and millions of supporters. MADD Canada's mission is to stop impaired driving and to support victims of this violent crime. MADD Canada, as an organization, has a number of central beliefs:

- Our primary reason for existence is to eliminate the killing and maiming caused by impaired driving.
- Equally vital to MADD Canada's existence is supporting victims of impaired driving.
- MADD Canada is a grassroots organization that draws on its strength, energy and leadership from its volunteers.
- Active participation in MADD Canada Chapters' activities is productive for the community and encourages healing for many victims of impaired driving.
- An aggressive legislative and public policy advocacy program is a must to achieve MADD Canada's mission.
- A National Victims' Bill of Rights must be established to ensure victims' interests are protected.
- A balanced program of public awareness, education, legislation and aggressive enforcement by police, Crown attorneys and the courts is essential to eliminating impaired driving.
- While an individual's decision to consume alcohol is a private matter, driving after consuming alcohol is a public matter.
- Impaired drivers and others who directly contribute to the crime of impaired driving must be held accountable for their behaviour.
- Proactive rehabilitation of impaired drivers is essential.
- Driving is a privilege, not a right.
- Impaired driving crashes are not accidents.

One of the unique aspects of MADD Canada, which differentiates it from other like-minded advocate groups, is its commitment to supporting victims and their families. There is a profound commitment to advocate for justice for families whose loved one was injured or killed by an impaired driver. MADD Canada believes that a comprehensive approach to ending impaired driving must be taken. This approach, which includes public awareness and education, and strict enforcement by police, also includes doling out appropriate penalties to those members of society who commit this violent and senseless crime, many of whom are repeat offenders. Holding the criminal-justice system accountable for its role in the apprehension and prosecution of impaired drivers is indeed a grand task.

Impaired driving is one of the biggest threats to traffic safety. Despite reported declines in impaired-driving incidents over the last decade (Tremblay & Kemeny, 1998), it is by far the leading criminal cause of death in Canada. A 1997 Health Canada study reported that 1,680 people are killed each year in alcohol-related crashes in Canada (Beirness, Mayhew & Simpson, 1997). This represents a figure almost three times greater than the number of homicides in Canada in 1997. Every six hours, a Canadian is killed by an impaired driver and hundreds more are injured.

Impaired driving is a complex problem. Some believe that impaired driving is an illness, a combination of an addiction to alcohol with an addiction to driving. In this view, impaired driving is condition to be "treated," not punished. Some members of the judiciary continue to view impaired driving as an unfortunate accident where offenders are not seen as "true" criminals, but instead, are the product of a misguided notion or the victim of an unfortunate and tragic set of circumstances. At a 1999 Ontario Provincial Court (*R. vs. Schrader*) sentencing hearing of a young man convicted of driving with over 80 milligrams of alcohol in his body, the judge remarked,

> you are twenty-one and a half years of age. You have no prior criminal record. You are a young man who seems to have a productive life. You are the sort of individual that the court usually only sees before it for drinking and driving charges. What I mean is that you are not here for a crime of violence. You are not here for a crime of dishonesty. You are not here for disrespecting other people or their property ... You are one of the tragedies of our society because you have been convicted of a Criminal Code offence for driving with more than 80 milligrams of alcohol in your system.

This young man was involved in a crash in which he struck a vehicle, killing one individual and seriously injuring another. His blood alcohol reading 100 minutes after the crash was 0.141. His sentence was two months in custody and a two-year federal driving prohibition.

Impaired driving is a technical charge for the police to lay and for the courts to prove. Consequently, many impaired-driving charges are not laid or followed through. In 1999, Carroll and Solomon undertook a review of the

1996–97 statistics for impaired driving in Ontario. Their review revealed not only major data gaps about the enforcement, prosecution and sentencing of drinking and driving cases, but also a number of serious and disturbing practices. Carroll and Solomon found that few impaired charges of driving causing bodily harm and impaired driving causing death, 536 and 74 respectively, were disposed of, despite the reported figures on the number of injuries and fatalities that were alcohol-related (15 to 30 percent of 89,572 traffic injuries and 41.3 percent of 1,164 traffic fatalities); that a large percentage of those charges laid were stayed or withdrawn (42 percent, or 225 of 536, and 40.5 percent, or 30 of 74), which they presume were in exchange for a guilty plea to a lesser charge; that there was a large percentages of withdrawals or stays in other offence categories (impaired driving, 38.4 percent; "over 80," 59.2 percent; failing to provide samples of breath or blood, 45.8 percent); and that a significant number of repeat offenders were sentenced as first offenders (approximately two-thirds of drinking and driving cases involve repeat offenders; however, collectively only 27 percent of those guilty of impaired driving, "over 80" and failing to provide samples of breath or blood received a jail term which is mandatory upon second, third and subsequent convictions). A similar finding was revealed when Canadian statistics were examined. Transport Canada reported that 1,350 Canadians were killed in alcohol-related crashes in 1998, yet in that same year only 103 people were charged with impaired driving causing death (Sauvé, 1999).

Members of MADD and other collegial groups are frustrated with the way impaired-driving charges are laid and with the lenient sentences imposed by the courts once a conviction is obtained. The maximum penalty for impaired driving causing death is fourteen years' incarceration. No Canadian has ever been sentenced to the maximum penalty. The average sentence for a first-time offender convicted of impaired driving causing death ranges between two and four years incarceration. The families of men, women and children who are killed will suffer a lifetime of pain and anguish; their loss is forever.

Injured victims and their families suffer their own losses: loss of dreams, aspirations, independence, physical and mental functions, social contacts and the ability to care for themselves. One can understand the frustrations for families when property crimes yield harsher penalties than a charge of impaired driving causing death. The combination of the significant number of people affected by drinking and driving, the frustration with the legal system and the ease with which technical defenses can be used, coupled with troubling complacent attitudes and lenient sentences, motivated MADD Canada to take action in the form of court monitoring.

■ The Court-Monitoring Initiative

MADD asks for volunteer action from victims and concerned citizens who share its mission and beliefs. These volunteers monitor the courts in their communities. Court monitoring is one way to study how impaired-driving charges are dealt with in the courts. It is performed by observing proceedings in the courtroom for offences that involve victims and those that affect others, or by reviewing court records outside of the courtroom. MADD Canada encourages monitors to have a physical presence in the courtroom, in the belief that their actual presence in the courtroom can make a difference to the outcome of impaired-driving cases. A volunteer's presence in the courtroom speaks of keen interest and action; it is not passive. Others notice this presence. MADD's hope is that "being there" means that they cannot and will not be ignored.

Several other organizations have undertaken the court-monitoring programs, also known as court watch, in order to effect positive change in their communities. For example, the American Judicature Society (AJS) conducts court monitoring using non-lawyer volunteers who observe and evaluate courthouse facilities and proceedings. The goal of this program is to improve the administration of justice. Achievements have included the establishment of in-court child-care facilities; the installation of court information kiosks; the enhancement of audibility during the proceedings; and a mandatory civility training program in response to complaints that court personnel were insensitive to the public. AJS reports that as a result of the increased credibility of its court-monitoring program, its volunteers are frequently called upon by court administrators to monitor projects or problem courts.

The Texas Citizen Action organization also conducts a court-watch program. The program tracks litigation that affects Texas consumer and environmental issues. Furthermore, the program studies court decisions and issues, and alerts both the media and other groups when key cases, including cases on appeal, are being heard. Similarly, the Court Watch program initiated by the Ohio Alliance for Civil Justice is made up of businesses and organizations that monitor cases with the goal of protecting tort reform.

Courtwatch of Hillsborough County conducts a program that most closely resembles MADD Canada's. Their Courtwatch program monitors domestic-violence cases. The organization reports its findings to the public and to those involved in judicial proceedings. Collected information is used to make changes or improvements to the system and in future proceedings involving domestic-violence crimes.

MADD Canada court monitors track impaired-driving charges through the courts and report on the dispositions of cases. The program can address specific concerns within the system. For example, if a particular jurisdiction disposes of a significant number of cases through plea-bargaining, the Chief Crown or Director of Crown Operations would be alerted.

There have only been a few studies of the impact of court monitoring on drinking and driving cases (Probst, Lewis, Asunka, Hersey & Oram, 1987; Shinar, 1990). Probst et al. studied data from two groups dedicated to ending impaired driving: a MADD chapter in a large Nebraska county (pop. 4,000,000) and a RID (Remove Intoxicated Drivers) chapter in a smaller Tennessee community (pop. 30,000). They compared court dispositions (guilty, not guilty, dismissed) and case outcomes (jail, fine, licence suspension) between two locations with court-monitoring programs and two locations without court monitoring. They also compared the case dispositions and outcomes in locations before and after court-monitoring activities began. The researchers concluded that well-organized court-monitoring programs could change the handling of a DWI (driving while intoxicated) offender and that both MADD and RID programs brought about an increase in the severity with which DWI offenders were treated. However, the study involved a very small number of court monitors who were able to monitor their courts only "partially." Further, the effects of court-monitoring activities were measured only by comparing convictions and outcomes on a community-wide basis rather than on a case-by-case basis, where individual cases that were monitored could be compared against cases that were not. Additionally, during the study Nebraska State DWI laws were changed to include minimum jail, fine and licence suspensions.

The study conducted by Shinar (1990) did not experience the methodological problems of Probst et al. Using a database of 9,137 charges, Shinar studied the effectiveness of MADD court monitoring on DWI adjudication (case by case) in Maine within the 1987 calendar year. There were 397 monitored cases and 8740 non-monitored cases. At all monitored cases, the volunteer court monitor was physically present during at least one court appearance, introduced him/herself (before trial) to the district attorney (DA) and stated his/her affiliation. Shinar measured the impact of court monitoring in two categories: court disposition and case outcome or sentence. The results showed that the likelihood of dismissal in non-monitored cases was 11.4 percent, compared to 6.1 percent for monitored cases; the likelihood of a guilty verdict was 87.3 percent for non-monitored cases versus 92.4 percent for monitored cases. Therefore, monitoring court cases for DWI offences reduced the likelihood of the case dismissal and increased the likelihood that the accused would be found guilty.

Penalties for guilty drunk drivers typically combine fines, jail time and licence suspensions. Shinar found that court monitoring had a significant effect on the likelihood and length of the jail term, with only a marginally significant effect on the amount of fine. For monitored court cases, the average jail term was 30.9 days; it was 50 percent shorter for non-monitored cases. Shinar found that across all cases, monitored and non-monitored, the likelihood of no jail time for guilty drivers was 25.3 percent. He found that the likelihood of no jail or a minimum jail term (1 or 2 days) was greater when the case was not monitored (65.1 percent) than when it was (50.1 percent). The likelihood of jail terms of ten days or more was consistently higher when the case was monitored (29.2 percent) than when it was not (17.7 percent). The likelihood of guilty offenders receiving a fine and licence suspension as part of their sentence was extremely high for both monitored and non-monitored cases (99.2 percent and 98.9 percent for fines, and 99.7 percent and 99.5 percent for licence suspensions). The average fine for monitored cases was only slightly higher ($407.70) than that for non-monitored cases ($393.58). There was no statistical significance between the average licence suspensions for monitored and non-monitored cases (176.9 days vs. 165.2 days).

In the study conducted by Probst et al. (1987), there was an indication that court monitoring may have more of an impact and effect on the disposition of repeat offender cases. To test this, Shinar conducted a separate analysis of first-time and repeat offenders (those convicted of DWI within the last six years compared to those with no DWI convictions in the last six years), in which a relatively small number of cases was analyzed (99 cases were monitored and 1695 cases were not monitored). The presence of court monitors in cases of first-time DWI drivers yielded higher guilty rates and lower dismissal and not-guilty rates. A high number of guilty drivers with a previous DWI conviction received a jail sentence, and the presence of a court monitor did not make a difference in these cases. Shinar reported, however, that there were significant differences in the magnitude of sentences (jail time, fine and licence suspensions) between first-time and repeat offenders. Shinar's research revealed that while there was a general lack of statistically significant monitoring effect on the sample of repeat and first-time offenders, more severe penalties were given to the monitored drivers compared to the non-monitored drivers.

Shinar also tested the hypothesis that court monitoring has an impact on DWI enforcement—more specifically, that officers are more likely to apprehend DWI drivers "knowing they will have a friend in court." After comparing DWI citations in different Maine counties to the level of court-monitoring activities in those same counties, he did not find support for this hypothesis. Shinar does not rule out the potential effectiveness of court monitoring on DWI arrests as only a weak test of the hypothesis was possible. It is important to note that the district attorneys in Maine screen police citations and decide to lay DWI charges. Although Shinar's examination of this potentially biased factor was reduced (Maine DAs charged 92 percent of DWI drivers), it is a point for further research consideration.

Shinar reported that repeated court-monitoring attendance is likely to be more influential than sporadic monitoring and concluded:

> court monitoring is an effective tool in affecting the adjudication process [in DWI cases]. In the presence of court monitors the conviction rates of DWI offenders are higher than those of drivers not court-monitored. Furthermore, once convicted, the likelihood of a jail sentence is higher and the length of the jail sentence is longer for court-monitored DWI drivers than for non-monitored drivers.

Similar research on court monitoring has not been conducted in Canada and careful consideration should be given when transferring the success of court monitoring from the US experience to Canada. Most American prosecutors (and judges) are elected officials; their terms as elected officials may make them more sensitive to public opinion, and thus court monitoring may have more influence on the decisions they make. Additionally, although not a stated component of Shinar's research, the American justice system allows the practice of jury polling, which is not permitted in Canada. Jury polling involves the practice of surveying jurors after a trial and asking their views about such things as the judge's performance during the proceedings, and the conduct and strength of both the defence counsel and prosecutor. This information could give the court monitor important insight as to what influenced the jury most, as well as provide important feedback to prosecutors and judges.

Research into the effectiveness of court monitoring in Canada is necessary. The Canadian legal system and the players in the legal system differ from those in the US, most notably, in the appointment of crown attorneys and members of the judiciary. However, anecdotal research in Canada reveals some results similar to US reports. Some court monitors report that their presence in the courtroom makes a difference and they are gaining respect and credibility in their communities. For example, the MADD chapter in Digby, Nova Scotia, received the support of an RCMP officer who stated that he "found the court monitoring initiative of MADD Canada [to be] effective; it is a program that I give my full support and must be continued." Furthermore, the officer recommended that other members of his RCMP detachment contact the chapter prior to court appearances so that chapter court monitors could attend. While unsure their presence has directly influenced the sentences offenders received, some court monitors believe their presence influences how the judge handles the case and results in victims being treated more compassionately. They also report that the judge treats the accused, and the nature of the offence, more seriously, often lecturing him/her about his/her behaviour.

Impaired driving is one of the biggest threats to traffic safety, and court monitoring has some proven positive effects on the outcome of drinking and driving cases. One hopes that impaired-driving offenders who attend court will get the message that drinking and driving is unacceptable behaviour. The knowledge that organized, ordinary citizens in the community are monitoring courts may have some influence on other citizens to conform to social norms and adhere to a community "code of conduct." It would be interesting to study the impact that court monitoring has on communities' members in terms of attitudes and beliefs about drinking and driving. If there were a significant impact, research could look at how it translates into crime statistics. If the community were to have a true effect on its members, one positive outcome would be that community pressure influences members to abstain from drinking and driving.

An additional positive effect of court monitoring is its ability to put some power in the hands of ordinary citizens—ordinary people who are concerned about traffic safety. Court monitoring may be one activity that makes all parties in the criminal justice system, and in political arenas, aware that the general public recognizes the seriousness of the crime and is examining their response to the problem. Many court monitors, who have never before stepped inside a courtroom, come to realize that they have some power to effect change in their communities. The realization that ordinary citizens can make a difference to an often overwhelming and complex system is in itself powerful.

■ Components of an Effective Court-Monitoring Program

A well-organized court-monitoring program can be effective in the adjudication of DWI offences. Probst and Lewis (1987) developed a comprehensive manual for groups interested in establishing and conducting court monitoring in their communities. A key element in organizing an effective program is a planned approach including a realistic design of the program based on available resources. In other words, taking into account the number of courts to monitor and the number of volunteers who are interested, able to attend court during the day and appropriate for court monitoring. Court monitors are expected to behave and dress in a professional manner at all times. To assist them, volunteers are given a training manual which includes, among other things, a list of do's and don'ts. Volunteers must also be educated on the criminal-justice system and court environment, including becoming familiar with legal terms; the roles of police, crown attorney, defense counsel; the defendant's rights; victims (if applicable), witnesses, and judges; and probation and parole.

Volunteers must be educated on impaired driving laws in combination with basic legal procedures and practices.

Recording and reporting the information collected is also a critical component of an effective court-monitoring program. MADD Canada volunteers are supplied with a recording form (see Appendix A) on which they are directed to record pertinent information about the case they monitor. Completed forms are sent to MADD Canada's national office and the information is examined. To date, MADD Canada has not undertaken any research to study the specific effects of its court monitoring activities and has, instead, implemented the program based on the court-monitoring successes achieved by MADD US chapters.

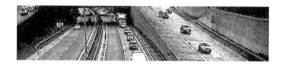

GIVEN THE EXTREMELY HIGH NUMBERS of deaths and injuries in impaired driving crashes, coupled with legal frustrations related to the crime, court monitoring represents one activity aimed at closely watching and reporting on how the criminal-justice system handles Canada's impaired drivers. Included in that strategy is the need for our criminal justice system to impose appropriate sanctions and meaningful consequences for those who drink and drive.

The effectiveness of court monitoring has been demonstrated in the, albeit limited, American research literature. While many Canadians are concerned with justice, few feel they can do anything that will actually have an impact on decisions made. Actively participating in making their communities safer is a task that ordinary people can accomplish. Volunteering to be a court monitor is a valuable job, a job that makes a difference. It can be expanded to cover other traffic-related trials that include major breaches of traffic laws.

■ Appendix A

Information to be recorded on the MADD Canada Court Monitoring Form includes the following elements.

MADD Canada Court Monitoring Form

Name of Monitor _____

Chapter _____ Date _____

The Court

Location _____

Name of Judge_____

Name of Crown Attorney _____

Name of Defence Attorney _____

Arresting Officer_____

The Accused

Name _____

City/Town _____

Age _____ Sex: ☐ M ☐ F

Marital Status _____ Alcohol Problem?_____

The Charge

☐ "Over 80" ☐ Impaired ☐ Refused breath/blood

☐ Impaired Causing Death ☐ Impaired Causing Bodily Harm

BAC _____ Roadside breath test? ☐ Y ☐ N   Blood Test? ☐ Y ☐ N

Driving while suspended? ☐ Y ☐ N

  ☐ First Offence ☐ Second Offence ☐ Third or subsequent

The Plea   ☐ Guilty   ☐ Not Guilty

The Disposition

☐ Charges Stayed or Withdrawn   ☐ Guilty   ☐ Not Guilty

Sentence: _____

Licence Suspension: ☐ Y ☐ N   For how long? _____

Other (community service, interlock, etc.): _____

If acquitted, on what grounds?

☐ No probable cause? Why? _____

☐ Problem with breath testing? _____

☐ Too long getting to breath test?_____

Plea Bargain? ☐ Y ☐ N If so what? _____

Was a victim-impact statement entered?   ☐ Y ☐ N

Comments

Please use back of page if necessary.

12

FROM WORKPLACE
TO COMMUNITY

WALTER BARTA

TRAFFIC SAFETY HAS NO BOUNDARIES. The impact of collisions, morbidity and mortality reaches beyond the individual and affects such institutions as family, community, government and economics. So far, little has been done to address the impact and its consequences in these areas, and we are just beginning to come to terms with the pervasive, far-reaching costs associated with mobility.

We are starting to realize that the costs associated with traffic trauma are much greater than repairing damage, replacing property and recovering lost time. These tend to be more immediate, micro-level costs—costs that directly affect the individual. The institutional, macro-level costs spread like tentacles through society to include the cost of lost or impaired life, rehabilitating life, lost productivity and revenue, insurance (life, property, disability, workers' compensation), and legal and infrastructure costs (police, ambulance, medical). At this level, the public seems to be far more aware of the threat and cost of AIDS, cancer or heart disease than that of driver and traffic safety. The paradox is that the cost of traffic trauma considerably exceeds the societal costs of AIDS, cancer and heart disease, while the resources necessary to deal with traffic safety are far less. We need to expand our thinking to include the true costs of traffic safety: that is, property loss, lost wages, ambulatory and medical costs, pain and suffering, the social costs of rehabilitation, and the most priceless, the cost of life—a complete and full life.

173

■ The Costs of Traffic Safety

According to the National Highway Traffic Safety Administration (NHTSA, 1998), 37,081 fatal crashes, 2,029,000 injury collisions and 4,269,000 property-damage-only crashes occurred in the United Sates during 1998. Of this number, 24,729 drivers were killed and 2,048,000 injured, while 10,519 passengers were killed and 1,014,000 injured. The economic cost of these traffic crashes (last calculated by NHTSA in 1994) was $150.5 billion (Blincoe, 1994). These statistics reveal a very slight and consistent downward trend over the last ten years in both injury and fatality numbers. Fatal crashes dropped slightly (0.7 percent) from 1997 to 1998, and the fatality rate remained at 1.6 fatalities per 100 million vehicle miles of travel in 1998, the same as in 1997. The injury rate per 100 million vehicle miles of travel decreased by 6.9 percent from 1997 to 1998. What is particularly interesting is that the ratio of fatalities to injuries and property damage has remained consistent (less than 1 percent fatalities, 32 percent injuries and 67 percent property damage only) over the last ten years, even though the overall numbers fell slightly.

□ *Societal costs: willingness to pay*

The numbers examined by NHTSA (Blincoe, 1994) were the economic costs that result from goods and services that must be purchased or productivity that is lost as a result of motor-vehicle crashes. They did not represent the more intangible consequences of these events to individuals and families. Numerous studies have been undertaken to measure the dollar value of those consequences by estimating values based on wages for risky occupations and purchases of products for improvements in safety. These "willingness-to-pay" costs can be several orders of magnitude higher than the direct costs of collisions. Most authors currently agree that the value of fatal risk reduction falls in the range of $2 million to $5 million per life saved. (Blincoe, 1994)

While Miller (1995) calculated the economic costs for collisions in 1994, he also produced a separate estimate of "comprehensive costs" that contain the values for "intangible" consequences of collisions. When we combine the economic costs with the comprehensive costs, we come up with a more realistic cost of collisions, approximately $336 billion—more than double the strict economic costs.

In their 1986 research into traffic safety, Lave and Lave identified both macro- and micro-level barriers to safety. They defined macro-level barriers as "aggregate-level collective judgements and actions ... manifested through voting or media reports" (1990, p. 78); they include mandatory seat-belt use laws and regulated speed limits. Micro-level barriers "result from individual actions" (p. 78); for example, individuals choose to exceed the posted speed limit while not wearing a seat belt, knowing they are wrong. Still, they make micro-judgements regarding their own measure of traffic safety. Hence, macro-level safety initiatives are affected by micro-level individual judgements and occasionally the two are in conflict.

Lave and Lave (1990) identified two particular troubles with macro-barriers: first, governments have difficulty prioritizing safety laws and adhering to them since they are overloaded with legislative bills calling their attention to societal problems; and second, it is difficult to change the public's behaviour, especially when the individual is the agent posing the most risk. Traffic safety is often offered a band-aid solution instead of a cure. For instance, engineering designs to make vehicles safer are more readily accepted than programs that attack the societal problem of impaired driving; laws are implemented rather than awareness or education campaigns, and road design is changed instead of driver attitudes. While it is generally agreed that behavioural factors are contributory in approximately 85 percent of collisions, we also know that driver behaviour is very difficult to change. Any traffic-safety initiative must recognize that the greatest challenge lies in addressing the micro-level behaviours that are so often in conflict with macro-level interventions.

■ Toward the Workplace

An essential component of micro-level economics is the workplace. A short overview indicates that motor-vehicle crashes, on and off the job, are the primary cause of death and injury in Canada and the US. And according to a US Bureau of Labor Statistics publication, *Issues* (1996), highway travel claimed more lives than any other work-related activity. In 1995, approximately 1,300 workers died in work-related highway accidents. At 21 percent, these workers represented the largest single cause of workplace death and injury. The macro-level costs are captured in organizational costs.

Although truck drivers outnumber by far any other occupation involved in highway fatalities, most victims of fatal work-related highway accidents did not operate trucks or other motor vehicles for a living. Rather, these casualties routinely drove, or rode, to various locations to perform work activities. They included nurses caring for the infirm in their homes; sales representatives visiting prospective buyers or current clients; managers and administrators attending meetings or monitoring job sites; protective service workers responding to fires and other emergencies or investigating crimes; and farm workers driving tractors to their fields. Truck drivers (and others operating motor vehicles as a profession) made up only two-fifths of all highway fatalities. According to Workers' Compensation Board Alberta statistics, the largest single cause of work-related deaths (23 percent) is traffic trauma (Cameron, 2000).

Whether on the job, on the way to the job or in the pursuit of leisure activities, motor-vehicle trauma is a major cost to organizations and to society alike.

Organizational costs accrue in a variety of ways: lost time, sick leave, temporary worker costs, insurance costs, short- and long-term benefits, lawsuits, property damage claims, lower efficiency, lower productivity and lower morale. Each type of motor-vehicle incident carries with it a unique collection of costs that affect the person, the family, the organization and society at large.

1. LOST TIME: When workers are in collisions on or off the job, there are almost always lost-time implications. The more serious consequences include time in the hospital, time at home recuperating and time visiting doctors and rehabilitation specialists. Even when the collision is minor, time is lost to medical visits, vehicle repairs and investigative interviews. Some companies continue to pay employees who are off work; others do not.

2. SICK LEAVE: Sick leave may seem to have little to do with work missed from traffic trauma. But the response to traumatic incidents—even minor incidents—often includes periods of emotional and physical stress (post-traumatic stress syndrome) and related physical symptoms. These symptoms look like illness but are actually another legacy of the collision. The costs associated with sick leave resulting from crash-related illness are rarely included in crash statistics.

3. TEMPORARY WORKER COSTS: Most organizations today run very lean operations with little staff redundancy. Every worker is required to do a specific job for which they have specialized training. When employees like these are involved in collisions, on or off the job, any resulting lost time or sick leave must be covered. The worker may be replaced by clever juggling of staff, but productivity may suffer since people are working in unfamiliar areas. The worker may also be replaced by a temporary worker. This also reduces productivity in the area of the replaced worker and may also affect overall productivity, depending on the industry. Putting aside the up-front cost of a temporary worker, the resulting reduced productivity carries a considerable cost.

4. INSURANCE COSTS: Insurance represents protection against future mishap or loss. Under an insurance plan, individuals, businesses and other organizations pay premiums in exchange for compensation for losses resulting from certain perils under specified conditions. Although insur-

ance costs are predictable and relatively low, they can rise significantly when incidents occur (depending on the number or severity of at-fault collisions), and the likelihood of an incident is relatively high. Insurance costs are a variable factor, depending on drivers of diverse ability, knowledge and emotional state.

5. LAWSUITS: Employers bear a special responsibility for the actions of employees driving on the job. Whether the employee drives in the city or the country, in fair or inclement weather, employers share the risk. This vicarious liability puts the organization at risk for loss. In the aftermath of a collision, a lawsuit is a very real possibility. Lawsuits happen when people have been injured in some way and believe that negligence or missed contractual obligations are to blame. Sometimes, after an injury, victims are not sure that the employer is legally at fault, but they feel that the organization should pay anyway. Occasionally, victims may threaten litigation (a whiplash claim, for example) to gain benefits to which they may not be entitled. We know much more today about soft-tissue injuries (whiplash, back pain, stretched ligaments), how they occur, when they manifest themselves and how long they take to heal. Such injuries don't require a large collision to occur, and they often turn up in lawsuits. The impression of deep corporate pockets makes filing a lawsuit an attractive proposition. Every time an employee is driving on the job and a collision results, there is a real risk of lawsuit and significant financial loss.

6. REDUCED EFFICIENCY AND PRODUCTIVITY: When people miss work, when positions are vacant or when replacements (internal or external) are brought in, the flow of work is disrupted. As in all groups, time and experience are necessary before work teams can function together effectively. Over time, they develop lines of communication, relationships and expectations. When a replacement worker is brought in and when an absent worker returns, a period of adjustment occurs, with all its inefficiencies. As a consequence, efficiency, quality and productivity may fall.

7. REDUCED MORALE: When a lost-time event occurs in the workplace, those associated with the employee, either though friendships or work affiliations, feel the loss. The loss of morale is directly related to the severity of the precipitating event. Lower morale is sometimes accompanied by depression. In cases like these, it is not unusual for corporations to hire psychologists to address the workers' emotional trauma. All of this carries a cost and also contributes to lower efficiency and productivity.

8. CORPORATE IMAGE: Million-dollar advertising programs, image and brand loyalty initiatives can be quickly nullified when members of the general public see company vehicles driven unsafely or irresponsibly. Being passed, cut off, tailgated or obstructed by a company driver may cause members of the public to wonder about the integrity of the company. The corporate image conflicts with the on-road reality; when faced with conflicting evidence, most individuals rely on what their experience, not advertisement, tells them.

Each of these factors is significant in itself, but when they effect each other synergistically, forming an intricate web of behaviours, the true cost of collisions is likely to be under-reported. One NHTSA study (Miller, 1995) found that in 1992 almost 3,000 people died and another 332,000 were injured in work-related traffic crashes. More than half of those injuries resulted in lost time at work. A later NHTSA study (1998) revealed that American employers pay an estimated $55 billion annually for motor-vehicle crashes and injuries on and off the job. These costs fall into three broad categories: health fringe-benefit costs, non-fringe-benefit costs and wage-risk premiums.

Health fringe-benefit costs are the costs of benefits paid because of illness and injury. They include contributions to workers' compensation, sick leave, social security (social insurance), and health, disability and life insurance, as well as insurance administration and overhead. Non-fringe costs include motor-vehicle property damage and liability insurance, crash-related legal expenses and the costs of vehicle damage and replacement. These costs also include taxes that help fund police, fire and ambulance services, lost productivity when employees suffer injuries preventing them or their co-workers from working at full capacity, and recruitment and training costs resulting from deaths and long-term disabilities. Wage-risk premiums are paid to workers for accepting risky jobs. Individual workers and their families, however, bear the non-monetary losses associated with workplace injury. This wage premium for risk-taking is often viewed as payment in advance for possible future losses (Miller, 1995).

Clearly, employers are significantly affected by collisions. Collisions drive up the cost of benefits such as workers' compensation, social security, and private health and disability insurance, and they increase company overhead involved in administering these programs. Recent statistics from NHTSA (1996) show that when a worker is involved in a motor-vehicle crash on the job that results in injuries, the cost to the employer is more than $24,000, while an off-the-job crash that results in injury costs the employer more than $18,000 (US).

The Network of Employers for Traffic Safety (NETS), through data collected by NHTSA, has identified the cost to employers per on-the-job crash and injury. Employers in the US pay approximately $15,200 for each crash and

TABLE 12.1

Annual costs to US employers, motor-vehicle crashes and injuries, on and off the job

$ 18.4 billion	Health fringe-benefit costs
2,550 million	Workers' compensation (medical & disability)
8,100 million	Health insurance and self-pay
570 million	Disability insurance
580 million	Life insurance
1,110 million	Insurance administration
1,330 million	Insurance overhead
1,560 million	Social security disability
2,680 million	Sick leave
$ 24.8 billion	Non-fringe-benefit costs
	• Motor-vehicle property damage and liability insurance
	• Crash-related legal expenses
	• Unreimbursed vehicle damage and replacement
	• Taxes to fund police, fire and ambulance services
	• Lost productivity (injuries prevent workers from working to capacity)
	• Recruitment and training costs (from deaths and long-term disabilities)
$ 11.6 billion	Wage-risk premiums
$ 55 billion	Annual costs to US employers

Note: Figures from NHTSA, 1998

$74,800 for each injury. Whether on or off the job, the costs and losses employers experience through motor-vehicle collisions are unacceptably high and result in both tangible and intangible loss to people, property and organizations. People are valuable in a company, but the real value of people extends beyond the wage paid to them or the actual costs of replacing them. Their value extends from the actual work that they do to the expertise they bring to the work in question as well as the workers around them.

■ Employer Responses to Traffic Trauma

Driving, the area that results in the greatest threat of harm to employees and cost to the organization, receives the least corporate money, time or energy. When the issue does warrant attention (usually in reaction to an incident), it is addressed in the simplest, most minimal way.

What is wrong with most traffic-safety interventions is that they consist of one-day, classroom-based defensive driving or driver-improvement courses. These courses are taken at three- to five-year intervals and are usually highly structured and unchanging in content. The participant's experience focusses primarily on cognitive processes. Large amounts of information are delivered in a programmed-learning approach that is inflexible, curriculum-centred and unresponsive to changes in the corporate or leisure driving environment. When employees take the course three to five years later, they receive the same information in much the same way, leaving them cynical and unaffected. The result is a whole-learning, mass-practice approach to training—a "silver bullet" vaccination for traffic safety that has yet to be proven effective.

Employers usually consider implementing such approaches for strictly economic reasons. At some level, whether immediate or delayed, short- or long-term, employers realize that traffic trauma costs money. Traffic-safety initiatives are offered either proactively as an investment that recognizes the future payoff through reduced collisions and losses (such as a training program, educational sessions or awareness messages) or reactively as solutions imposed on the company as a result of crashes. An insurance company or regulatory agency may insist on an intervention to avoid increased premiums. A lawsuit may also force management to make changes to policy and practices.

☐ *Workplace wellness*

On the positive, proactive side, workplace wellness has become a popular organizational concept. While relatively new in Canada, its benefits have already been realized. The costs of wellness programs per employee per year vary depending on whether a comprehensive approach or a single program is presented, but for companies that have evaluated their wellness programs, cost benefits have increased. A review of worldwide wellness studies by Dr. Ray Shephard found that workplace wellness programs have a return on investment of between $1.95 and $3.75 per employee per dollar spent (Dyck, 1999). Canada Life insurance company developed a health-promotion program in 1978. Independently evaluated over a ten-year period, the program showed a return of $6.85 per corporate dollar invested, based on reduced employee turnover, greater productivity and decreased medical claims (Dyck, 1999).

Workplace wellness has two components: organizational wellness and personal wellness. Organizational wellness involves managing both business functions and employee well-being in a manner that allows the organization to be more resilient to environmental pressures. Personal wellness involves managing both psychological and physical issues in response to environmental stress, including one's work environment.

Companies that adopt reactive approaches (such as attendance, disability, accident, employee assistance programs, staff turnover rates and costs) tend to focus their resources on controlling "failure costs"—costs that occur after an incident. These costs accrue when prevention systems break down (such as workers' compensation claims costs resulting from an injury). Companies that focus on proactive approaches generally use detection and prevention activities. These systems focus on identifying concerns and issues before they become problems (e.g., health and safety audits, incident or "near miss" investigations), and then avoiding or eliminating the concerns through special programs (e.g., fitness, smoking cessation, stress management, nutritional counselling) so they do not result in failure costs (Dyck, 1999).

☐ *Due diligence*
According to the Canadian Centre for Occupational Health and Safety, "due diligence is the level of judgement, care, prudence, determination and activity that a person would reasonably be expected to do under particular circumstances." Applied to occupational health and safety, due diligence means that employers take all reasonable precautions to prevent injuries or accidents in the workplace. This duty applies to situations that are not addressed elsewhere in the occupational health and safety legislation. To exercise due diligence, an employer must develop and implement a plan that identifies possible workplace hazards and carries out appropriate corrective action to prevent accidents or injuries from occurring (Canadian Centre for Occupational Health & Safety, p. 1).

The standards of due diligence have risen steadily. To prove due diligence for employees who drive, a company must establish an effective system (like an employee traffic-safety program) that prevents offences; monitor the results of the system (develop and administer a program evaluation), and evaluate and improve the system if collisions continue to occur (program monitoring). Some key factors for determining whether due diligence was exercised are the likelihood of harm, the level of potential harm, the alternatives for prevention, the skills an employee requires for the work and the extent to which the company could control worker risks. The greater the likelihood of mishap occurring and the more serious the mishap, the more stringent the system for monitoring and controlling risks must be.

In strict legal terms, concern about due diligence relates to companies trying to reduce their exposure to liability and accompanying litigation. Company executives are also well aware that issues of due diligence affect the organization's profit. As indicated previously, this economic view of due diligence argues strongly for the value of workplace-focussed traffic-safety initiatives.

■ Employer Costs Extend Beyond the Company Door

As in any complex system, cause and effect are seldom simple and are rarely constrained to any one domain (workplace, home or recreation). Family issues (an argument with a spouse) often "leak" into work activities (like driving) and occasionally contribute to a collision. Although the police report may list "following too close" as the cause of a collision, its antecedents are likely much more complex. Similarly, work issues affect family life. A bad day at the office can become a bad commute and a bad evening at home. Even though the drive to and from work takes place on the employee's time and is not directly connected to work, the employee-as-driver may be affected by work concerns and costs the company significantly if a traffic incident occurs. Although there is no direct employer responsibility for off-the-job crashes, the effects are nevertheless far-reaching. Employers must cover the missed time, worker benefits, replacement costs and lost productivity—significant costs. Lost-workday injuries include those resulting in an inability to perform wage, salary or household work.

In 1999, a survey was conducted at two large US organizations: the American Automobile Association and Nationwide Insurance. The survey indicated that the productivity of 40 percent of employees was negatively affected within the past 12 months by collisions involving themselves, family members or close friends. In addition to lost time, most reported that the quality of their work was adversely affected. According to the survey, the average time away from work per employee was 5.3 hours. The cost of traffic trauma to these organizations was significant: number of employees x 0.40 x 5.3 hours (NETS, 1999). Clearly, employers have more than a passing interest in the safety behaviour of employees both and off the job. It is abundantly clear that employers are in a unique position to influence a large portion of the population through their own workers.

■ The Workplace: An Opportunity

Mission Possible is a provincial traffic-safety initiative for Alberta, Canada. Based on experiences in traffic-safety awareness and fleet driver education, we concluded that there was a need for a comprehensive, integrated, long-term and scaleable employee traffic-safety program. We looked at the limitations of other programs and considered the opportunities that research and practice presented to us. From this thinking grew a traffic-safety initiative that extends beyond the workplace—that addresses the worker's traffic-safety concerns, commute, leisure driving and family driving. We geared the program toward corporate benefit by working with employees. An educated worker who feels good, has broader knowledge of the issues and feels part of the corporate culture is likely to be a safer worker and more in alignment with corporate needs and goals. In the US, NETS came closest to offering this kind of program through its support of corporate traffic-safety programs focussing on awareness, education and special-events materials. Even with the support of NETS, however, companies wishing to develop traffic-safety programs are still left on their own, with a very limited understanding of the complex issues surrounding traffic safety.

☐ *Identity and the workplace*

People work out of either economic necessity or career aspirations. Work gives people identity, purpose, meaning, social status and social interaction. Moreover, in our urbanized lifestyles (whether big-city or small-town), the workplace is one of the few settings where people from disparate backgrounds meet and relate on a daily basis. It provides an opportunity to discover other perspectives, learn new skills and test ideas. It offers a place to broaden perspectives, observe other behaviours and discover different ways of doing things. Full-time workers spend anywhere from six to twelve hours per day and from four to seven days a week on the job. This is more time than most people spend with their families. Since most workers spend much of their time together, they naturally form relationships that may cross over into their personal lives. They are more likely to discuss matters and influence each other's behaviour. The workplace, therefore, provides an ideal setting for an injury-prevention initiative.

Employers can see the effects of stressors, like the loss of life due to automobile crashes (Rice, 1995). From the employer's perspective, putting employees together in structured but informal settings to discuss traffic-safety issues has merit. Our challenge is to educate and to make the learning and instructional process interesting and engaging. Additionally, the quality of a workplace can be improved through documented policies and procedures. Using the power of the printed word is one of the most cost-effective ways to achieve change in the workplace.

■ A Fresh Approach to the Workplace

Mission Possible @ Work (MP@W) was developed as a response to the alarming escalation of traumatic traffic incidents. It recognizes the workplace is an excellent meeting ground for many people. While most models of behavioural change focus on individuals or groups, it is becoming clear that positive changes may be much more effectively accomplished when directed at social settings (like work) in which individuals are involved and through which they define themselves.

MP@W is a low-cost traffic-safety program designed to "heighten traffic safety awareness among employees, increase awareness of driving hazards on and off the job, promote traffic safety information-sharing among employees, motivate employees to drive safely on and off the job, and reduce both the number and severity of motor-vehicle collisions in which employees are involved." The program addresses the increasing importance of road trauma, both on and off the job, and tries to meet the traffic-safety needs of organizations. It was structured according to a set of sequential guidelines:

- Sessions are designed around themes relevant to motor-vehicle trauma (speed and speeding, inattention and distraction, aggressive driving, drowsy driving, winter driving, animal hazards, holiday driving, occupant restraints, driver impairments).
- A special launch session starts the program and begins the process of behaviour change with awareness-building information (a motivational objective).
- Awareness sessions are designed to generate an appreciation of the scope and consequences of traffic collisions (an affective objective).
- Education sessions follow topically similar awareness sessions and help participants develop prevention and accommodation strategies concerning the topic (a cognitive objective).
- Sessions are conducted with regularly scheduled staff meetings to increase ease of delivery and reduce costs.
- Sessions are short to allow easy and interesting presentation of information and to avoid interference effects.
- Sessions are facilitated by peers to encourage participation and discussions, and to keep session topics relevant.
- Sessions are interactive and promote discussion to allow participants to work through all the issues presented in the sessions.
- Sessions use affective and emotional materials (stories and video) and use the principle of flashbulb memory to anchor important concepts in each participant's memory.

- Sessions use multimedia to make topics more relevant and learning activities more engaging.

MP@W is, to some degree, a wellness program that uses prevention and accommodation strategies to help employees deal with the most common driving issues. The program uses an established model of behaviour change and proven principles of adult education. It touches on systems thinking and embraces many aspects of modern learning theory through the use of media, affective learning and process education. Special attention is paid to group discussions, part rather than whole learning, meaningful rather than rote learning, distributed rather than mass practice, and flashbulb memory.

□ *Wellness*
Like wellness programs, we approached problems from a proactive position and listened to employees to understand their needs and challenges in the work-place. Instead of waiting for problems to occur and addressing them later, MP@W examines the scope of the problem and provides information to understand it better. Later education sessions (in keeping with the principles of distributed practice) build on that understanding. Education sessions focus on how drivers can deal with the issue—how they might effectively prevent the problem from occurring near them, or how they can accommodate the problem should prevention strategies not work or be practical.

□ *Behaviour change*
As a theoretical model of behaviour change we chose the transtheoretical/ stages of change model (Miller & Rollnick, 1991) because of its relative simplicity, its ability to deal with resistant or habitual behaviour as well as relapse and its expression in more discrete elements (precontemplation, contemplation, preparation, action, maintenance, relapse). Most drivers are not well prepared for the many issues they face on the road despite the often serious risks presented; behaviour is often based on ignorance or erroneous assumptions. Awareness sessions in MP@W address the precontemplative, contemplative and preparative condition of most drivers. Drivers are often unaware of the scope, severity and consequences of driving problems in certain situations. Education sessions in MP@W address the action, mainte-nance and relapse aspects of driver behaviour. The sessions are offered in sequence at relevant times and supplemental support materials (posters, fact sheets, surveys, etc.) are provided to help drivers effect real change in their driving behaviour.

□ *Systems thinking*

MP@W takes a systemic approach to program development and intended audiences in that it is integrated into already-existing organizational structures. Topics are threaded together in various forms to create synergy with training activities. In designing MP@W, we integrated the worker's family through the use of outreach activities. After all, if learning is to take hold, it needs to be supported. Family and friends reinforce learning through a family-outreach kit that facilitates the same concepts and topics in a family-friendly format.

"Systems thinking is a discipline for seeing wholes, recognizing patterns and interrelationships, and learning how to structure those interrelationships in more effective, efficient ways" (Senge & Lannon-Kim, 1991); in simpler words, it means seeing the forest, not just the trees. Systems theory is related to the recently developing "sciences of complexity," including artificial intelligence (AI), neural networks, dynamic systems, chaos and complex adaptive systems. The systems approach distinguishes itself from the more traditional analytic approach by emphasizing the connectedness of components in a system. Although in principle the systems approach considers all types of systems, in practice it focusses on more complex, adaptive, self-regulating systems, which we might call "cybernetic." MP@W uses systems approaches in blending and connecting its components. Discussion opportunities in staff meetings constitute the complex, adaptive, self-regulating aspect of the program.

Systems theory suggests that real systems are open to, and interact with, their environments, and that they can acquire qualitatively new properties through emergence, resulting in continual evolution. Rather than reducing an entity (e.g., the human body) to the properties of its parts or elements (e.g., cells or organs), systems theory focusses on the arrangement of the parts and relations between the parts that connect them into a whole.

□ *Process education and discussion*

There has been considerable uncertainty about the effects of many educational and behaviourally oriented countermeasures targeted at traffic safety. The group discussions, which form the core of MP@W, were designed with guidance from the theories of adult and process education. This highly interactive environment ensures that awareness and educational activities are relevant and are geared to the level of interest and ability of the participants. According to a recent Swedish study (Gregersen, 1996), group discussion and driver training successfully improved accident risk and reduced accident costs. Compared with campaigns, financial reward or driver training, the best approach was group discussions. The study speculated that discussions were likely to serve as an important means of exchanging information about possible dangers and ways of avoiding them in traffic. The study further suggested that the group setting provided an opportunity for participants to make personal decisions about their driving, which became the cement that joined intention and action.

□ Adult education

Adult education principles played a large part in designing MP@W. First, we deal with adults in the workplace. Second, and perhaps more importantly, we know that adults learn best when they are able to use their previous experiences. In 1970, in *The Modern Practice of Adult Education*, Knowles suggested four adult teaching principles where adults move from dependency to self-directedness; draw upon their reservoir of experience for learning; are ready to learn when they assume new roles; and want to solve problems and apply new knowledge immediately. Knowles also wrote, "at its best, an adult learning experience should be a process of self-directed inquiry, with the resources of the teacher, fellow students, and materials being available to the learner but not imposed on him." This assessment of an ideal adult-learning experience ideally describes the MP@W staff-meeting sessions.

□ Affective learning

Emotions have an important connection to memory. They help to store information and trigger its recall (Rosenfield, 1988). According to Caine and Caine (1991), participants learn best in an supportive emotional climate marked by mutual respect. The recognition of the importance of emotional and affective approaches in the pursuit of durable learning among adult participants of MP@W sessions is an anchoring concept. The use of video, case studies, participant stories and self-assessment activities is designed to exploit this concept. Caine and Caine further suggest that "Content that is emotionally sterile is made more difficult to understand ... To teach someone any subject adequately, the subject must be embedded in all the elements that give it meaning" (1991, p. 58). People need to relate to material in terms of personal importance, acknowledging both the emotional impact and deeply held needs and drives. Creating a sense of emotional tension and discomfort around topical issues is a key strategy of MP@W. The principle of flashbulb memory anchors learning to intense affective experiences. The emotional tension of these experiences translates into heightened motivation to resolve the tension and gain better information, resulting in more personal involvement on the part of the learner.

□ Learning

We know that the way one learns and practises simple things makes little difference. However, for complex issues (like driving), part learning and distributed practice are best. Information and learning are stretched out over time, and issues are presented in small pieces. This piecing makes learning sessions more effective and reduces the interference effects of previous or later learning. By partitioning learning and distributing practice, the learner is better able to reflect on the topic and related issues and can associate the material with many different contexts rather than the single context afforded by mass practice.

☐ *Prevention and accommodation*

When we look at the issues that affect drivers, we quickly see that there are two general themes for intervention. Prevention activities are generally more desirable, effective and efficient. For example, by taking steps to avoid being drowsy, aggressive or distracted, we engage the best and most effective solution.

However, when drivers find themselves in situations where they become angry, tired or bored, they need to know how to deal with the problem at the moment; that is, they need to accommodate the issue. MP@W provides employees with accommodating strategies to help employees deal with fatigue while driving, aggressive driving (in self and others) and a wandering or distracted mind. The program approaches each issue from both prevention and accommodation perspectives.

☐ *Media*

Staff-meeting sessions are designed to encourage discussions that are engaging, meaningful and memorable. Through the use of video material such as public service announcements from the Traffic Accident Commission in Victoria, Australia and the AAA Foundation for Traffic Safety, participants are exposed to lifelike depictions of issues. The traumatic, gripping drama that often accompanies motor-vehicle crashes creates a sense of concern or unease in the participants.

Topical poster materials, bulletins, fact sheets and self-assessment instruments are also included in the sessions. These materials are strategically distributed throughout the department (in the cafeteria, work area or hallway, for example) to provide a persistent reminder of the topic and to encourage on-going discussion.

☐ *Format*

MP@W uses four basic behaviour-modification tools—awareness, education, enforcement and reinforcement—to promote change. The program avoids driver training, leaving that to professional trainers for specific employees in special situations (for example, on-road training sessions for employees who drive in hazardous environments).

Awareness activities are designed to occur frequently (weekly or monthly) and in a variety of formats. The messages must be accessible across all company levels and functions (departmental and regional). Awareness messages should be sent through existing communication channels. Although regular and pervasive, they are presented in novel and stimulating ways to avoid desensitization. Messages are grounded in facts relevant to the organization and the local community. For example, the crash-involvement rates of employees relative to local and national averages (along with information about monetary and psychological costs) would be good starting points. As program components proceed, evaluation information is collected and disseminated. The broader perspective (assuming it is presented in ways available to local employees) is most desirable. The use of peer influence and interaction is an important part of awareness sessions.

Educational activities are designed to take place monthly or quarterly, depending on job function, exposure to risk and departmental resources. As with the messages, these activities must be accessible, relevant and appropriate across all company levels and functions. The length and intensity of the educational activities themselves are geared to the type of exposure to collisions that the employees normally experience, but for the most part, they are short, focussed and relevant. The educational activities are designed to provide some degree of knowledge and skill improvement while reducing the tendency toward overconfidence. The use of engaging and provocative media and ample group interaction are key ingredients in making sessions more effective.

Company expectations are enforced through codification that also spells out consequences of violation. Policies should be highlighted during appropriate opportunities at company and department levels. The review and communication of traffic-safety policy is effective in increasing awareness of traffic safety and it reinforces concepts already presented. Policy needs to be clearly, positively and consistently communicated to and by all employees.

Reinforcement of company expectations and guidelines occurs through a blend of awareness, education and evaluation, and through a fair system of punishment and reward. Sample traffic-safety policy guidelines are provided in program materials. Evaluations also take place at various times each year and across all company levels and functions. These evaluations examine qualitative, quantitative and process issues. The results of the evaluation activities are most effectively used as awareness-generating opportunities. The measurement of any change in driver behaviour is important for increasing awareness and providing positive reinforcement. Evaluation measurements occur at the level of individual program components and for the overall organization.

■ How the Program Works
The strategy behind MP@W is based upon a view of human development contained within an ecological systems model. Human beings are more than autonomous self-contained individuals; they exist within a context of rela-

tionships and communication. This model states that self-concept and identity are determined not only by intra-individual factors but also by inter-individual factors such as the familial, community, sub-cultural and cultural groups in which the individual participates. Effective change initiatives must be simultaneously directed at social levels that help constitute and support individual persons. For example, child-safety programs are most effective when families, schools and peers are involved. Anti-drinking and driving initiatives are most effective when they are directed toward general social attitudes.

At the heart of MP@W is the notion that group interaction promotes employee involvement and permits information sharing. This interaction is important in both involving employees and allowing information to be shared. It also helps keep sessions and topics relevant. Session materials are presented to employees through regularly scheduled staff meetings. The staff meeting takes advantage of the collegial atmosphere that already exists. This venue is used so that staff can learn about traffic-safety issues in an atmosphere that promotes knowledge-sharing. Short, snappy MP@W presentations are added to the end of these meetings. Presentations by experts (driving instructors or traffic-safety professionals) are strongly discouraged. Managers and supervisors are encouraged (and supported through program materials) to present the sessions to their own staff. Their relative inexperience with the issues may encourage participation and sharing among participants. The staff-meeting setting was also chosen to help keep group sizes small and appropriate (ten to fifteen people) for proper group discussion and interaction.

MP@W has been built through expertise but is designed to be delivered at the grassroots. The program encourages non-expert employees to lead, which ensures a sense of equality among participants and creates an open atmosphere for discussion. A traffic-safety expert would likely dampen interaction and create a passive learning environment. Employee facilitators do not need to have any subject matter expertise; they simply need to lead a staff meeting. Sufficient support for delivering MP@W sessions is provided in the program materials and, if necessary, facilitators can contact experts (such as the MP@W coordinator or the Alberta Motor Association).

Discussions about the material usually continue at coffee and lunch breaks. Employees are likely to discuss personal experiences and new learning, because the materials are thought-provoking and intended to create an emotional response.

□ *Scope*
The scope of the program is broad and inclusive. Employees are exposed to program elements regularly throughout their time with the company. The program addresses awareness and educational opportunities along a number of

dimensions. It presents activities in a variety of ways and to various employee groupings, including family and friends. It addresses the issue of intensity, presenting activities with a high degree of focus and detail at times (such as the topical self-assessments included in some sessions); at other times, the activities are subtler and broader, featuring general-awareness information. The program is designed to respect the diverse nature of a working population and accommodate that diversity by presenting similar messages in many different ways.

■ Why Mission Possible @ Work Succeeds

Since the workplace is primarily made up of adults, the program uses the principles of adult learning. These include the use of techniques such as dialogue and involvement, shared experience, and peer support (positive and peer-sanctioned behaviours). Adult learners are seen as generally self-directed learners who "borrow" the assistance of a more knowledgeable resource person. Adults approach any educational experience with a wealth of life experience that informs both the learning process and the teaching process (Knowles, 1980). In MP@W, participants already have an understanding of driving. Since employees are part of the traffic environment every day, their learning can be applied immediately.

Employees are part of their workplace, geographical community and social network. One employee may be involved with local sports; another participates in various hobbies, while another enjoys the arts. Their lives are connected through a variety of networks, which provide opportunities for significant communication and influence. MP@W provides an opportunity for all employees to speak more confidently about their traffic knowledge and experience.

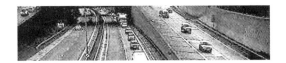

FOLLOW-UP, SUMMATIVE and formative evaluations showed that some participants changed their driving behaviour. Participants documented that they have slowed down while driving and now keep a greater distance behind cars. Some stated they have become more aware of distractions created by other roadway users and have changed how they use cellular phones in the car. Others started to scan the roadway for possible problems. The program has motivated some to discuss issues among staff members during breaks, at incidental opportunities (in the parking lot, work area and hallway, for example) and with family and friends away from the workplace.

The workplace provides an opportunity for awareness campaigns to reach the bulk of the population at low cost—especially when compared with the equivalent cost of reaching this group through mass media. It also provides opportunities for discussion, feedback and reflection in a friendly, peer environment. Since work is a necessary part of life, it makes sense to implement a traffic-safety program in the workplace. Employers and employees can work together to create a safer traffic reality in their communities, large and small.

13

REVISITING COMMUNICATIONS AND TRAFFIC SAFETY

JORGE FRASCARA

MOTOR-VEHICLE ACCIDENTS ARE a major health and safety problem. In the last decade, 51,300 people died in road crashes in Canada; another 2,342,300 were injured, many of them permanently disabled. Road crashes are now the leading cause of death to people under the age of 45 and a major cause of injury (Road Safety and Motor Vehicle Regulation Directorate, 2). In Canada, traffic injuries kill twice as many people under 35 as cancer and heart disease combined; however, whereas research on cancer and heart disease prevention is substantially funded, little funding is dedicated to the study of strategies aimed at reducing the traffic-injuries epidemic. In the United States, "Injury research expenditures are estimated at $160 million for fiscal year 1987 compared with expenditures for cancer research by the National Cancer Institute of $1.4 billion. The National Heart, Lung and Blood Institute spent $930 million for cardiovascular research in fiscal year 1987" (Rice et al., 1989, xxxvii). The difference between funds directed at cancer and heart research and those directed at traffic-safety research is staggering, and it does not include the millions of dollars invested in research and development of cancer- and heart-related drugs by the pharmaceutical industry.

Wars always attract public attention, create heavy reactions and mobilize the press, but "if every war since 1776 is taken together, no instrument of death—flintlock, repeating rifle, machine gun, tank, plane or bomb—has resulted in as many American fatalities as has the motor vehicle. From 1910 to 1985, there were more than 2.5 million traffic fatalities" (National Committee for Injury Prevention and Control, p. 118). In 1991, 43,500 people died in car crashes in the USA, and 1,600,000 suffered disabling injuries (an injury disabling the person beyond the day of the accident). Of these, 130,000 were left with permanent impairments (National Safety Council, p.1).

It is impossible to quantify the human costs inflicted upon individuals and their families. Spinal cord, brain and other severe injuries mark people for life, reduce their potential contribution to society and often contribute to other future ailments. In most severe collisions, the health care and suffering do not end the day of the crash. In addition to the human suffering, the cost of traffic crashes is enormous. The direct cost in the US for 1991 was $96.1 billion, including medical expenses, wage loss, insurance administration, motor-vehicle damage and uninsured work loss (National Safety Council, p. 2). Seen from the perspective of the economy, happiness or life expectancy, traffic collisions are a major burden for human life and public administration.

This chapter proposes to reduce the problem through the development of a cost-effective communication campaign that targets specific groups so as to be more effective than generic campaigns. In order to confront this problem, the campaign must be conceived of as a cluster of promotions addressed to different groups recognized as over-represented in the collision statistics.

■ The Communicational Power of Driving

For many people, driving equals power: the power to do some things, to enjoy others and to achieve comfort. People get used to using the car and the roads, take them for granted and believe it is their right, not their privilege, to use them. A character in a story by Milan Kundera manages to convince a Paris policeman that she has the right to park her car illegally, since the city does not offer drivers enough parking facilities. As it is her right to go shopping, it is therefore the municipality's fault, and not hers, that she has to park illegally to go shopping. Something similar happened to me in Spain, when I was riding a train. I was in a non-smoking car and a lady lit a cigarette. When I called her attention to the prohibition, the man sitting by her explained to me, irritated, that, "She went to the car behind, and it's forbidden, she went to the next car, and it's also forbidden! OK! Smokers have to smoke!"

People use things without consciousness of the needs of others or the processes of production. The well-known separation of use from production has resulted in the belief in infinity of resources: the only limit is set by what we can afford to pay; sometimes, beyond that, we feel we should have enough money to buy even what we cannot afford. Having access to things gives us the feeling of freedom and power. For example, some contemporary artists paint using gallons of acrylic gel. They do not mix the colors; they just buy the gallons. Jan van Eyck would never have conceived of producing a painting three centimetres thick: getting the pigments and preparing the colours was a major task; colour was precious. If we had to dig for petroleum and refine it, we would think twice before using the car to go to buy bread two blocks from home, as most North Americans do. People fear any restrictions on the use of the car as a potential reduction of freedom and power, and therefore resist it.

From the auto industry's point of view, use generates consumption, which generates business. The auto industry is highly interested in promoting the use of the car: lots of use, intense use. More use means more demands for more quantity. More quantity means more business. In order to promote that intense use, people must fulfill deeply felt needs: transportation is not enough. Power and freedom are better. Driving has to be glamorous, desirable, hot. A revision of car culture that would foster a less-glamorous perception of driving would remove motivation and result in a reduction of use. This might reduce business, and will, therefore, be opposed by industry and commerce.

Industry and commerce (and, to some extent, people) seek to control governments. Therefore, a revision to the use of the car that would be opposed by people, industry and commerce will create difficulty for government, resulting in no hope for legislation that supports meaningful change. Reducing the road toll demands attention to people, business and government, three reluctant areas of power. One would have to think about the three areas, developing an appropriate understanding of each one.

■ People, Business and Governments

It would be difficult to devise a good strategy to promote a revision of driving among people, since people move according to more complex systems of decisions than business (which fundamentally moves along the uni-dimensionality of short-term profits), and reaching a substantial number of people to effect significant change is an almost-impossible task. Business must see an advantage in order to engage in a revision, and we will need innovative ideas to build that argument. Governments today, to a great extent, make their decisions in response to pressures from business and voters; while they provide strong, accessible centres of control, they will not initiate dramatic changes without support.

A revision of traffic culture that begins by addressing people on the basis of an obvious sense of responsibility will find that responsibility is not a strong sentiment compared to individual rights. Similar to the story written by Kundera, an Edmonton man took the Province of Alberta to court after being charged for not wearing his seat belt while driving. Seat-belt enforcement was suspended for several months until the courts supported the Province in its action. The man's argument was that mandatory seat-belt use was against his constitutionally guaranteed individual rights and freedoms. He did not acknowledge that, if he got injured, his medical costs would be paid by the

Province (to the tune of $300,000 for the first year of spinal-cord injury) and that in an emergency situation he was more likely to lose control of the vehicle without a seat belt on and would therefore be more dangerous to others.

The truth of the matter, however, is that the great majority of drivers do very well. Even in the segment that is responsible for more collisions per driver (males 18 to 24 years of age), there are normally about 3,500 injury collisions per year, in a universe of over 120,000 drivers. Most drivers drive safely. On average, about 3 percent are involved in one collision every year in the 18–24 age group in Alberta, and of them, possibly only 1.7 percent are at fault, rather than victims. We might recognize that we have at least two types of driver: one that frequently appears in collisions and another that only occasionally appears, usually as a victim. The severity of crashes defines another possible difference. A study I did in 1992 concentrated on repeat offenders (drivers with at least one licence suspension) and drivers who had been involved in injury collisions. In this study, several of the subjects interviewed had been in more than ten collisions. In another study I did in 1998, selecting drivers randomly among the driving population, I was somewhat surprised to find that among the 30 subjects interviewed, 19 collisions were reported, 3 subjects having been involved in 10 of them. None, however, was reported to have been a severe injury collision. We face, therefore, different kinds of drivers. We need to look further into the details, in order to determine the kinds of actions needed to increase safety on the roads and the limits that communications face when dealing with certain sectors of the driving population.

Responsibility in the use of the car, to the eyes of the public at large, opposes the right to use it and the carefree attitudes promoted by the mass media; it is thus perceived as negative. To make responsibility acceptable, it must be connected to a value that people hold dearly. We need to find the values that the public supports strongly and shift the meaning of these values. For instance, if driving carelessly gives people a sense of freedom, control and power, the important thing is not driving carelessly but the feelings it evokes. It would be very difficult to make people relinquish those feelings. The challenge and the opportunity consist of shifting the meanings of concrete actions, so that driving responsibly becomes source of feelings of freedom, control and power. In addition, it should be possible to provoke a change in attitudes in a second group of people who hold responsibility as a high value. These people, who would most likely be community leaders, could take on a conscious attitude and set new models of behaviour. A large third group of people will adopt the new notion through imitation of the behaviours of the leading class and follow the new models.

Having proposed a context that recognizes three different groups of people, and having begun discussing how a revision of driving culture could be supported, we should think about actions that should not be perceived as a reduction of freedom, power and control, but the opposite. This calls for a change in the symbolic meaning of certain actions that people perform in order to project a given "image" in their social environment.

■ Ethics and Communication

From a strategic point of view, the promotion of a public change in attitude requires a recognition of the multiplicity of people and an ethical communications approach, wherein people become active partners in the process. When dealing with responsible, intelligent, active people—who form the group we need to approach first—there is no hope for campaigns that communicate things to people; we need to communicate with the people about things, particularly when these things require their action. This difference merits elaboration within a discussion of ethics and communication.

Every situation of human communication falls within the field of ethics. That is, a situation can be ethical or unethical, but it cannot be a-ethical. The basic tenet of ethical communication is the recognition of the Other—the so-called receiver of the communication—as a subject (a person) and not as an object. By recognizing the Other as a subject, one recognizes the Other as an independent, thinking person with a specific way of understanding, evaluating and integrating experiences and information.

In ethical communications, one communicates with someone about something: one does not communicate something to someone. Ethical communications presuppose a similarity between the communicating subjects, unlike military communications, where a superior communicates something to an inferior. He transmits an order, which is received passively, not allowing for differing interpretations. Only the severe discipline of the military can repress one's natural resistance to such annihilation of the self. One certainly cannot base a public-interest campaign on the military model: the campaign must be ethical. In the public sphere, one must recognize persons to work with, not subordinates to talk at.

In ethical communications, Shannon's popular terminology, borrowed from electronics and information science that defines the poles of the communication chain as transmitter and receiver, is untenable. In a universe of people engaged in communications, it is more fitting to talk about producers and interpreters of communications than about transmitters and receivers, terms which do not allow room for context, history, expectations, goals, intentions, values, priorities, feelings, preferences and differences of intelligence. Since ethics implies the recognition of the Other as an independent, thinking person—as someone different—the first step to be taken in any communicative attempt is to learn, to understand and to use the languages of the people one wants to reach, and then to actively engage them in the dialogue.

■ The Active Viewer

Using the language of the audience is not enough: the audience has to speak. Mass media usually renders the audience passive; the entertainment industry is based on moving enough things on the TV screen so that people in front of it don't feel the need to move at all. Other aspects of culture also encourage this passivity. According to an article published in *Vogue* magazine, fat people cannot lose weight without the help of drugs. It seems as if people had lost the notions of willpower and discipline, and the ability to make choices and efforts. All that is left is a magic pill that takes away from us the responsibility for our weight, our mood or our intelligence. Athletes use drugs before competitions, students use drugs before exams, and business people use drugs before meetings. This progressive deterioration of the ability to use willpower goes hand in hand with the passing of one's control on to someone else who must solve the problem. The pharmacist should solve the psychological problem, the plastic surgeon should solve the physical beauty problem, and the government should be blamed for everything that goes wrong in the country. All are aspects of a passivity that is both allowed and promoted by culture and the media.

This general passivity, which characterizes every aspect of the news and entertainment industry, extends to intellectual passivity. Media narratives are normally based on short storylines and organized as clusters of content juxtaposed against one another. The media tend to avoid long lines of logically organized sequences, and therefore don't contribute to the development of people's ability to think, particularly in terms of understanding the interconnectedness of systems. Advertising is no different: it usually pushes the audience to be active in only a prescribed way, to go and shop, without thinking, and promotes the development of a magic relation between products and human values.

With a few exceptions, business, government, education and the mass media converge in constructing "the consumer," a person whose job provides no satisfaction whatsoever and who is trained to look forward to retirement to arrive finally at the perfect situation of only consuming without producing. The passive viewer is the communicational counterpart of the passive citizen. Without an active viewer there cannot be an active citizen, there cannot be active understanding of responsibilities and rights, and there cannot be active understanding of a revision of anything.

According to Robyn Penman of the Communication Research Institute of Australia, the notion of citizenship we hold is reduced to being a mere descriptor of nationality. However, quoting Bryan Turner, she argues that "Citizenship may be defined as that set of practices (juridical, political, economic and cultural) which define a person as a competent member of society, and which as a consequence shape the flow of resources to persons and social groups" (Turner, 1993, p. 2). Penman adds, "One of the key ingredients to the practice of citizenship is participation in public life. And this act of participation is a communicative one. It is in our public communication processes that practices are enacted that define a person as more or less a citizen. And it is the quality of the practices that counts. Good practices bring about good citizens." Referring to a study of government communications in Australia, she continues, "We identified three dominant themes that are not conducive to citizenship: the growing tendency to treat citizens as consumers in an information market place; the reliance on social science "experts" to monitor and mediate in the "market place"; the use of communication as a simple selling tool" (Penman, 1994, pp. 1–2). If we want people to understand the need for a revision of driving, we have to engage them in activity and make them good citizens of this revision so that they actively contribute to its development.

■ The Structure of the Communicational Engagement
In order to conceive of ways in which a revised idea of driving could be promoted among other groups of people, we must review our own process of change of perspective, arrive at a new conception through reflection, and exchange information and discussions in a partnership that occurs within a shared cultural value system, and with a sense of purpose and importance. Those of us who share a more responsible notion of driving and are interested in promoting it should acknowledge the above process as a model and consider that if we are to succeed in the promotion of our idea, it will have to be done in a situation of active partnership. Further, it will have to become the idea of the Other, and in the process it will have to suffer a number of transformations.

□ Values and motivations
While it is difficult to know what makes people accept a given notion of driving within their culture, it is easy to assume that people have conceptions of driving that serve as means to achieve the comfort—physical and social—they aspire to. Driving seems to give some people a sense of freedom and power, and therefore pleasure and self-confidence; it gives them prestige among their peers; it can be thrilling and stimulating; it gives people a sense of being in control; and it can be entertaining. To implement changes in an area that provides people with a feeling of self-worth, we need to offer something important in exchange: technical arguments lack the strength to promote a change if that change is perceived as a loss. We need to offer a positive cultural

value for the behaviour we promote, a positive cultural value in the terms of the very people we want to reach. We must therefore understand their values and see how those values can be adopted to support a revision of driving.

To promote our ideas, we have to understand that, although we are interested in safe driving, many people are not. Therefore, we cannot start from our evidence but from the interests of our audience. Their interests vary widely. Politicians want to remain in power: they are interested in job creation and in balanced finances. Business people are interested in personal gains and short-term profits. People at large are interested in comfort, leisure and freedom. Nobody is interested in restrictions in the use of anything. Our task is to define a way to revise driving so that it can be seen by politicians as helping them stay in power; by business people as a possibility for personal gains and profit; and by people at large as providing more comfort, more leisure or more freedom. (There might be a few people who could be moved by something that appears morally right, but when it comes to massive changes, this might not be a reliable strategy in our culture, beyond the group that I defined before as leaders.)

□ *Would fear be a possibility?*
People are selective concerning what they want to fear and what outrages them. The Vietnam war, where 50,000 Americans died in ten years, was a source of enormous political tension, suffering and scandal in the USA. The same number of people die not every ten years, but every year in traffic collisions in the USA and few people care. In the USA, every year, 130,000 people are left with a permanent disability as a consequence of a traffic collision. Four hundred and sixty-six people are being injured in traffic collisions in the USA during the forty-five-minute reading of this article, and forty-five of them are being hospitalized. If nobody is horrified by this, can we think that fear would work to make people revise their driving habits?

□ *Would money be a possibility?*
The Australian Transport Accident Commission of the state of Victoria, which operates third-party liability insurance, decided in 1989 to launch a traffic-safety campaign, after noticing that the amount of money being paid for traffic-collisions insurance was rapidly increasing (Harper & L'Huillier, 1990). They implemented better speed controls by installing high-technology speed cameras; new police buses were dedicated to random controls of drivers' blood alcohol content. They also launched a media campaign aimed at both announcing the new measures of control and promoting safe driving. After one year of implementing the campaign—which was conceived by Grey Advertising with the assistance of research by Robert Sweeney—and having spent $6 million in media space, the results showed clearly the value of the program:

- a 30-percent reduction in the road toll;
- 230 lives saved, compared to previous year;
- $118 million less than the previous year paid in insurance, an estimated saving of $361 million for the community; and
- 98 percent support by the public independently surveyed.

The campaign and the measures have continued and so has their effect. The trigger to create it was money. The effect was quite important, particularly for those 230 people that might have died and the 670 who might have been permanently disabled, if things had remained as they were.

It is surprising that the motor vehicle enjoys so much freedom of movement. In the US, the direct cost of car crashes for 1991 was $64 billion, including only medical costs, insurance administration and vehicle damage, and without counting loss of wage, police and courts costs, stress on the family and loss of productivity in the workplace, where 200 million working days were lost due to car crashes in 1991. It is surprising that in such a pragmatic country so much can be accepted without serious countermeasures. What benefits must accrue from a change in the driving culture in order for it to make people and governments act? Should everything have a price tag? Should we conceive of a revision of driving that is "sold" on the basis of cost benefits? Would money create a common field of relevance?

■ Communications, Individuals and Relevance

Any group is formed by different individuals, with different characteristics, and it is not advisable to overgeneralize or oversimplify when describing large groups of people. Any communication system will have to be formed by a wide spectrum of arguments and approaches so as to reach different conceptions and interests, and will have to include producers and interpreters in the formulation of the communicational engagement. In every case, we must create a common field of relevance. Relevance prompts attention and prepares reception. Without perceived relevance, there is no communication. Communication comes to exist on the basis of intention; without both parties being intentionally connected, there is no hope for change-generating communication.

The creation of a field of relevance and the meeting of intentions can sometimes take place on the basis of an emotional appeal. One of the strengths of the Australian traffic-safety campaign was that it touched the viewer. Research conducted before the development of the campaign generated the following recommendations:

- Don't concentrate solely on twisted metal;
- Don't overdo statistics;

- Don't lecture;
- Do be as shocking as you like;
- Do be as emotional as possible; and
- Do ensure that they come away from any communication thinking "that could happen to me." (Harper & L'Huillier, 1990, p. 193)

The latter was not done on the basis of the fear of being killed in a car crash, since all of us tend to think "it's not going to happen to me," but on the basis of the fear of becoming responsible for the pain of another person—particularly a loved one—apparently a more believable possibility.

People tend to believe that their own pain is their individual problem and that it is their own business if they crash their cars. The Australian campaign seems to have touched people by making the point that they might survive, but in a wheelchair, and become dependent and burdensome for others; or that they might survive, but after killing or maiming someone else, facing court charges, losing their license and ending up in jail for drunk driving causing death. Legal consequences and the pain of others seem to have managed to do what the threat of one's own death had not managed to do before.

The Australian campaign brought the issue of collisions away from statistics and down to the personal level, and entered it in the public agenda. Journalism became interested and served as a multiplying force. During the first 50 days of the launching of the campaign, the press responded with 17 major articles and 84 other media references in the state of Victoria; this continued for the rest of 1990, with 869 recorded media references. The campaign managed to outrage, shake and upset the people into reviewing their notions of driving.

■ Reaching People

Penetrating the public agenda is not easy, but there are several ways. Hollywood created American history from the conquest of the West through to the Vietnam War passing by the Civil War and, more than anything, World War Two. The cartoon character Popeye is said to be the brainchild of a high officer of the American Food and Drug Administration who made a creative leap to promote the use of vegetables in the American diet.

Other than these campaigns, launched from powerful bases in a top-down way, the way to work from the ground up is to begin with the immediate community. National governments have become so removed from the life of people that it is no longer possible to reach them. Neighbourhoods and small towns offer a better possibility for community action. The "nuclear-free zone" signs in small Italian towns seem ridiculous but, upon reflection, it becomes clear that this is the only way small communities can oppose national policies, the only way in which people could affect national policies.

Certain professions can offer other points of entry. Doctors offer a localizable, prestigious and powerful community-size group, as do other colleges of professionals that, one way or another, have a measure of power. Educators certainly have the possibility both to understand and to disseminate a revision of the notion of driving; but in order for the educational system to subscribe to the notion, government must be supportive, which bring us back from the ground-up approach to the difficulties of the top-down approach, with all the vote-seeking and in-fighting that this implies. A revision of the notion of driving incorporated in the educational system calls for a revision of several aspects of the system, including the notion of the learner as an active partner in the educational process, and must hinge on the notion of responsibility.

■ Change of Behaviours, Change of Attitudes

Much can be learned from the Australian experience on traffic safety. Two things should be clear: communication was not all; enforcement supported the change. (It seems more people were afraid of being surprised by a police officer than of losing control of the car.) Behaviours changed, but on one occasion, when the media budget was spent and the transmissions were interrupted, traffic fatalities went up immediately, from 39 to 70 per month, suggesting that attitudes had remained essentially untouched. How long is it possible to sustain a change of behaviours without a change in attitudes? What would it take for a change in behaviours to become a change in attitudes? Would a change in attitudes happen through sheer repetition of behaviours?

Repression through fear of facing emotionally taxing situations of guilt, coupled with police control of speed and alcohol, and the fear of losing one's driver's license, has proven useful for the immediate reduction of collisions and for a sustained effect over years. Will the public become used to the campaign and the measures, and little by little slide back into dangerous behaviours requiring more and more repression? Would it be possible to maintain a constant growth of these systems to compensate for the increase of habituation to their messages?

To what extent is the fight between the way people are and the way the Transport Accident Commission wants them to be—or between the prevailing messages of the culture, including those of the mass media, and the messages of the TAC? Put this way, we see that we are not talking about a conflict of positions between the nature of people and the campaign of the TAC, but between two campaigns. One campaign is led by advertising and entertainment, and promotes the excitement of sensorial experiences, information overload, assertion, courage, violence, exploration and the primacy of the individual to the point of total self-centredness; the other proposes restraint, consideration of others, no-nonsense pragmatism and control, so as to be able to react properly to surprise situations. But if a change of attitude were generated by one campaign, could it ever stop broadcasting, so long as the other campaign continued pushing people in a different direction? Examples of the promotion of dangerous driving abound in car culture. As an example, above a picture of a super-charged white sports car, the front page of a car magazine reads: "At 179 miles per hour all that you hear is the pounding of your heart."

Our question is this: is it the nature of people that leads to an abusive and irresponsible notion of driving, or is it certain messages in our culture that promote that abuse? If so, which are the active messages of our culture that promote the notion that has to be revised? Which could be the counter-messages that must be conceived? We cannot look exclusively at advertising as the source of the conflict. Many other aspects of the culture, including everyday language, remove responsibility from the picture and create constructs within which situations of abuse become acceptable.

☐ *Language, culture and the car*
The first and most important problem created by language in the universe of car-related horror is the word *accident*. Accident implies a chance occurrence and frees everybody from responsibility. I worked with a focus group of men who had been repeatedly involved in collisions, and asked them whether their "accidents" helped them prevent others in the future. One put the answer very clearly: "Surely not! That's why they are called accidents!" (While I prefer to use "crash" or "collision," I used the word "accident" with the focus groups in order to avoid creating a ridge between my language and theirs.) We know that traffic collisions are not really accidental; rather, they are the result of wrong decisions, mistaken perceptions, failed adjustment to conditions, errors and distractions, and only in three percent of cases are they the result of unforesee-able mechanical failures, some of which nevertheless could be avoided with proper car maintenance.

In addition to the word "accident," other constructs result in the same lack of responsibility. "The weather was a factor," "Road conditions were poor" and "Heavy fog contributed to the accident" are all expressions from police reports and are commonly quoted by journalists (to a certain extent constructed to avoid blaming someone before formal charges have been laid). These expressions lead one to assume that the drivers could not notice bad weather, road conditions or fog while driving, and thus could not adjust their driving accordingly. One report on a crash read this way: "An Edmonton couple were killed instantly when their car plunged 100 meters down an embank-ment near Lake Louise. RCMP said the accident happened about 7:15 pm Friday when a Chevy Cavalier failed to make a curve and drove off the road and down a huge drop." So it seems that the car had a will of its own, did not want to make the curve, drove off the road and finally killed the innocent couple.

A emphasis on pain rather than responsibility appears in another newspaper report about a collision where four teenagers were killed and one was seriously wounded as a consequence of failing to observe a yield sign. A subtitle on the front page read "'ROAD CONDITIONS, Gravel road surface wet from rainfall occurring most of the day'—RCMP report." The article, loaded with sentimental statements about the sadness of the mourning crowd, quotes a pastor saying, "I studied in a seminary to find answers to hard questions like why people die before their time." In this case, the answer was easy: they drove through a yield sign and got in the way of an oncoming pick-up truck, not only killing themselves but endangering the life of the truck driver, whose vehicle rolled over as a consequence of the collision, and his family. The newspaper concentrates on how nice these youngsters were, without a word of outrage about the driver's lack of responsibility, perpetuating a common belief about the mystery of "accidents" and maintaining the possibility for more traffic tragedies to happen.

In its statistical reports, Alberta Transportation also obscures the issue. In 1990, for instance, it reports that 47 percent of drivers involved in casualty collisions were driving properly, leading to the conclusion that one can be driving properly and cause a serious collision. But this is not the case: the text says "involved" and not "causing." Quite likely, 47 percent is the number of drivers who were hit by the other 53 percent, who otherwise tend to run into light poles, parked vehicles and trees. However, when we look at the leading causes of collisions in the Alberta report and find that the top "action of drivers involved in casualty collisions" is "driving properly," we are led to believe that in almost half of the cases, traffic accidents happen without human error.

These are examples of structures of language that must change to alter people's perceptions and their notion of responsible use of the car. In order to understand the use of the car in our culture, in addition to looking into the language that surrounds the use of the car (and that not only affects journalism and advertising, but that also shapes values and attitudes), we must consider the car itself as language, the object as symbol and its use as communication.

☐ *Driving as communication*
When asking subjects in the focus group what they liked most about driving, they tended to talk in a matter-of-fact way about the freedom to go from A to B at any time according to their needs and wants. It took some prompting to get to other ways of using the car, such as going at 170 kph down a winding road (Groat Road) in the city of Edmonton at three in the morning, or going for a drive in the country, or speeding to scare a girlfriend, or doing figure-eights and

donuts in a snowy parking lot. The practical aspect of freedom as experienced when "going from A to B" later gave way to a use of the car whose purpose was the enjoyment of freedom itself, a notion of play that resulted in a sense of control, power and excitement. It seems that, for many people, the use of an object is boring if it is not attached to an imagined dimension, as in children's play. When a child has a broomstick, he imagines it is a horse. But having a horse is not the point. When he has a horse, he pretends he is a cowboy. Playing for children and using things for adults frequently involves imagined dimensions. A car is not a means of transportation: it is a means of communication. When I asked my focus group subjects whether they thought the car they drove expressed themselves, they initially said no. They said that the car they used to own did, but then they destroyed it in a crash, their insurance went up and they could no longer afford that kind of car. All this without acknowledging that the car they now owned did express their true existence. But they did not perceive their true existence as truth; they actually thought the symbol was wrong and, up to a point, felt unable to realize themselves until they once again got the right object to live through it.

The magic power of objects has been skillfully promoted by advertising, and not only in relation to cars. In one ad for running shoes, the text reads, "When you move the world slips away from your mind and the strength slips into your life, and you are free, you are free you are absolutely free, strong enough and sure enough to do anything ... It has attitude. It's strong. It's sure. Like we said: it can do anything." The same encompassing promise given by this brand of running shoes is given by a shampoo: "Hair so full of sensual energy you can feel it down to your toes."

In addition to the symbolic dimension of the car as an object, driving is a cultural activity, a social activity and, therefore, an act of communication. As such, when norms become stereotyped, they develop into an aesthetic; that is, functional actions become loaded with a sense of the beautiful, the ugly and the desirable. In our culture, driving a car is an aesthetic act; it must flow, as beautiful lines flow, and anything that disrupts that flow will be resented. This is the reason, when I asked the focus group what they disliked most about driving, that what came up was "bad drivers" and "the lack of courtesy of other drivers": the subjects always put the obligation for courtesy on the other driver, to make room for themselves to continue their fast flow.

The cultural task ahead is to modify the aesthetics of driving, as the aesthetics of smoking and hockey helmets have been modified among some groups in Canada. Smoking used to be a symbol of glamour. Now it is a symbol for self-destructive, anti-social behaviour among radicals; it has become, in general, a small nuisance to put up with in some public places. It is certainly no longer an image-booster, at least, not after outgrowing adolescence. Playing hockey without a helmet used to be a sign of manliness. Professional players resisted the notion of using a helmet until it became mandatory; thereafter, the helmet became a symbol for manliness. In addition to changing the aesthetics of car driving, we must work toward reducing the emotional investment and dependence that many young people place on driving. This might reduce the likelihood of unsafe driving behaviours performed more in response to self-image-building needs than to the traffic reality. The task will also consist of moving the driver's focus of attention from the axis that links the driver with the car to the axis that links the car with the traffic.

□ *Understanding and acting*

Understanding is a cognitive process; acting is a social process. As an idea that has to do with action, the revision of driving will have to be understood; then it will have to be adopted, and then it will have to be acted on. That is, the idea must affect people's knowledge, attitudes and behaviour in order to succeed. Communication, even ethical, active, partnership-based communication, might not suffice, given that we are dealing with a revision that might be anti-thetical both to the temperament of humanity as it has been expressed since the beginning of civilization and to the general tone of the media. The success of the TAC campaign of Australia was partly due to communications, but communications were supported by legislation, control, enforcement and penalties.

■ **Summing Up**

Further to this discussion, we can pose several questions.

- How can a change be created in the symbolic function attached to some aspects of driving, so that, without attacking strongly held values, change could become desirable?
- What can we learn from the existing experience about the design of communication strategies that can help us affect people's knowledge, attitudes and behaviour in relation to driving?
- How can we recognize leaders, followers and our potentially most supportive partners?
- How can it be possible to work simultaneously with government, people at large and the business sector toward a revision of driving?
- How can we constantly increase the circle of partnership involved in the process?

- How can we develop this partnership in order to deal ethically with a revision of driving, so as to ensure as a consequence the active participation of all partners?
- What are the specific actions that will promote a revision of driving, materialize that revision and establish new cultural paradigms?

☐ *Recommendations for a communication campaign strategy*

My analysis of the two focus groups lead to recommendations in which some principles are applicable to all the population but different strategies are required in order to address the different groups involved. A large group of people does not necessarily include a majority of subjects who share specific traits and concerns, but instead is formed by a large number of "minorities" who suffer among them, for different reasons, a similar problem—in our case, a vulnerability to collisions. Any communication strategy aimed at road users will have to include a variety of messages, so that the different clusters involved can recognize themselves in the communications. My studies suggest a number of common elements that may apply to any of the groups studied, but specific recommendations relating to the high-risk driver need to be considered.

A number of social values have to be affected by a communications campaign if it is to succeed. The objectives to be achieved should include the following:

- O N R I S K : to reduce the social value of risk-taking and to teach risk-perception and risk-reduction skills.
- O N P E R C E P T I O N O F R E A L I T Y : to increase road users' ability to assess their driving skills properly, the car's ability to manoeuvre and the severity of the risks faced.
- O N P E R S O N A L V A L U E V E R S U S T H E V A L U E O F T H I N G S : to persuade people to value themselves independently from their car and their driving style.
- O N T H E V A L U E O F R E S P O N S I B I L I T Y : to promote the ideas that driving is a responsible act and that responsible driving has a high social value.
- O N C O M P E T I T I O N V E R S U S C O O P E R A T I O N : to discourage competitiveness and aggressiveness in driving and to encourage cooperation toward a better traffic flow.
- O N T H E E M O T I O N A L C O M P O N E N T O F D R I V I N G : to reduce the emotional involvement that dangerous drivers invest in driving.

Recommended implementation methods include the following:

- Decision-makers involved in the implementation of the campaign should be brought into the production team as early as possible to ensure their cooperation at the appropriate time.
- The campaign must be sustained, intense and multi-channel, using all media appropriate for the target audience. This is not to be seen as a "shotgun approach" but as one that considers the most important emerging characteristics of the different members of the target group and the specific media they interact with.
- The campaign should seek favourable news coverage and gain the support of the entertainment industry for the promotion of its goals; it should aim at making traffic safety part of the social agenda, gaining support from both government and the private sector.
- The campaign should be complemented by a revision of legislation, and the enforcement and publicity thereof.
- The campaign should include a long-term plan divided in distinct phases, each having achievable, specific and measurable objectives.
- Each phase of the campaign must concentrate on one point. Each conceptual point might require a number of specific pieces of communication. (see Frascara, 1997)

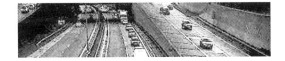

MY STUDIES OF DRIVERS suggest that there are at least two clusters of drivers: the high-risk driver and the general driver. Each of these clusters includes a variety of components, and two different types of high-risk drivers can be distinguished for the purpose of designing a communication strategy.

One type of high-risk driver seems to suffer from excessive personal invest-ment in driving. This driver's collisions seem to be the result of cultural values, and result from an overestimation of the driver's information-processing capacity, reaction times and vehicular performance. Any communication campaign directed at these drivers should offer them something they desire if it intends to remove the thrill of sensorial load and adrenaline flow. These drivers could learn from their collisions but are unwilling, always believing that next time they will be able to avoid the crash, or that the pleasure of freedom and speed is worth the risk. Communication campaigns directed at such drivers must be motivational, aimed at affecting the exteriorization of their value systems or their value systems themselves, not an easy task.

Another type of high-risk driver seems to suffer from an inability to assess risks. This driver does not drive aggressively on purpose but dangerously out of poor judgement. This driver is repeatedly involved in collisions without really understanding their causes, and assumes they are accidents. Social conditions, lack of general education and the nature of the daily job create a context of low mental development that cannot be counteracted by a traffic-safety campaign. Mass-media communications directed at these drivers would have little effect, since they will not be easily able to adopt new behaviours on the basis of their experiences in crashes or information directed at them.

General drivers are normally safe but suffer from a lack of experience and knowledge that makes them vulnerable to a large variety of traffic hazards. Mass-media communications could centre on information, since these drivers already agree with the importance of safety and are able to adopt new behaviours on the basis of both experience and information.

☐ *Future action*
To complete the campaign plan, it will be necessary to develop a survey to find out media preferences of the target group. Further, it will be necessary to develop a series of campaign themes and test prototypes. Finally, a campaign concept, media strategy, and production and deployment budget will form the key elements for actual implementation. For the campaign to be effective, the budget must at least match the level required to launch a new consumer product in the region, and the campaign must be supported by legislation and policing.

14 DRIVER SKILL
Performance and Behaviour

LAWRENCE P. LONERO

THIS CHAPTER ATTEMPTS TO contextualize the role of skill in drivers' on-road performance and behaviour. It is primarily conceptual and theoretical, based on earlier literature reviews in support of exercises to develop a driver-education curriculum, as well as a certain amount of practical experience in driver preparation. It briefly touches on the fundamental human capacities that underpin the diverse skills of driving. It presents a conceptual model of ten categories of drivers' skills and offers an overview from three different conceptions of skill: traditional pre-industrial, modern "human engineering" and postmodern "human re-engineering." It draws a hierarchical distinction between real-time driving skills and broader driver skills. Finally, this chapter attempts to sketch a future direction for a skills perspective on drivers, as smarter highways and vehicles become available.

■ What Is Skill?

A skill is a learned ability to perform some task effectively and efficiently. Traditionally, abilities called skills involved relatively simple physical manipulation of tools and materials toward some objective product, as in arts, crafts and industrial trades. These are "perceptual-motor skills," in which the skilled person perceives critical aspects of the task and performs just the right motor actions to accomplish it (e.g., Welford, 1968).

Modern interest in skill derives from industrial psychology and human-engineering research. These disciplines broadened the traditional definition of skills, and mental processes and abilities came to be seen as trainable skills.

More recently, the human-growth movement has broadened the definition of skill again, as great faith has developed in the "re-engineering" possibilities of human perfectibility. Just about every human trait now seems to be viewed as a trainable skill, starting with social skills and including communication skills, thinking skills, decision skills, managerial skills, and life skills, among many others. The concept of skill may have become so inclusive that it has lost useful meaning, as has happened with attitude. Office posters and coffee mugs proclaim that "attitude is everything." Similarly, if everything is a skill, the concept becomes meaningless. Nevertheless, a skills perspective can be useful, so long as we remember that the same activity may also be usefully viewed through different perspectives, such as motivational, cultural or ethical/legal.

Clearly, driving is a skill, in both the old and new senses. A traditional skills perspective on driving has been used since the early days of road safety and driver education. Driving researchers and educators argue that driving is a complex skill and present the idea to non-experts as a reason for taking driving more seriously However, to many non-experts, who may have taught themselves to drive, driving seems as simple and natural as walking. Of course, walking is also complex when viewed in scientific detail, and its performance may be enhanced through learning and practice. Nevertheless, most people are content with their own driving skill and performance, and it is hard to induce change in either (Lonero & Clinton, 1998). As part of a complex performance, driving has both continuous skills (such as tracking) and discontinuous skills (such as gear shifting). With much practice, many aspects of perceptual-motor skills become automatic, requiring little attention or thought. Indeed, performance is labelled "skilled" when it becomes automatic (Rasmussen, 1987). The skills of making the car go, keeping it between the lines and stopping before hitting anything are individually mastered very quickly. However, smooth integration of control skills takes much longer.

In the modern, human-engineering sense, driving skills also involve the purely mental activity needed to maintain situational awareness and manage vehicle systems in a wide range of conditions. In the postmodern, human-re-engineering sense, there is more than driving skill involved in driver skill, including the life, social and consumer skills required, as well as self-control and values-management skills, if skills they truly be.

Driving skills also exist in different degrees. As individuals learn, they climb a learning curve, and not all driving skills will be honed to the same level of excellence, even in the same individual. Routine skills are carried out so frequently that they are highly over-learned, no longer improving with further practice. Not all drivers top out at the same level either, of course. Some skills, such as emergency handling, are rarely needed and may degrade or never be learned in the first place, especially in an otherwise "good" driver, as they almost never have an emergency to react to. Certainly an important issue is whether we should focus on the skills of normal, routine driving or on errors, failures and emergencies that lead to crashes (Ranney, 1994). For lack of information on routine driving, this chapter is necessarily biased toward the errors and failures that form the "flip side" of the driver skills record.

■ Basic Human Capacities Underlying Driving Skill

Driving skill is built on a broad foundation of basic human abilities. The underlying capacities (and limitations) are complex and not always well understood. Two aspects of fundamental capabilities are important and often forgotten. First, human information-processing capacities, even in a highly capable individual under optimal conditions, have fundamental limitations that may be exceeded within the range of predictable operational demands. Second, these basic sensory, mental and psycho-physical capacities vary greatly between individuals and within the same individual at different times.

The human engineering perspective on driver failure focusses on the fact that driving demands may exceed a driver's mental capacities at a given moment. As a classical expression of this view, Svenson (1978) wrote,

> Risk stems from the fact that drivers have to conduct their vehicles in situations producing an overload of their information processing and motor capacity, either because of difficult external conditions (e.g., darkness) or because of deteriorated functioning. (p. 267)

Much early research work was devoted to finding relations between stable individual differences in drivers' basic abilities, as measured by lab tests, and their crash risk. In early work, various measures of perceptual style and certain aspects of attention typically showed positive but weak correlations with prior accident history. In his excellent review of driver models, Ranney (1994) concluded,

> Individual differences research has focussed almost entirely on predicting accident rates. To the extent that this research has used performance limits on information-processing tasks as predictors, it implicitly assumes that pre-crash behaviours represent the limiting capabilities of drivers. The questionable validity and the restricted focus on the set of behaviours that precipitate crashes are likely the reasons for the lack of success of efforts to identify predictors of safe driving. (p. 740)

Recently, "useful field of view," a measure of the early stages of visual attention, has shown promise as a tool for understanding driver performance, although primarily for elderly or cognitively impaired drivers in whom this ability may have degraded significantly (Owsley, Ball, Sloane, Roenker & Bruni, 1991). Elander, West and French (1993) also extensively reviewed research on factors related to drivers' differential crash involvement. They point out that research has looked at two categories of skills, "those related directly to driving and more general aspects of information-processing ability that may underlie components of the driving task" (p. 285). They conclude that fundamental abilities that account for some differences in crash risk likely include speed of hazard detection, speed of detecting figures embedded in a complex background and ability to switch attention rapidly.

General abilities underlying driving skills may themselves be trainable. For instance, Gopher (1992) showed that Israeli fighter-pilot trainees learned attention-management skills playing a specially designed computer game and successfully transferred the skills to the cockpit. However, as we will see below, at least some skills are fairly specific to situations and do not readily transfer.

Experience in training "generic" decision skills indicates it is possible to train some aspects of these cognitive skills, but the generic skill does not necessarily transfer to new problems or environments. The use of realistic, relevant and specific subject matter in training enhances the transfer to real decisions. Transfer also depends on the fidelity of simulation of conditions, such as time pressure. There is more to being a skillful real-world decision-maker than just learning a good normative analytic process (Mann, Harmoni & Power, 1989).

■ Looking for the Whole Driver

Many task demands must be met to operate a motor vehicle safely and efficiently. Indeed, the widely respected driving-task analysis done by James McKnight and his colleagues nearly thirty years ago identified as many as 1,500 task requirements (McKnight & Hundt, 1971). Paradoxically, there is no equally comprehensive model of the driver that would explain how we are able to meet these demands most of the time. Many different partial models give us fragmentary glimpses of diverse parts of the driver, similar to the fragmented understanding developed in the parable of the blind men and the elephant. In the parable, the blind protagonists each try to figure out what an elephant is by grasping a different part of the beast's anatomy (Mintzberg, Ahlstrand & Lampel, 1998). Until we have a comprehensive model, we have to make do with examining component parts, but it is important to keep in mind that it is the whole driver that is safe and efficient—or otherwise.

One way of finding out what parts of the driver's skill are more or less critical is to investigate differences between groups with differing crash risk. Addressing collision-causing driver failures, the landmark Indiana in-depth collision investigations study indicated the importance of attention and scanning in crash causation (in Dewar, 1991). The failures shown, in order of prevalence, were improper lookout; excessive speed; inattention; improper evasive action; internal distraction; improper driving technique; inadequately defensive driving technique; false assumption; improper manoeuvre; and overcompensation. Dewar summarized the importance of attention and visual skills as "looking in the right place at the right time," clearly a cognitive skill.

Rothe (1986) reviewed the literature on young, inexperienced drivers' failures, identifying failure to keep in proper lane, running off road; failure to yield right of way; speeding; driving on wrong side of the road; failure to obey traffic signs; reckless driving; inattentiveness; overtaking; fatigue; and poor equipment. McKnight and Resnick (in Young, 1993) summarized frequent youth violations as speeding, sign non-observance, equipment defects, turning unlawfully, passing unsafely, right-of-way violations, major infractions and alcohol. Trankle et al. (1990) reviewed predominantly European research and concluded that young drivers are over-represented in only a few types of crashes: speed related, loss of control, and nighttime. Inappropriate speed in curves and cutting curves were frequent factors. To what extent these failures represent the skill deficiencies of the inexperienced or the excess enthusiasms of youth are still not clear.

What is clear is that experienced drivers as a group have important skill advantages (e.g., West & Hall, 1994). In particular, while on the road, they appear better able to control and distribute attention, automate and integrate the various simple psychomotor-control skills, extract the full richness of information available in the environment, detect and recognize hazards at a safe distance and make driving decisions quickly under pressure. Similarly, based on an extensive review of the driver research literature, Mayhew and Simpson (1995) identified research support for eight individual traits as being related to the excessive risk of collision for young, inexperienced drivers: steering control; speed control; parallel processing/multitasking (skill integration); visual search/scanning; hazard detection; risk assessment; decision-making; risky lifestyle and risk-taking. The first seven of these traits would be seen as skills in either the traditional perceptual-motor sense or the more modern mental-skills sense, and all would seem fair targets for education and training. However, the last in the list, risky lifestyle, seems more reflective of motivation or cultural influences in both the traditional and modern perspectives. A broad, postmodern conception of skill might suggest addressing the last trait by re-engineering "lifestyle-management skills."

High-level self-management skills aside, research findings indicate that weakness in the basic driving skills causes at least some of novice drivers' crashes (Jonah, 1990). It may also be that some driving skills cannot be developed or consistently used until others are (Gregersen, 1994). A model that provides a perspective on the role of skills in drivers' performance thus seems necessary.

■ A Taxonomic Model of Driving and Driver Skills

In aid of developing objectives for new approaches to driver education, Lonero et al. (1995) emphasized the central importance of drivers' cognitive skills among a number of distinct "educable driver qualities." As seen in slightly modified form in Table 14.1, we presented a taxonomic model of drivers' sensory, mental and psychomotor functions. This was an attempt to move beyond the overly simplistic IPDE/SIPDE (identify, predict, decide, execute/scan, identify, predict, decide, execute) models as a basis for developing objectives for driver education. The targeted categories in this model mainly represent stages of information processing and outputs that take place while driving. Immediate, real-time processing takes place continuously, in routine situations, and discontinuously, as the occasional detection, perception and evaluation of potential hazards, and the decisions and actions taken in response. These categories can be seen as families of related skills, that serve related purposes and call upon related underlying capacities. The model also attempts to account for motivation, a common failure in earlier information-processing driver models (Ranney, 1994).

This model attempted to identify major chunks of information processing broken up by steps where critical failure is likely to take place. For instance, a potential hazard might be visually fixated and detected, but still not perceived in any meaningful way, perhaps for lack of understanding of its identity or meaning. These potential failure points are promising intervention sites for education and training. A process model adding hypothetical links to the taxonomy is shown in Figure 14.1.

☐ Knowledge

Driving knowledge consists of a wide range of information stored in both long-term and short-term memory. It includes rules and principles, scripts, schemata, performance routines, recognition templates and expectations. Knowledge builds up continuously as drivers receive instruction and experience driving in the system. Distinguishing knowledge from skills, which are also learned, requires some fine hair-splitting. Perhaps it would be useful to think of knowledge as the content or raw material used by the cognitive and mental skills.

As Fuller (1992) pointed out, experience can be a double-edged sword. We learn bad habits and risky behaviours at the same time as we become wiser about the operation of the system. As we learn the details of how the system

TABLE 14.1
Driver skill categories

Skill Category	Definition	Importance
Knowledge	**Cognitive/memory**: Experiences, facts, rules, principles and expectations stored in long-term memory	Provides the background against which all the perceptual and cognitive functions take place
Attention	**Cognitive/perceptual**: Controlling, dividing and switching focus	Real-time management of cognitive resources and perceptual channel-capacity, screening out distractions
Detection	**Sensory/pre-attentional**: Fixation, formation of images	Identifies changes in the environment that may need identification and evaluation
Perception	**Sensory/cognitive**: Processing images to extract meaning and produce schemata	Creates awareness and understanding of constantly-changing situations
Evaluation	**Cognitive/affective**: Risk analysis of situation to produce outcome expectations, attributions	Estimates consequences and probabilities of alternative actions in the situation
Decision	**Cognitive/affective**: Matching options and motives	Selects optimal response: risk acceptance or rejection
Motor Skill	**Perceptual-motor**: Integrating control actions	Execution of intended manoeuvres
Imagination	**Cognitive**: Safety margin, anticipatory responses	Time, speed and space choices
Motivation	**Affective/social**: Transient objectives, drives, needs, emotions	Prioritizes and balances a large and often conflicting set of goals and values
Responsibility	**Cognitive/affective/cultural**: Executive "policy" skills	Chooses goals and values, directs self-monitoring, consistently controls transient states

FIGURE 14.1
Process model of skill categories

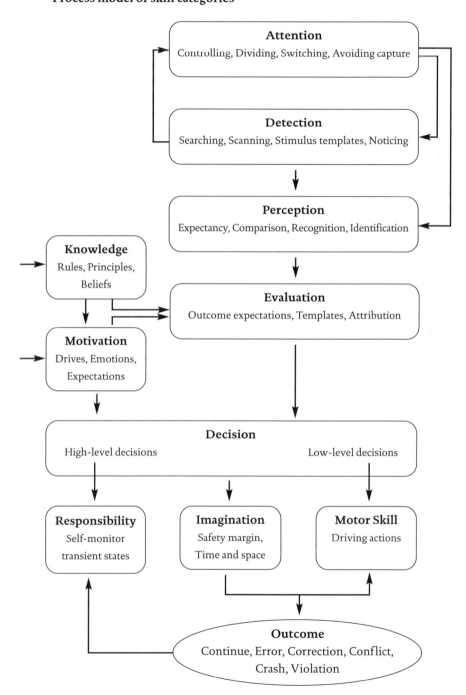

works and other road users behave, strong expectations are established. Critical errors often occur when expectations are violated. The importance of driver expectancy is recognized in highway design (e.g., Alexander & Lunenfeld, 1986). Crude attempts to modify expectations have been undertaken through exhorting drivers to "expect the unexpected," although it is not clear if this has ever been helpful or if drivers can deliberately "manage" their own expectations in the manner suggested.

Knowledge has pervasive enabling influences on skills and other driver qualities, as reflected in the process model. As in most cognitive tasks, a wide range of different types of knowledge may be implicit in the performance (e.g., Resnick, 1987). However, it is also important to keep in mind what knowledge cannot do. For instance, it does not necessarily create motivation for behaviour change, as has been assumed by many ineffective, traditional safety education programs (Lonero et al., 1994a; 1994b).

☐ *Attention*
In the model, attention is meant to include the states of vigilance, alertness and mental arousal, essentially the "internal" predisposition to interact with the environment. It directs and focusses searching, scanning and noticing, and it determines how our limited supply of mental processing capacity will be allocated. Attention is both automatic and controllable by deliberate action. The prolonged, disciplined alertness that driving requires is one of those task demands we humans are not inherently good at, and we have to develop attention management as a skill.

The key skill factors in control of attention involve pre-attentional screening of irrelevant targets and events; allocating attention over the many driving tasks conducted simultaneously; and switching the allocation of focussed attention in appropriate ways. Attention must be allocated among different spatial areas (e.g., ahead versus behind) and different conceptual categories of objects or information (e.g., objects in the road versus vehicle instruments; see Allport, 1992). Training and experience place a stimulus in a category that gets attended to. Drivers must learn what needs attention and how much of their limited resources each task item demands or deserves. There is evidence that attention control is trainable (Gopher, 1992), as well as being improved and eventually automated by experience (e.g., Shiffrin & Schneider, 1977). Attention must not only be directed to task components and the immediate environment but to all the important factors that make up the driver's situation. These include what is known, what is unknown and even what is imagined.

Critical errors can result from any failure of attention, and there is evidence that control of attention is related to collision experience (Arthur, Strong &

Williamson, 1994; Dewar, 1991). It is possible to be "paying attention" and still miss important information in the environment, for a number of reasons. First are the fundamental limitations of attention channel capacity. Second is the many possible mental-processing failures "downstream" because of sensory, scanning or other detection or perception limitations. The model assumes that proper attention is necessary but not sufficient for the detection of visual targets and other information input.

□ *Detection*

Detection skills primarily involve visual searching, scanning and noticing things that are relevant. Also important at times are inputs from the other senses, such as hearing a siren, feeling a change in pavement texture with the kinesthetic (muscle) senses or feeling an incipient skid with the vestibular (balance) senses. Our senses are built to detect change and contrast. With our sharp central vision, we fixate "targets," objects that are moving or otherwise contrast with the background. With our peripheral vision, we are particularly sensitive to moving targets; we use peripheral vision with exquisite precision to orient ourselves in space, detecting changes in lateral position on the road and very fine changes in heading (yaw).

As with attention, detection skills have limitations. It is possible to "look but fail to see," a frequent reported occurrence in crashes. Little is known about these detection failures, and what seems to be a failure of detection could also result from "upstream" failures in attention or "downstream" failures in the further processing of detected data. However, the visual system has distinct limits as to how much information it can take in (e.g., Moray, 1990) and is highly variable in how much information it does take in.

At the basic sensory level of the visual system, the eye must fix on a target to view it clearly. Unfamiliar and unexpected objects are less likely to be detected. It may be that a sort of "pre-recognition" template is necessary for an object to be reliably fixated. The model suggests that attention and detection interact in both directions: what is detected may also affect attention, altering its distribution in space or over categories of potential targets. The issues of where the filtering processes of attention take place (blocking irrelevant stimuli that are not attended to) are still not resolved in basic research (e.g., Allport, 1992). We could theorize that the attention-detection loop is the source of both the filtering and the "looked but didn't see" errors. Weakness of skills in this area could also mediate novice drivers' slow reaction to potential hazards (e.g., Fuller, 1990; Rumar, 1990). Novices have not yet developed effective attentional distribution and scanning, and they may miss memory templates for visual targets that should be fixated.

Night driving is a particular challenge for detection skills. Drivers cannot detect a target if it is out of range of their headlights on a dark road. Even many experienced drivers do not recognize the visual limitations of driving with headlight illumination only (e.g., Leibowitz & Owens, 1986), and insight into these limitations needs training. Anticipating and responding to sensory detection limitations is perhaps another of the hypothetical high-level self-monitoring and management "skills."

☐ *Perception*
Perception consists of mental organizing and processing of patterns of data from the senses, turning data into information. Perception is largely the comparison of detected patterns to known patterns or templates, resulting in the recognition and identification of potential hazards, opportunities and other relevant information.

The process model reflects the fact that perception is itself influenced by cognitive knowledge, experience and expectation (e.g., Ranney & Simmons, 1992; Shinar & Drory, 1983; Shinar, Rockwell & Malecki, 1980). Some comparative knowledge, in the form of schemata or templates, is needed to see the situation with understanding. Endsley (1995) points out,

> In addition to affecting the selection of elements for perception, the way in which information is perceived is directed by the contents of both working and long-term memory. Advanced knowledge of the characteristics, form and location of information, for instance, can significantly facilitate the perception of information ... That is, one's preconceptions or expectations about information will affect the speed and accuracy of the perception of that information. (p. 42)

Expectancy may operate through some memory patterns and templates being more readily available than others. Perception errors include failure of timely recognition or misinterpretation of what is seen. Unless it cannot be recognized, a detected target is identified and stored knowledge about that type of target is added. A pattern of perceptions, both current and recent ones stored in memory, contribute to "situation awareness," another complex skill concept, which has proven useful particularly in combat pilots, whose targets are heavily armed and hostile.

☐ *Evaluation*
In this model, enriched perceptual information is output to an evaluation skills category, where higher "thought" processes can evaluate it for opportunities and risk. Evaluation of situations is also shown to be influenced by knowledge,

in the sense that rules and principles are needed to predict outcomes and are built up mainly from experience (e.g., Wilde, 1994). As with most other driver skills, evaluation becomes virtually automatic and "unconscious" for routine driving.

Evaluation is a complex cognitive skill, and as such it is strongly affected by impairments such as alcohol and fatigue. As reflected in the process model, evaluation is also influenced by the driver's motivational states. For instance, if the driver is hurried or angry, a small gap in traffic may seem less risky. Endsley (1995) summarized these motivational effects as follows:

> SA (situation awareness) is largely affected by a person's goals and expectations, which will influence how attention is directed, how information is perceived, and how it is interpreted. This top-down processing will operate in tandem with bottom-up processing in which salient cues will activate appropriate goals and models. (p. 49)

Evaluation errors could result from lack of knowledge about likely outcome, because of the evaluation being distorted by some transient motivation or impairment, or by some consistent, systematic bias (Colbourne, 1978). Examples of the last might be excess optimism (optimism bias) or "attribution bias." Attribution bias is the tendency to attribute one's own errors to situational factors, while attributing the errors of others to malicious intent or fundamental character defect, a bias that may be a major contributor to "road rage." In the model, evaluation produces predictions as to how the current situation is likely to unfold and passes them on to real-time, on-line decision-making skills.

☐ *Decision*

Given a particular situation evaluation, final authority for action (or inaction) rests with the driver's decision skills, which weigh the optional courses of action, selecting and timing responses. Decision skills are pivotal in this and any other plausible driver model. A clear definition of decision making is provided by McWhirter et al. (1994):

> Decision-making is a goal-directed sequence of affective and cognitive operations that leads to adaptation of behavioural responses to external and internal challenges or demands. A clear link exists between deficits in decision-making skills and high-risk behaviour. (p. 192)

Decision skills include identifying and weighing optional courses of action, and selecting and timing responses to optimize the driver's personal benefit–cost equations. Although strongly connected and influenced by evaluations, decision skills are clearly distinct and autonomous; we might choose a different action in two identically evaluated situations, perhaps for some "good" reason outside the situation.

In real-time driving continuous, evaluation and decision are seen as necessary because few of the elements that are perceived require any action. But continuous real-time driving decisions are only a part of the driver skill picture. Drivers' decision skills can be seen as a hierarchy with various levels ranging from the operational to the strategic (Ranney, 1994). From the human-re-engineering perspective, it is clear that they even reach beyond into the realm of self-management decisions and values-consistency skills.

Even the real-time decision skills are based in complex, highly variable cognitive processes. They depend on and are influenced by the driver's knowledge and motivation, and they are strongly affected by impairments such as alcohol and fatigue. Clearly, the motivational influence on decision-making is critically important (e.g., a consistently evaluated hazard may be acted upon differently if we are angry). In recognition of this importance, a major portion of intensive, high-performance training (as in military and commercial aviation) is to practise decision-skill responses so heavily that they become less susceptible to disruption by transient motivational and emotional states.

The driver's motivation will influence not only the choice of action but also the timing of action. A risk-accepting, inappropriate choice will often result. Since many potential hazards do not develop, we often choose to delay response. This may be a kind of skill in its own right; it would be inefficient, and maybe even unsafe, to react to every possible hazard as soon as it is perceived. A critical failure of this skill occurs when a decision is delayed until safe correction of the problem is no longer certain or even possible. Both the choice of appropriate response and the choice of appropriate timing of response are critical skills.

□ *Motor skills*

Drivers must have a certain amount of traditional perceptual-motor skill to execute an intended action properly. The required motor skills can develop over a wide range of levels, from the basic ability to steer and control speed to high-performance, stunt and emergency crash-avoidance skills. Basic, individual control skills are relatively simple and quickly learned. More critical, and requiring more practice, is the integration of the basic skills into smooth, coordinated, simultaneous automatic operation (Mayhew & Simpson, 1995).

Eventually, the individual skills and their integration become consistent and automatic in routine driving. In effect, they are pushed to the periphery: in a figurative sense when they can be performed simultaneously with other tasks and place little demand on higher mental resources, and in a literal sense, such as lane positioning and tracking becoming based on peripheral vision.

We must also recognize that drivers do not accomplish manoeuvres alone: they are dependent on the response of the vehicle to their control inputs. Higher levels of motor skill involve perceiving feedback from vehicle response through all the senses and having the ability to correct control inputs quickly in real time during manoeuvres. Given that the vehicle responds as intended, the outcome will still depend on how much of a "safety margin" has been left for manoeuvring.

□ *Imagination*

The amount of safety margin that is chosen and maintained is the result of a higher-order mental skill process that takes place at some time ahead of any obvious hazard or risky situation. It is in effect a preparatory response for possible situations and scenarios that cannot yet be seen but must be imagined. It is, therefore, an abstract mental skill, which we have previously called safety margin but from a skills perspective might better be called imagination.

This highly abstract skill is probably not practised too strenuously even by good, experienced drivers, as we usually do not prepare for even fairly obvious low-probability situations. Imagination skill may be especially difficult for novice drivers, who appear to be more bound by what they can actually see and who lack the experience to know all the possible hazards that could appear with little warning. They also lack the "spare" mental capacity to devote to such an abstract effort.

In real-time driving, safety margins are manifest primarily through choice of driving speed and placement of the vehicle, although other preparatory responses, such as "covering the brake," have occasionally been taught and practised. The amount of time and space available will determine whether an intended action can be successful and whether there is time to try something else if the first choice does not seem to work. The outcome of the situation provides feedback and contributes to the growth of the self-managing driver skills.

□ *Motivation*

In the model, motivation is the internal "affective" or "emotional" force compelling the individual to seek satisfaction of personal needs. It consists of the appetites, drives, emotions and utility-maximizing efforts that energize behaviour and direct choices. In part, motivation comes from within, driven by personal needs or norms (Parker et al., 1992) and the need to reduce uncertainty. It also may be driven by external factors such as incentives and disincentives (e.g., Wilde, 1994), as well as more social and cultural forces such as "active caring" for the welfare of others (Geller, 1991, 1996). The driver model shows that individual motivation affects many aspects of skilled driving performance. It activates and directs behaviour toward the immediate objectives.

The question of whether is it is useful to view motivation as a trainable skill brings us back to the arguments about postmodern conceptions of human re-engineering versus intrinsic motives and cultural influences. This argument should be resolved more on pragmatic than logical grounds. The health-promotion field has had some success in enhancing healthy behaviours through this broad skills perspective (Lonero & Clinton, 1998). Related approaches have been used in some driver-improvement efforts, such as training in anger-management skills for "road rage" perpetrators.

☐ *Responsibility*

Responsibility in the model is defined as the driver's top cognitive management, a sort of rational executive process focussed on the highest level goals and values. As with any successful manager, there are skill components, in this case presumably mostly the postmodern, life-re-engineering skills. Responsibility is based on the values and internalized norms that influence individual motivation and character, as well as ethical, pro-social conduct.

Responsibility helps energize and direct behaviour toward goals beyond the personal and immediate, requiring a commitment to helping meet social objectives beyond those of the individual. It requires acting in accordance with good practices based on risks identified over whole communities, even if the risk seems too small to worry about for each individual.

Responsibility shapes and monitors shorter-term motivation, requiring the capacity to assess one's own performance on the road and to keep it in line with personal and social values. It provides the basic self-correcting and self-control needed for safe, mature, efficient and socially responsible use of the roads. There are legitimate questions as to whether responsibility is "trainable," even though it can probably be influenced in some systematic ways. In practice, individuals are most likely to take on responsibility when they are persuaded or induced to become actively involved in the issue, as in Geller's (1991) active caring model, or as "transmitters" of persuasion (Parker, Manstead, Stradling & Reason, 1992a; Parker, Manstead, Stradling, Reason & Baxter, 1992b). Perhaps these "involvement" activities are in fact higher-order, skill-building training and practice. As Wilde (1994) suggested, this may be what we mean by education, as opposed to training.

■ How Important Is Driving Skill?

Drivers' bottom-line outcomes, in terms of safety and efficiency, result from their performance capability (driving skills and whatever else determines what they are able to do) and their actual behaviour, which includes what they choose to do (Lonero et al., 1995; Naatanen & Summala, 1974). Both amount to more than just skill, at least as traditionally conceived. Bower (1991) points out that the alternative to the human-factors view of the driver is "to view the driver as a bundle of motivations" (p. 10). This view was expressed by Fuller (1984):

> It is the driver's own actions which determine the difficulty of his task. Driving is essentially a self-paced activity. Because of this it may be argued that the driver's motivation is at least as important, if not more so, than limitations of his perceptual-motor capabilities. (p. 1139)

Presumably he includes the resulting skills as well.

One way of studying the role of skill in driver performance is to look at what happens when certain skill components are improved. Lonero et al. (1995) reviewed evaluations of advanced driver-training programs. Advanced training, of both the defensive-driving and collision-avoidance types, holds out attractive possibilities for skill improvement. However, until recently there was little evidence that skill-improvement training had any positive effect on crashes, at least given the skills targeted for improvement (e.g., McKnight, Simone & Weidman, 1982; Lund & Williams, 1984; Whitworth, 1983).

Evaluations of specialized car-handling training suggest the counterintuitive conclusion that raising levels of these skills may lead to a higher crash risk (e.g., Glad, 1988; Jones, 1993; OECD Scientific Expert Group, 1990; Siegrist & Ramseier, 1992). Williams and O'Neill (1974) found much earlier that licensed amateur race drivers, as a group, had poor on-road driving records, despite presumably superior skills in car-handling. Around the same time, Naatanen and Summala (1974) concluded that a more comprehensive approach to driver improvement was needed. Otherwise, there is a clear danger that "increased skills raise the level of aspiration in driving (higher speed, more frequent overtaking, smaller margins of safety, etc.)" (p. 243). The OECD Scientific Expert Group came to similar conclusions (1990).

There may be a mutually supportive effect of safety motivation and cognitive/perceptual skills, as suggested by Gregersen's "insight" training to sensitize the driver to the limitations of skills (Gregersen & Berg, 1994; Gregersen & Bjurulf, 1996). Insight may emerge as a critical high-level driver skill. But not every skill-training attempt is actually effective in increasing the targeted skill, let alone some downstream measure of safety performance. This is supported by Gregersen's slippery-road training work with young drivers, who showed increases in confidence even without any actual increase in skill (Gregersen & Bjurulf, 1996). Most training evaluations have not looked at intermediate effects, such as the effects on skill or confidence, but looked at downstream safety records.

When the landmark DeKalb County study was followed up over six years, it was found that a lower-skilled group trained in a minimal curriculum had fewer crashes (6 percent) than the untrained controls (Weaver, 1987). Lund et al. re-analyzed the DeKalb data and concluded that the lower skills of the minimal curriculum students led to slower licensing and more caution in driving after they were licensed (Lund, Williams & Zador, 1986). Mayhew and Simpson (1997) provide an excellent recent review of the DeKalb experiment and its sequel.

Improving driving skills may be necessary but not sufficient for improved safety, because situational factors, motives and higher-level driver skills are clearly important. If crashes result from what drivers choose as much as from what they are able or unable to do, we must consider a whole hierarchy of driver skills, ranging from "simple" control to coordination of controls, through a range of higher mental skills, perceptual, cognitive and "meta-cognitive."

■ Driver Skill and Preparation in the Future

It is interesting to speculate how emerging trends in driver task demands and skills might influence alternative futures. Driver preparation is not immune to the influence of broader societal trends, such as demographics; social/cultural trends and movements; economic globalization; brands, relationship marketing and industry consolidation; and the movement to quality and standardization. To provoke thought and discussion, I will briefly point out some directions of likely change.

In the past, drivers have occasionally had to learn to use innovations, such as electric turn signals and controlled-access freeways. In the future, technology-forced task changes will occur much more rapidly. Even fairly basic skills will be affected by accelerating technical changes in vehicles, as has already been seen with airbags and anti-lock brake systems. Whole new skill areas will develop in response to "intelligent vehicle and highway systems" and other developments, such as vision enhancement systems (Gish, Staplin & Perel, 1999). How drivers learn will also likely change, as emerging trends reshape driver training and testing. Particular needs of target learners can be addressed by adaptive instructional technology. More individualized and self-paced instruction, with active involvement of peers and parents, is crucial (Mann et al., 1989).

In the twenty-first century, trends in organization, technology and standards may converge with increased sensitivity to produce real progress; or else they may diverge to produce a nightmare of bureaucratic and technical chaos. The current backward state of driver preparation provides an opportunity for a leap forward, perhaps analogous to less-developed nations' skipping straight to wireless technology for their communications. Organization and management of service delivery is less exciting than technology, but serious change is needed, likely in the management of driver training and testing as well.

Much change in the training of driving skills will be technology-driven. Micro-computer technology has made a start in changing the delivery of instruction and testing services, and driver education is available on CD-ROM, through the Internet, and in "virtual reality." Intelligent vehicle and highway systems will change the driving task and force more effective and efficient training applications, perhaps even for experienced drivers. Computer-based instruction and simulation will be consolidated into seamless, proprietary training environments for lifelong learning, which will be needed to operate in the intelligent vehicle and highway environment. Simulation will be used for training higher-level cognitive skills, such as risk-management decisions and attention management (e.g., Brock, 1997; Decina, Gish, Staplin & Kirchener, 1996; Gopher, 1992).

Drivers' mental workload will perhaps increase unduly through lack of coordination among the sources of even relatively simple highway and vehicle technologies, each of which is individually intended to aid the driver. On-board vehicle technologies will likely progressively exceed current driver capabilities, and drivers will require training in new skills. Check rides and maybe even "type ratings" will verify that drivers have the skills needed to pilot their new cars safely and efficiently (Sharfman & Lonero, 1999).

Just how much of a problem even simple technologies may present is just now becoming widely recognized. Industry equips vehicles with innovative and sophisticated technology, but people must be taught to understand and use it. An example is smart airbags with sensors in the front seats. Drivers can inadvertently defeat this technology, in a dangerous manner, simply by placing their groceries on the front passenger seat. This has profound implications for vehicle design and manufacture, as well as for the training, education, testing, certification and upgrading of drivers' skills. A major bottleneck to automotive progress may occur in drivers' skills—and in the product developers' abilities to understand and accommodate them.

Even relatively simple innovative technologies require thoughtful driver preparation for their potential to be fully realized and for negative side effects to be minimized. The recent examples of problems with car phones, airbags and anti-lock braking systems show that technical mismatches with driver skills must be anticipated and managed. Increasingly complex vehicles imply lifelong learning for drivers. People are *necessarily* unfamiliar with innovative technology. Newly available and soon to be available vehicle technologies include satellite-based (GPS) navigation systems; traffic information and route planning systems; multimedia entertainment systems; on-board video game units; radio-based data system; on-board e-mail and Internet connectivity; integrated, centralized control for driver inputs to vehicle systems (touch screens); multiple-zone climate conditioning; in-car shopping, reservations, banking and bill-paying; electronic brake-force distribution to supplement ABS; electronic yaw-stability systems; radar proximity sensors, smart cruise control and collision-warning systems; video-based collision prediction, warning and active avoidance; active anti-roll suspensions; infrared night-vision enhancement; heads-up displays; sonar parking guide systems; on-board data recording and crash reporting "black box" systems; highway–vehicle data communications; emergency call systems and breakdown diagnosis/assistance; two-way satellite communications; run-flat tires; passcard keyless entry; automatic road toll transponders (and "ports" in coated glass for them); higher average engine performance capabilities; tall, heavy sport-utility vehicles and personal trucks; and smart all-wheel-drive systems.

These, and systems not yet imagined, will have serious implications for vehicle usability and for driver skills and preparation. Some technologies will tax skills, knowledge and even perhaps fundamental mental "channel capacity," at least initially. For example, ABS pedal feedback at first apparently scared drivers, who then released the brakes inappropriately. Time and education efforts may have fixed this initial problem, but all may not be well with ABS even now. The AAA Foundation for Traffic Safety and Insurance Institute for Highway Safety found that the combination of ABS, the car's responsive steering and drivers' inappropriate emergency-steering reactions seemed to send cars off the road out of control. A substantial research program has been undertaken by the US National Highway Traffic Safety Administration (NHTSA) to verify these findings. Other new systems with the driver "in the loop" will also undoubtedly interact in unexpected ways.

The main bottleneck on the route to "smarter" highways, cars and drivers will be in the driver's head. The critical issue for innovation is driver knowledge: that is, both what the technology innovator knows about drivers and what drivers know about new technology. It is far from clear who will invest in the research and development to advance the general driver performance knowledge required for meeting these needs and develop the necessary content, methods and training/testing services.

Changing driving skill requirements and rapidly advancing technologies for delivery of training and testing will demand more valid, credible content for driver education. As demands become more critical and effective training becomes more technically feasible, driver preparation will be under more pressure to teach and test the right things. A large body of empirical research data and limited explanatory theories already exist on driver performance and behaviour, but major areas of ignorance about crash causation and especially about normal driver performance remain. Better use of current knowledge and faster, more efficient creation of new knowledge is the key to progress. Creating the required knowledge will place a great demand on driver research and development services. However, the data-gathering abilities of intelligent vehicles and highways will help answer the age-old questions of what drivers are capable of and what they actually do in "normal" driving. The massive data of integrated training and testing systems can be used as "development machines," leading to effective training and valid testing of driving skills.

Arguably, the highest-level driver skill performance is that of a concerned, active citizen, motivated and able to ensure that the driving world becomes a better place for mobility, safety and equity. The need to justify regulation and to support competitive claims for privatized services will generate a lively, contentious evaluation research environment. The need to show that restrictions on liberty are reasonable and effective has been better honoured in principle than in practice. However, for our future driver-citizen, political expediency and common-sense ideas of "what ought to work" should not be good enough. If the quality trend really catches on, even governments may have to evaluate their driver testing and other programs. Skillful driver-citizens would demand equally skillful and transparent governance of the roadway system. "Something must be done" would be replaced with "Something *effective* will be done."

15 — BREAKING THE CRYSTAL BALL

*Participatory Action Research
and Traffic Safety in the School*

CLAY LAFLEUR

*I am conscious of the world as consisting of multiple realities ...
Among the multiple realities there is one that presents itself
as reality* par excellence. *This is the reality of everyday life.*
(BERGER & LUCKMANN, 1966, P. 35)

*You argue that a man cannot enquire about that which he knows or about that
which he does not know; for if he knows, he has no need to enquire; and if not,
he cannot; for he does not know the very subject about which he is to enquire.*
(MENO'S DILEMMA, CITED IN PETRIE, 1981, P. 2)

I VIVIDLY REMEMBER a colleague (Boomer, 1985) saying "To learn deliberately is to do research." In a sense, participatory action research in classrooms and schools breathes life into the antonym of this statement—that is, "To do research is to learn deliberately." It is my premise in this chapter that students and teachers who perform participatory action research on social issues like traffic safety are intimately connected to learning—learning that is relevant, meaningful and connected to the reality of everyday life. As Petrie (1981) indicates, the dilemma between inquiry and learning is "to alternate in a constantly adaptive way between what we already know and what we do not yet know. It requires us to act in the world as well as think about it" (p. 223).

Participatory action research is a social and practical form of inquiry. It is a way of thinking and acting that supports evidence-based conversations designed to bring about social change that reflects a significant community concern. More specifically, students and teachers who engage in systematic and intentional inquiry are acquiring knowledge and skills that are integral to life-long learning. By engaging in a heuristic process that involves the posing of questions, the gathering of good data, the analysis and interpretation of those data, critical dialogue and planned social action, these individuals are being groomed to become informed and responsible members of society. They are internalizing the ethical, virtuous, responsible and practical approaches to everyday activities, including traffic safety.

It is not my intention to limit my comments in this chapter to traffic-safety issues only. While I will use a number of examples related specifically to traffic safety, it is important to realize that the assumptions supporting a culture of inquiry in classrooms and schools transcends any particular topic or field of study. The approach I am advocating follows a recursive cycle of planning, studying, acting and reflecting (e.g., Carr & Kemmis, 1986; Cochran-Smith & Lytle, 1993; Heron, 1996). There is an increasingly large number of Internet resources (e.g., Schafer, 1998; Dick, 2000) that can be used to enhance understanding and social action in a variety of areas that individuals encounter in daily living.

I particularly value several noteworthy characteristics of participatory action research.

- Individuals are no longer marginalized. Their knowledge about their own local context is acknowledged and legitimized.
- Teachers and students must negotiate and construct what counts as knowledge. Participatory action research is a powerful way to understand how the curriculum is constructed and reconstructed.
- Individuals are empowered. They choose issues that are important and engage in inquiry that is meaningful to them in their situation. Inquiry is guided by issues and concerns based on their own practice. Research is no longer a privileged activity of others, done only by experts or to individuals.
- The recursive and cyclical nature of participatory action research— planning, studying, acting and reflecting—promotes individual growth. It promotes reflection-in-action, reflection-on-action and

reflection-for-action (Brubacher, Case & Reagan, 1994). In addition, it helps individuals develop their own living theories of day-to-day practice.

- Participatory action research is a social enterprise. It involves working collaboratively and cooperatively with others.

- Participatory action research is ideally suited to working in a world where change, uncertainty, turbulence, intensification and fragmentation dominate. There is a mutual sharing of roles and responsibilities. The iterative design provides ongoing feedback that promotes public conversations, problem-solving and decision-making.

- The inquiry process invites the use of multiple perspectives (Rothe, 1990) and a wide range of complementary qualitative and quantitative research methods. The focus on complementarity (Rothe, 1981; Lafleur, 1990) allows the portrayal of inside and outside perspectives of a situation or phenomenon.[1]

- The focus is on informing local practice rather than making generalizable truth statements.

- Participatory action research is educative. The knowledge and skills acquired become essential to solving problems; they support and nurture lifelong learning.

■ Participatory Action Research as Systematic Inquiry

Participatory action research is a form of inquiry that integrates ideas and practices from a variety of different disciplines. As such, the integration of subject matter, the adoption of multiple perspectives and the use of complementary research methods are integral to the inquiry process. Individuals play a crucial role in creating the reality that surrounds them. In addition, the social, cultural and historical contexts provide authentic support for the creation and substantiation of their reality.

The *World Book Dictionary* (1983) describes inquiry as "the act of asking; a search for information, knowledge, truth; a question" (p. 200). This definition helps situate general inquiry within a context devoted to posing questions and solving problems. In other words, there is a predisposition to finding things out. There is also a concern with collecting data and interpreting evidence in such a way as to make knowledge claims—claims that enhance and advance understanding.

What do we typically do when we engage in inquiry? Let me share a couple of everyday examples. We are going about our daily routines and the car won't start. We are pulled up in our tracks as we experience a *discrepancy* between our practice and our expectations. Out of our need for the car to work, a question arises: "Why is this so?" We have a look at the piece of equipment, perhaps involving a little piece of hands-on *participant observation* fieldwork. Perhaps we also do some *secondary analysis* as we consult the manufacturer's manual. We may then develop a hunch (hypothesis) and draw some conclusions. Then we try it out in a form of a *naturalistic experiment* and "give it a go." The car starts and we carry on. Or, the car fails to work and we once more stop in our tracks, ask our question, do further fieldwork to develop yet another theory and try yet another tack, and so on.

Here is a second example. We are looking for our car registration after a police officer has pulled us over for speeding. We review previous *historical data* (memories of earlier experiences) as part of planning our *research design*. We generate several hypotheses and move quickly into the *field* to involve passengers and gather new data to test them. We use some *observational anthropology*. Two brief interviews with our passengers result in reports of failed hunches: the registration papers aren't in the glove compartment or panel door pouches. We interview ourselves, asking aloud where the papers could have been stored as the officer witnesses the activities. Then *secondary analysis* of the previous day's timetable generates a further hunch: it was Sports Day and the papers fell out of the wallet, were picked up and were placed somewhere. Subsequently, an additional round of observation reveals that the registration papers are in the side panel of a sports bag in the trunk.

These trivial events contain a structure that ironically begins with *stopping*. In other words, we do not begin to inquire until we suspend our current action because of the raising of a question. The question prompts us to plan ways to find answers. We now begin a recursive cycle of planning, studying, acting and reflecting that leads to the planning of new and transformed actions.

In participatory action research, we are conscious of making an existing action or practice problematic. In many instances, the problem is the problem. Therefore, we must be explicit about identifying and naming the problem. This task is not easy. Human situations and problems have histories that must be considered. In the context of traffic safety, the process by which individuals identify alcohol and driving as a commonly accepted problem, for example, is the "distinctive subject matter of the sociology of social problems" (Gusfield, 1981). The way in which we view research and inquiry is intricately linked to how we have been trained to identify and solve problems. These filters to problem-solving and method also condition thinking about what is acceptable research and scholarship. Foremost in this discourse is the need to resolve issues such as those related to the meaning and process of knowing, the management of objectivity and subjectivity, the validity of knowledge claims, the generalizability of acquired knowledge and the rigour required.

We need to be deliberate about beginning a process of inquiry and involving others who could or should be involved in that inquiry, systematic and rigorous in our efforts to get answers, and careful in documenting and recording action. For example, a dangerous crosswalk near a high school may become a school problem worthy of inquiry. Students may become involved with the help of planners, engineers or the police. Planners may indicate the reasons for placing a crosswalk in that location. Town engineers may provide students with proper instrumentation on how to collect data on close calls. Members of the police department may provide information such as the number of crashes or violations that happen at the site.

Always skeptical, we must strive to ensure that our inquiry is comprehensive, employs multiple perspectives and uses complementary methods so that we can develop rich understandings about the situations, phenomena or issues we are researching. In this way, we can produce new knowledge that can be used to improve action and practice. Changing our actions is always part of the participatory action research process. And, in a continuing, cyclical way, we research further these changed actions. Open and public conversations that support clarification and reflection of our findings must be encouraged. While consensus may never be reached, it may be possible to move toward a clearer understanding of differences and similarities.

Over the course of many years, I have discovered first-hand that individuals who engage in participatory action research achieve the following:

- gain a better understanding of the situations and issues related to their inquiry;
- feel more empowered and confident in their effort to understand and to implement actions related to the focus of their inquiry;
- view the skills learned during the process as helpful in other areas of their lives;
- have opportunities to serve as project leaders or mentors for less-experienced colleagues;
- develop further leadership skills;
- contribute to the development of a broader community of learners;
- share the results in various ways (e.g., summary reports, storefronts or posters) so others have learned about the results and the processes;
- serve as resources on specific topics for other individuals.

■ Creating a Culture of Inquiry in Public Schools

In a delightful book, Handy (1995) indicates that turbulence and paradox are features of life. Paradox, he writes, is "inevitable, endemic and perpetual. The more turbulent the times, the more complex the world, the more paradoxes" (p. 7). He continues, " There is no perfect answer in a changing world. We must therefore be forever searching" (p. 59). Mutual commitment in this endeavour lays the foundation for a culture of inquiry. Handy's message is, indeed, an optimistic and challenging one:

> The world is up for reinvention in so many ways. Creativity is born in chaos. What we do, what we belong to, why we do it, where we do it— these may all be different and they could be better. Change comes from small initiatives which work, initiatives which, imitated, become the fashion. We cannot wait for great vision from great people, for they are in short supply at the end of history. It is up to us to light our own small fires in the darkness. (pp. 270–271)

Education today is apt to be characterized by chaos, non-rationality and zones of uncertainty. Furthermore, social systems are much more open, mobile and interactive (Urry, 2000). The integration of time, place and self in contexts of relatedness, complexity, interconnections and subjectivity, for example, provide new temporal-spatial patterns and possibilities. Learning often occurs when teachers and students are ready—when past experiences and the anticipation of future visions are unified in the present. In Slattery's (1995) terms, we need to understand time as proleptic; that is, the past and the future have meaning only in the context of the present. For example, having students relate their own personal and family history to a current science, history or traffic-safety project and creatively explore future possibilities helps them develop significant connections. In this sense, time offers an opportunity for curriculum to have meaning for students and to unfold in an environment of unpredictability, dynamic change and natural flow of learning activities.

I believe that classrooms and schools must develop a culture of inquiry if they truly wish to be learning organizations (Senge, Kleiner, Roberts, Ross & Smith, 1999). A culture of inquiry can help each of us embrace different ways of knowing. It occurs when individuals become increasingly more collaborative and participatory during the inquiry process. As I have indicated elsewhere (1995), in such a context "we will be better able to reflect critically on our own assumptions and practices, meaningfully and openly engage in dialogue and participate as responsible members of a community of learners" (p. 19). In other words, a culture of inquiry becomes the catalyst for the mobilization of meaning-making and meaning-shifting. When we choose to work collaboratively and cooperatively together and in a way that promotes commitment, encourages consensus and enhances self-efficacy and understanding, then we are collaborating on our journey in making a difference. We are better positioned to participate in meaningful public conversations, reflect on what we believe and value, and take appropriate social action.

I am convinced that inquiry should be nurtured through participation and result in informed decision-making that improves practice. It is important for student inquiry not only to be concerned with the generation of new knowledge but also to be an educative enterprise and a learning experience for those with a stake in the inquiry. The collection, interpretation and use of comprehensive data are key to making quality decisions, setting directions and creating appropriate programs. In an era of increased accountability, participatory action research has the potential to contribute to inquiry-minded schools and to increase confidence by having public conversations that are based on good evidence and quality research.

I want to advocate passionately for the inclusion of various modes of inquiry as a personal and collective way of meaningfully influencing the roadway system, increasing socio-political awareness and improving learning. Inquiry fosters collaboration and collegiality, questioning and curiosity, reflection related to practice, and searching for better alternatives. Inquiry promotes understanding and provides the foundation for learning. For a culture of inquiry to be maintained in classrooms and schools there must be an ongoing commitment to valuing curiosity, mutual respect, and support among and between individuals. There must be a willingness to try new ideas and practices. And there must be a determination to remain open to the unforeseen and the unexpected.

■ Participatory Action Research Applied to Traffic Safety

Developing a culture of inquiry, like most cultural change, does not occur overnight. It happens as a consequence of sustained efforts to foster and create the conditions necessary for successful learning and inquiry to occur. Inquiry, learning and curriculum go hand in hand. As Stenhouse (1967) says, "Curriculum translates itself into a social process in which learning takes place, discoveries are made and pupils come to terms with culture, and, we hope, learn to think independently within culture" (p. 57). As a guideline, I use seven key questions as a practical, moral and meaningful guide for doing collaborative and reflective inquiry:

- What are you researching?
- Why are you doing the research?
- What difference will your research make?
- Should you do the research?

- How can you make your research scientific and comprehensive?
- What are the equity issues related to your research?
- How can your research improve the situation?

These seven questions provide a framework for interrogating a wide range of topics related to traffic safety. The complexity of traffic-safety issues demands that all the nooks and crannies of each topic or phenomenon be carefully and critically examined. What may appear to be a straightforward research topic, for example, is frequently a much more complex phenomenon mired in controversy.

☐ *What are you researching?*
Since the problem in any research endeavour is usually the problem, knowing what is being investigated must be crystal clear from the outset. What, for example, are the safety issues related to crosswalks near schools? Is the problem related to the behaviour of drivers, e.g., those who fail to reduce speed and drive more carefully? Or are students inadequately educated about how to use crosswalks, e.g., do students fail to look both ways? Is jaywalking prevalent? In both of these instances, is there an element of stunting or risk-taking behaviour? Perhaps the problem is linked to inadequate supervision and lack of adequate patrols? Or maybe it has to do with environmental issues such as those involving road designations, commercial zoning, building density, poor visibility or the lack of adequate signs and road signals. Stopping, problematizing the situation and then posing good questions are the basics of the participatory action research process.

☐ *Why are you doing the research?*
Understanding why you are doing the research is also important. If the inquiry is merely a course requirement or an expectation by local traffic professionals, then there is likely to be little commitment. If, on the other hand, the research is also connected to the lives of individual students and is intended to be used in some public way to improve safety conditions, then motivation is likely to be enhanced. For example, getting students involved in researching speeds near a kindergarten workplace would be enhanced if students are involved in a cross-age tutoring program with the kindergarten children or if the local media present the findings. Awareness of the problem is raised and city officials may be stirred to investigate closer. Making inquiry and the findings of that inquiry personal and public is not only engaging but is also a form of accountability. Part of understanding why you are doing the research is also to understand whom the research is for.

Students need time to ponder significant happenings in their lives. When they have wonderment about a topic, issue or phenomenon, a willingness to do inquiry over time, a commitment to take action and a determination to modify their own behaviour based on the evidence they gather, then the opportunities presented by participatory action research are open-ended. I often reflect on Dearborn's dictum (see Bronfenbrenner, 1977) as a rationale for the inherent value in engaging in inquiry. At root, it says, "If you wish to understand the relation between the developing person and some aspect of his or her environment, try to budge the one, and see what happens to the other."

□ *What difference will your research make?*
It is important to consider what difference your research will make. Participatory action research helps individuals examine important social issues collaboratively and make evidence-based decisions that lead to responsible action. It challenges people to be responsible producers of knowledge and not just consumers of information.

When students and teachers are involved in critically examining social issues, they become more aware of the implications for and impact of these issues on their own lives. In the case of traffic safety, for example, this can involve a range of circumstances related to historical, financial, health, social and situational matters. Participatory action research is a value-added approach to learning that features generic, lifelong skills along with problem solving and responsible social action. Through such inquiry, students and teachers learn how to gather quality data as a way of engaging in consensual decision-making that makes a difference about high-stakes issues. For example, one traffic-safety issue is reliance on witnesses and their actions after a crash. Students may investigate the issue and, in the process, learn first-aid manoeuvres, traffic control and other collaborative involvement required by the police and paramedics.

□ *Should you do the research?*
Inquiry often includes a number of moral and ethical issues. Suppose you are investigating dangerous driving conditions that include such topics as driving at night or in poor visibility, speeding, driving through red lights at intersections, driving under the influence of alcohol or drugs, or driving in a risk-taking manner. If you are going to talk with or interview people, what constitutes informed consent? How do you ensure confidentiality of participants? To what extent is a person's right to privacy violated by the use of surveillance devices such as photo radar or video cameras? What do you do when someone admits to breaking the law? What are your obligations to

others, especially if what you discover during your research falls within "duty to report" legislation? Inquiry related to traffic safety can open a Pandora's box of moral and ethical issues. For example, how do you handle "presentation of self" during your inquiry? Undoubtedly, a range of psychological or sociological needs related to such factors as power, control, affection, belonging, self-worth and identity litter the inquiry landscape.

"Should you do the research?" is a question that is not only integrally connected to your understanding of the problem but also related to the rights of others and the trust that is required. And, of course, your own skills, resources, values and support must be in top working order. Furthermore, in some instances it may be necessary to follow organizational protocol and obtain the necessary authority and mandate before you proceed.

In many instances, those who do research have responded in a practical and eclectic manner to changing preferences as well as socialization. For others, it has become a conscious choice based on the assumptions we make about knowledge, our views about the nature of reality and our appraisal of what is ethical and valuable in thought and action.

☐ *How can you make your research scientific and comprehensive?*
There are many resources and strategies for making your traffic-safety research scientific and comprehensive. Following the canons of accepted research practice, regardless of your paradigm or methods, is sound advice. Here are a few general tips:

- create a plan in advance;
- ensure you have support, including one or more critical friends, before beginning your project;
- consider using complementary data sources or research methods;
- keep your questions in mind when analyzing your data; and
- consider using innovative reporting strategies for different audiences.

Seeing establishes our place in the world. And there are many ways of seeing a roadway situation, phenomenon or problem. As Berger (1972) says, however, "The relation between what we see and what we know is never settled" (p. 7).

Open, public conversations that support clarification and reflection of these issues must be encouraged. While consensus may never be reached, it may be possible to move toward a clearer understanding of differences and similarities. Remember that disciplined inquiry can be distinguished from general inquiry in that posing questions and solving problems occurs in a context of agreed-upon assumptions and rules of procedure. For example, there are certain presuppositions or beliefs about the nature and limits of knowledge. Issues about how researchers approach the world, how they construct reality, how they distinguish knowledge from belief and how they know that they know assist in demarcating the boundaries of what has come to be called participatory action research. In a similar manner, those presuppositions and beliefs about how reality is defined and how to decide what is valuable also shape the terrain of disciplined inquiry.

☐ *What are the equity issues related to your research?*
Ensuring that your research is fair, just and bias-free for all participants and stakeholders can be a challenge in present contexts of diversity and complexity. Foremost among equity issues are topics related to gender, race, culture and age. In addition, inquiry related to traffic safety introduces a whole range of additional equity issues involving specific groups such as victims, caretakers, families, government, police, corporations, insurance companies, lawyers, drivers, ex-drivers, biker subcultures, and on and on. The rights and specific concerns of all individuals and groups must be acknowledged and considered during all phases of the participatory action research cycle.

Participatory action research is a collaborative and cooperative enterprise that involves people in the investigation of an issue, phenomenon or concern that affects their mutual lives. Since all participants are co-researchers and co-subjects throughout the entire process, the distinction between researcher and subject is blurred. Equity issues are everyday realities that must be faced and resolved.

☐ *How can your research improve the situation?*
The goal of purposeful research is action. When such research is done in a participatory and collaborative manner, then the shared purpose stems from the understanding people have mutually developed about what is of value. Participatory action research is uniquely positioned to provide good data for decision-making and improvement. From another perspective, however, such inquiry has consequences. Things inevitably change as a result of inquiry. The mere act of asking questions is an intervention in a situation; interaction—giving and hearing answers and making sense of them—inevitably brings about changes in those involved. Whether people then choose to continue as before or to change course determines the quality of the new situation.

Most individuals who choose to do participatory action research in traffic matters set out explicitly to study something in order to improve it. Such inquiry often arises from an unsatisfactory situation that those most affected wish to alter for the better—speeding or questionable police procedure. In some instances, the research occurs to improve further something that is already valued. Meaning is mobilized. Moving to improved action involves a creative moment of transformation. This involves an imaginative leap from a world of "as it is" to a glimpse of a world "as it could be."

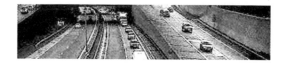

INQUIRY IS A WAY OF CREATING new contexts for interweaving beliefs and actions. In other words, webs of beliefs and actions continually reweave themselves, and inquiry becomes a way of recontextualizing ongoing change in the web of beliefs. I have suggested that inquiry is socially crafted and has implications for safety and the roadway system. More specifically, however, it is a systematic and disciplined approach to understanding and resolving problems. Motivated by values and curiosity, inquiry is a dynamic and highly contextualized process.

I believe there is merit in adopting a philosophy of participatory and holistic knowing. Skolimowski (1994), for example, articulates new insights and fresh perspectives in his theory of the participatory mind. He explains the essence of his ideas in the following passage: "Wholeness implies participation. Participation implies empathy. Participation and empathy in action, while we do research, implies entering the territory of phenomena on their terms" (p. 167).

Citing the work of Barbara McClintock, who received a Nobel Prize in 1983 for her work in biology, Skolimowski explains:

> She vividly describes the process of identification with the chromo-somes she investigated. What she describes is the characteristic method-ology of participation: "I found the more I worked with them, the bigger and bigger the chromosomes got and when I was really working with them I wasn't outside. I was part of the [system] ... it surprised me because I actually felt as if I was right down there and these were my friends ... As you look at these things they become part of you ... (p. 166)

Participatory action research is a way of thinking, feeling and acting. It is a research process that values systematic and scientific inquiry, respects all indi-viduals and honours individual experiences. Participants are involved in every stage of the inquiry: from the initial conceptual and planning stage to the determination and use of research methods to stage of making sense of the data to the taking of action based on the evidence gathered.

In doing participatory action research, collaboration may involve struggle and must engage commitment. Through collaboration, each person's contribution results in recognition of the whole. And recognition of the whole means that all parts belong together and all parts participate. The recognition of each person's contribution comes from a blending of beliefs, values, experiences and knowledge that enhance the process and products of the collaboration. Through conversation and hard work, each person's own voice becomes clearer and more articulated. Meaning emerges and is socially constructed. In this sense, collaborative inquiry contributes to personal growth and more informed social action. It invites productive use in traffic safety.

NOTES

1   For example, Collingwood (1956) refers to the task of the historian during inquiry:

> The historian, investigating any event in the past, makes a distinction between what may be called the outside and inside of an event ... His work may begin by discovering the outside of an event, but it can never end there; he must always remember that the event was an action, and that his main task is to think himself into this action, to discern the thought of its action. (p. 213)

SECTION THREE
TECHNICAL SUB-SYSTEMS

AN INTEGRAL COMPONENT of any system is its context. The environment in which a system exists serves as a boundary profile, the location in which physical features, and the design to better understand and control them, are noted. The focus of engineers is the design of roadways that enhance traffic safety—think of innovations like rumble strips, highway slopes and roadside reflectors. The changes are implemented according to features of the natural environment, social behavior, driver skills and qualities like age. Engineering feats do not exist outside of the natural environment and thus both deserve our attention.

In traffic, as in other systems, technology is the mediary that interacts with all sub-systems to produce change. When a technological innovation is introduced, sub-systems must adapt by re-designing to restore equilibrium. Although many technological innovations have been implemented, the latest and the most highly visible is the cellular phone. The use of cellphones has direct implications on a driver's psychological and social environment as well as on the law, economics, politics and electronic space.

Another area of technological change is policing. Techno-policing, exemplified in photo radar and red-light cameras, is creating major advances in enforcement. But we must consider the extent to which implementation of technology serves the common good and how it may affect the dignity of the individual.

To drive is not only to operate a vehicle but to master it. Drivers make situational decisions, use their skills and present demeanors that serve their own ends while fulfilling basic cultural and social norms. Mastery is intense driving: premeditated, planned action directed toward a definitive goal within the constraints imposed by political, legal, environmental, engineering and vehicular constraints. We need to work with drivers to regulate their actions according to the numerous sub-systems that form the roadway system. It is, after all, the structure of the roadway system that puts drivers into their roles. Its patterns allow drivers to adapt to changes so that, in its turn, the roadway system can adapt to emerging functions. In the face of new circumstances, such as rapidly changing technical innovations, we need innovative driving programs to help drivers, within their web of inter-connectedness, to manage ever-new expectations.

16

GEOGRAPHIC INFORMATION SYSTEMS, CASE-BASED REASONING AND SYSTEM DESIGN

Fixing the Normal Accident

NIGEL WATERS

ACCORDING TO THE Alberta Think and Drive program, most accidents occur between 4 p.m. and 7 p.m. But if we know *when* an accident is most likely to occur, we should be able to do something about it—something other than simply "blaming the victim," the driver. According to research (Arthur & Waters, 1997) and programs such as the Black Spot campaign of the City of Calgary Police Services, we know *where* accidents are most likely to happen. If we know where an accident is likely to happen, we should be able to do something about it. We should be able to intervene in the system and help the driver avoid making the errors that cause the collision.

This chapter begins by discussing case-based reasoning and its use in transportation research. It then suggests how a case base might be integrated with a geographic information system to form a smart, spatial decision support system. This tool could be used in both a predictive and prescriptive way to reduce the probable occurrence of accidents and to allow for more effective enforcement intervention strategies.

■ Speed Management and Traffic Safety

Traffic-safety literature is divided about the influence of speeding on accidents. Extensive reviews may be found in Arthur (1996) and the IBI Group et al. (1997); other recent examples may also be found in the publications of the

Transportation Research Board (see, for example, Elvik, 1997). The effect of speeding on the severity of an accident is unequivocal: the destructive force of the crash increases in proportion to the square of the speed. But the relationship between speed and the probability of accidents occurring is debatable. There isn't even a universally accepted measure for the speed variable. Should the measure be the average speed of traffic, the 85th percentile or some measure of speed variance—or indeed a composite of one or more of these measures? Enforcement strategies and the lowering of posted speed limits have also received a mixed response in the literature.

Although a Mission Possible (1998) discussion paper suggested that "studies have indicated that a reduction in average speed of just 2 to 5 km/ph can result in a reduction of up to 30% in injury and fatal collisions," others have been more cautious. After reviewing extensive evidence, the IBI Group et al. (1997) state that "it cannot be decisively concluded that changing the posted speed will result in a change in crashes. Where such changes are detected, the important questions of under what conditions changes in safety and speed occur and what actually caused the change remain largely unresolved" (p. S1).

A variety of confounding effects have been noted with respect to enforcement strategies. They include spatial "halo" effects and temporal "memory" effects. Such decays in the effectiveness of isolated enforcement strategies were noted early on by Hauer (1982). Some studies have suggested that the memory effect may be relatively long-lasting when informational and advisory strategies are used (Bowron, 1996). Increasing the complexity of the relationship between speed and enforcement strategies, on the one hand, and between speed and accident probabilities, on the other, is the likelihood of "pulses" or the "kangaroo" response (Elvik, 1997) to the visibility of police radar. A warning from a radar detector—or even just a sudden reduction in the speed of drivers ahead—may also result in erratic driving behavior. Again and again, the IBI Group et al. (1997) recommended the need for a comprehensive approach to changing driver behaviour to increase safety: " This indicates the limitations of enforcement and reinforces the need for an integrated approach including education, engineering and enforcement techniques" (IBI Group et al., 1997, pp. 3–10).

■ Case-Based Reasoning: A Way Out?

The Canadian Review of Safety, Speed and Speed Management (IBI Group et al., 1997) gives considerable praise to the traffic-safety programs developed in New South Wales and Victoria, Australia. Particularly impressive, according to the Review, is the comprehensive and integrated approach to speed management used by the Australians (IBI Group et al., 1997). This program included the following steps:

- data collection, including information about speeds, accidents, behaviour and attitudes;
- public consultation and education;
- review of road features and environment, and compatibility with safe speeds;
- realistic speed zoning and enforcement of speed limits;
- development of appropriate, complementary legislation or regulation reflecting community values;
- particular emphasis on reduction of speed-related crashes involving heavy vehicles;
- development of useful technology for speed management; and
- monitoring and evaluation of speed management program. (pp. 6–10)

Early in this study (p. S-3), the procedure for setting speed limits is referred to as "a knowledge-based system." This does not appear to be a formal knowledge-based system in which traditional knowledge-engineering techniques, such as asking experts, have been improved through the use of computerized rule-based expert systems. Perhaps this is as it should be, since such systems are notoriously difficult to develop and the knowledge-engineering process is frequently seen as a bottleneck even with the development of highly specialized, interactive elicitation software that can develop the rules automatically (see Waters [1988, 1989] for a review of some of the strengths and weaknesses of traditional approaches to knowledge-engineering).

During the 1990s, there was a movement away from traditional knowledge-based approaches that result in the development of expert systems and a movement toward the development of case-based reasoning (CBR) tools (Leake, 1996). CBR tools are similar to expert systems in that they assume that new problems are solved based on previous experience. CBR tools use previously experienced problem situations to solve new problems based on similar past cases (Aamodt & Plaza, 1998). The CBR software retrieves cases similar to the current problem and attempts to reuse the case in a new solution. When a new solution is found, it may be added to the case base, and in this way the case base may be considered a dynamic entity. Any individual case may include video, audio and mapped information.

It is important to note how CBR differs from other database and information-retrieval systems in its adaptation, information-retrieval and learning processes. The ability to adapt old cases to fit new situations depends on reasoning processes found in the CBR but not in conventional database and information-retrieval systems. Even in CBR without the adaptation facility, information-retrieval is quite different from other systems; CBR is more interactive (Leake, 1996). The dynamic, interactive search functions provided with most CBR programs quickly separate CBR from standard search engines in which users develop their own search criteria (see Waters, 1996, for a brief review and references). Most CBR research will use readily available commercial CBR software. Clayton and Waters (1999), for example, used software from Inference Corporation (1995) when integrating traditional environmental knowledge with a geographic information system (GIS).

Clayton and Waters note a number of difficulties with the application of CBR tools, but despite this, the last few years have seen an explosion of interest in CBR. Veloso (1994) provides additional how-to advice, and Veloso and Aamodt (1995) and Smith and Faltings (1996) include numerous studies from a variety of fields. None of the applied studies are GIS applications, but Haigh and Veloso's (1995) study of route planning and Bonzano et al.'s (1996) paper on the use of CBR to provide a support system for air-traffic control are in closely allied disciplines and come closest to our interest here in integrating CBR with accident databases and GIS. In the next section we consider how a single case from an accident case base might be used to inform subsequent decision-making once it had been integrated into a spatial decision support system (SDSS).

■ The Complexity of Traffic Accidents and Traffic Safety

The complexity of traffic-safety issues has long been acknowledged. Vahl and Giskes (1990, cited in IBI Group et al., 1997) suggest a variety of approaches for traffic calming. These include physical features, such as road humps, constrictions and bends; psychological features, such as paving materials, rumble strips and pedestrian-environment notices; visual features, such as pavement markings; social control, such as education for residents and users, consultation and "buy-ins" on adaptations; and legal controls, such as reduced speed limits.

The IBI Group et al. (1997, pp. 5–12) noted various factors that influence driver behaviour with respect to speed. These variables include the driver's age and gender, attitude to speed limits and knowledge of speeding risks; the number of vehicle occupants; the trip purpose and schedule; vehicle type, age and performance (top speed); prior accident and speeding history; and whether a driver had recently joined a road with a lower speed limit from one with a much higher limit. The importance of these variables was found to vary by jurisdiction, and it may be reasonably expected that many of these variables may be variously correlated with each other, making their use in statistical models problematic (see Arthur & Waters [1995] for a principal component analysis delineating the intercorrelations between characteristics associated with accident occurrence). One might also surmise that a lack of knowledge or awareness of the posted speed limit should influence speed choice. The temporal complexities and inadequate signing of, for example, Calgary, Alberta's school and playground zones make us wonder whether compliance is really the desired goal. This is perhaps an argument against "micro-management" of speed limits and certainly in favour of more standard and more visible signs.

Perrow (1984) has argued that systems that exhibit "interactive complexity," where unexpected and unanticipated interactions lead to system failure and where the system processes and events are "tightly coupled" (that is to say, things happen so fast that intervention to rectify the situation is not possible), are likely to have accidents. He refers to such accidents as "system accidents" or "normal accidents." Although Perrow does not examine automobile safety specifically, concentrating rather on systems that may lead to catastrophe (such as nuclear power stations and airplane travel), he does mention this topic briefly (pp. 304–05 and see Fig. 9-1, p. 327). he sees automobile safety as an area where the system might well be improved through better design. Norman (1992, 1993) echoes these thoughts in his long-term crusade for a better-designed world.

In the spirit of his comments, we might well ask why we design safety seats for babies that 90 percent of the population cannot attach correctly. Is it really a good idea to issue tickets to those who cannot install these seats correctly? Might it be a better idea to design a seat that is foolproof and installs correctly or not at all? Why design garage door openers with a clip for the car's sun visor if this is a hazard? Would it not be simpler to include a Velcro strip on the back of the garage door opener and another piece of Velcro with an adhesive backing that would allow the opener to be positioned where it was unlikely to impact the driver's head in a collision? Why design a car with a pedestrian-friendly, rounded shape if you then permit vehicle owners to install pedestrian killing bars on the fronts of their vehicles? We are not blaming the technology itself (Florman, 1981), although that viewpoint should perhaps also be considered, but rather the way technology is designed and implemented.

Let's look at how a single case might be used to inform accident specialists and those in charge of safety and speed management about a variety of difficulties with the system itself.

■ Princess Diana's Car Crash

What might one expect to learn from a single case? Perhaps the answer is not much; after all, anecdotal evidence is usually dismissed in scientific research, and indeed the goal of case-based reasoning is ultimately to use thousands of accident cases. But even a single case can be informative. If we consider the case of Princess Diana's fatal crash, we can see that a number of factors might be alleged to have increased the probability of the accident. According to a recent report in the popular press (Sancton & Macleod, 1998), the following factors may have played a part in the crash:

- THE CAR: although it was a Mercedes S-280, normally considered to be a relatively safe vehicle, it appeared to have been poorly repaired and may have had malfunctioning air bags (which appear to have deployed with explosive force) and a malfunctioning anti-lock braking system;
- THE DRIVER: Henri Paul was alleged to have been legally drunk, to have consumed two prescription drugs and to have had an abnormally high concentration of carbon monoxide in his blood; the driver lacked experience driving the poorly repaired vehicle (which was alleged to have a tendency to veer to the right—this tendency was found to be the most important contributing factor in the official report released almost two years later);
- ANOTHER VEHICLE: a slow-moving, white Fiat Uno was alleged to have precipitated the crash; the issues here are the interaction between the vehicles; speed variation between the two vehicles; the constrained physical environment in the tunnel; and the thirteenth pillar, which the Mercedes eventually smashed into; Sancton and Macleod (1998, p. 36) described it as "a dangerous stretch of road";
- THE ALLEGED INVOLVEMENT OF THE PAPARAZZI: presumably somewhat equivalent to such infractions as stunting or young drivers racing each other, although the photographers were later cleared in the official accident report by Judge Herve Stephan (this report was not made public but was summarized in many press reports);
- SPEED: from the amount of destruction, the speed appears to have been excessive;
- TIME OF DAY: night; and
- three of the four occupants were not wearing seatbelts.

One might assume that each of these characteristics increased the probability that an accident might occur. Taken together, they made it almost a certainty.

We can extract several lessons from such a case:

- speed kills—but usually in conjunction with one or more other factors;
- the physical environment, in this case the tunnel and associated pillars, may exacerbate the problem of speed;
- the condition of the vehicle is likely to contribute to the probability of a speed-related accident;

- the condition of the driver, the driver's experience with the vehicle and the road conditions may contribute to an accident;
- the time of day is likely to be factor; 4 p.m. to 7 p.m. may be when most accidents occur, but the rate of accidents per vehicle on the road is likely to be higher later at night when poor visibility, driver fatigue and poor conditions may aggravate the situation;
- others on the road may contribute, especially if their behaviour is sub-optimal;
- improper use or lack of use of safety devices will increase the severity and perhaps the probability of an accident; and
- learning from past mistakes can be made more efficient and effective through the use of such tools as case-based reasoners.

In the next section, we consider just one aspect of the safety problems the case-based reasoner might be used to mitigate.

■ Network Deficiencies in Calgary

If we concentrate on a single aspect of Princess Diana's crash, namely the environment, we can see how this might be used to inform decision-making concerning speed management in a city such as Calgary, Alberta. For example, anecdotal evidence indicates that we have many situations where the road and driving environment in Calgary exacerbates the problem of speeding. Here we can cite a few examples:

- On Crowchild Trail NW travelling south and east into the city between Shaganappi Trail and Northland Drive, a ninety-degree right turn is permitted (with no turn lane) to allow motorists to access the U-Haul, Java-to-Go and the Turbo Gas Station (it is interesting to note that these three businesses had existed for many years before the road was widened in the year 2000);
- Further along the Crowchild Trail, travelling southeast (toward the city centre), a left turn is permitted at the traffic light against oncoming traffic travelling at 80 kph (this too was recently changed after many years);
- Looking east down Campus Drive at the University of Calgary, the road runs between the parking lot and the building; pedestrians and those who have just parked their car are forced, unnecessarily, to cross the road;
- A bus stop on Scenic Acres Boulevard just to the west of 85 Street NW is so close to the intersection that it must cross traffic which has been advised by a traffic sign that it has the right of way;

- Travelling north on 14 Street NW towards Berkley Gate, a left turn is permitted into a parking lot at the base of Nose Hill Park, but there is no turn lane;
- Traffic turning off Crowchild Trail NW can cross Charleswood Drive and continue northwest into the shopping centre; although such traffic obviously has the right of way, it is almost invisible to left-turning traffic coming in the other direction because of the peak in the road; the left turn should only be permitted with a turn signal when the oncoming traffic has a red light.

A case base might use accident-occurrence forms to determine whether these locations had an accident history (the last example cited recently contributed to an injury accident).

■ Integration of Case-Based Reasoning with Geographic Information Systems

The case base of accidents can be integrated in a GIS. As a first step, we would expect the GIS to record as an attribute on each link, or each part of a link (if it is "dynamically segmented"; see Waters [1999] for an explanation), and at each node (intersection) any characteristics that might be perceived as dangerous (such as those listed above). These attributes might be used to flag potentially dangerous locations where remedial steps (such as lower speed limits) might be taken proactively to inhibit the likelihood of speed-related accidents in the future. This proactive approach would seem preferable to lowering the speed limits after the accident has occurred. In addition, the accident case base might be queried with respect to the GIS to help determine where design inadequacies contributed to the accident.

Integration of GIS and CBR is not a simple task, as Clayton and Waters (1998) have shown. An ideal configuration might be to have both the case base and the GIS available through a web-browser. A user-friendly interface would allow transportation planners and engineers to determine just exactly where network design is contributing to speed-related accidents.

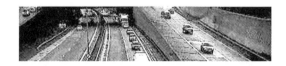

WE HAVE ARGUED HERE THAT ACCIDENTS are rarely the result of speed alone. Numerous other conditions, including driver and vehicle characteristics, the physical environment and the time of day, contribute both to the probability and the severity of an accident. If we are to increase traffic safety, we need an integrated approach, one adapted to each geographical location. As the IBI Group et al. (1997) state, "Program details can then be tailored to suit the individual jurisdiction" (p. 7–6; see also Catalano & Schoen [1997] on the topic of building consensus).

We have suggested that the best way in which to implement these changes is the use of CBR software in conjunction with a GIS. This would allow the detection of problem times and locations and of system deficiencies. Together with the use of other approaches, such as simulation models (see, for example, the work of Yang & Koutsopoulos [1996] and Koscielny et al. [1997]), it would also allow ongoing monitoring of any changes to the system. Finally, such a methodology might allow us to avoid taking the easy option of simply blaming the victim. As Hauer (1998) has stated, a driver does not deserve to die simply because he or she has made a mistake.

17

MODELLING HAZARDOUS LOCATIONS WITH GEOGRAPHIC INFORMATION SYSTEMS

ROBERT M. ARTHUR

AUTOMOBILE ACCIDENTS seem ubiquitous: where there is traffic, there are accidents. No matter where one lives and drives, some locations are reputed to be dangerous or to have a higher-than-average number of collisions: a stretch of rural highway, a busy intersection, a bridge deck. For whatever reason, collisions—especially those resulting in mortality or severe injury—occur at a high rate at these locations. Today we have methods to determine statistically exactly how hazardous these sites are.

Entrusted not only with designing and building our roadways but also with monitoring, maintaining and re-engineering them, engineers have developed numerous tests to determine which locations exhibit dangerous characteristics (Hauer, 1996). Once a site is identified as having an undue number of collisions, it can be studied to determine what can be done to improve its performance. Such solutions may focus on environmental design issues such as widening the roadway, adding another lane, dividing the two streams of traffic, or upgrading from stop signs to traffic lights. Such remedies attempt either to increase the efficiency of the roadway, thus relieving congestion and increasing flow, or to decrease the potential interaction of vehicles. But solutions are not always to be found in engineering. Research indicates two other methods of alleviating traffic collisions: education and enforcement.[1] These centre on the driver in an attempt to modify driver behaviour.

Geographic information systems (GIS) are used in the search for solutions because of their ability to process large amounts of data and to deal with

FIGURE 17.1

Layers in a geographic information system

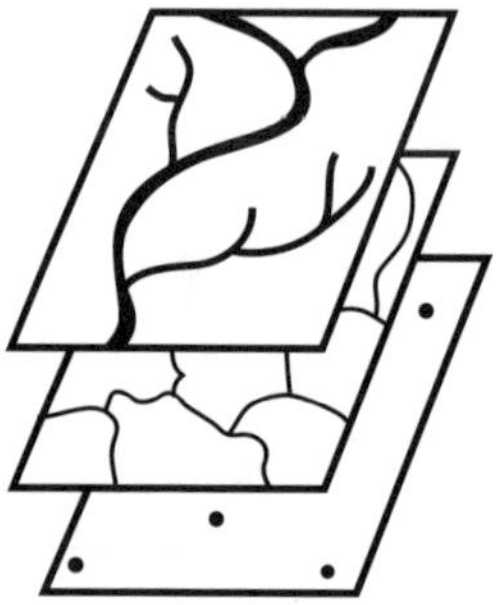

Layer	Object Type
River	Line
Soil Class	Polygon
Well site	Points

spatially organized information. Road networks lend themselves extremely well to analysis with GIS. While GIS is relatively new to the field of traffic-safety research, its use is intensifying (Spring & Hummer, 1995; Andaluz, Roberts & Siddall, 1997).

■ Geographic Information Systems

A GIS combines trained people, computer hardware and software. The system is designed for the acquisition, storage, manipulation, analysis and display of geographic data (Martin, 1996). GIS grew from the convergence of two computer technologies: computer-assisted design (CAD) and database-management systems (DBMS). The power of graphic displays coupled with the flexible data-handling capabilities of DBMS offers the GIS user an extremely powerful analytical tool. Structured Query Language (SQL) adds the ability to select specific variables or locations for study, as well as allowing the recombination of the data in sometimes novel ways. As the software has grown in sophistication, specific algorithms have been incorporated, many of them dealing with the unique spatial character of the data.

GIS uses raster and vector data models. The raster method arranges the data in a grid of small cells or pixels; this model is not used here. The vector model divides the world into objects of three types: points, lines and polygons. Each object type is drawn on a layer that normally contains only one kind of object. Intersections can thus be indicated by points, sections of roads by lines and buildings by polygons. Each layer can be overlaid on another, as if they were drawn on transparencies (see Figure 17.1). This overlay process allows us to create more complex maps and search for spatial relationships. The system allows as many layers as are required (Aldenderfer, 1996).

■ Study Area

The study area encompasses the City of Calgary, Alberta. The collected data spans the years 1993 through 1995. By 1995, Calgary had a population of 738,184 and covered 671.75 km² (Clear-View Maps, 1995). The city has a well-designed road network that does not experience the gridlock that plagues many other large modern cities. The entire road-network digital file was supplied by the City of Calgary. The file is extremely detailed, to the point that it includes alleyways. The file was edited to remove alleyways and residential streets, leaving collectors, major streets and highways as designated by the City of Calgary Transportation Planning Division. Using the mapping capabilities of the GIS, line thickness was adjusted to indicate traffic flow and line colour to indicate posted speed limit. Other attributes pertinent to the road network were added to the database, such as divided or undivided status. This then forms the "base map," the map to which other information was added. Water features and railways were also included because bridges and railway crossings are of interest. Communities were outlined and colour-coded by type: residential, industrial, reserve and park.

Once the base map was completed, another layer was created to indicate the location of all collisions that occurred over the time frame of the study. This information was gathered from Alberta collision report forms (under Alberta law, a form must be completed for every collision resulting in damage of $1,000 or more). The information was supplied by the City of Calgary Police Services and included a great deal of detail regarding each accident: for example, address of the collision, environmental and road conditions, driver action and condition, condition of vehicle, type of vehicle, age and sex of driver, and severity of the collision (fatal, injury, or property damage only). All data was "sanitized," meaning that information that might identify the individuals involved was removed.

The GIS had the capability to geo-code individual collisions. As each collision occurred at a specific location in Calgary, we needed to indicate its presence on the map with a symbol—a task that would be daunting if performed manually, as there are approximately 35,000 collisions in the data set. The GIS can match the address of the collision, contained in the collision database, to addresses contained in the base map, thus automating an otherwise arduous task. It was this capability that helped us decide to use GIS in our study. With the information spatially organized within the GIS, the search for hazardous locations was simplified.

While traffic collisions may occur at any time and at any place, research indicates that some locations are more hazardous than others (Hummer, 1994; Hauer, 1996; Arthur & Waters, 1997). Various methods have been developed for the determination of hazardous locations, "black spots" or "sites with promise," as Hauer (1996) has labelled them. By applying the multivariate statistical technique of principal components analysis to a year of traffic-collision data, we determined that intersections (this term is meant to include interchanges also) in general were implicated to a greater degree than "links" (intervening stretches of road) (Arthur & Waters 1995a). Further, subsequent analysis that compared intersections to links indicated that the severity of collisions occurring in intersections was greater than that occurring on the links (Arthur & Waters 1995b). While this is a reasonably intuitive conclusion, given the variety of collisions that can occur in intersections and the greater interaction of vehicles at these locations, it is reassuring to be able to confirm opinion with statistical values.

In order to concentrate on intersections and interchanges, we described a 100-foot radius for selected intersections. All collisions that occurred within the radii were selected for analysis. This employed a "buffering" routine in the GIS, a technique that draws a boundary (this size of which is determined by the researcher) around selected objects (Hummer, 1994). We then used the rate quality control method to compare intersections with each other; those exhibiting higher collision rates were identified. These sites were then flagged as targets for intervention. Hauer (1996), however, points out that sites need not exhibit higher rates to be candidates for intervention. He devised a methodology of viewing sites with a variety of statistics. Taking them all into account can identify sites where improvement is possible, whether they have been identified as "black spots" or not. This capacity, coupled with the ability of GIS to capture an entire city network, permits a more systematic and holistic survey of collisions within a municipal setting.

■ The Temporal Dimension

Temporality is a factor that has not been introduced in most engineering research. It appears only to be used in time-series intervention studies (such research compares the accident frequencies before some form of intervention and those after to determine if the desired change was brought about). I believe that the conventional statistics of average annual daily traffic flow (AADT) and collision rates (collision frequency divided by AADT) ignore the effects of the temporal dimension.

Such statistics propose a "snapshot" view of data, generally aggregated over a year. This view masks the diurnal and weekly ebb and flow of the traffic within a city. It is similar to viewing accident rates for an entire city or a single, complete road and concluding that such places exhibit either safe or unsafe characteristics. As the search for hazardous locations has shown, specific locations on a road or within a city exhibit higher or lower values. It is possible for the same location to show variation in time for collision frequencies. An obvious argument to support such a claim is that traffic flows vary considerably over the course of the day, with a secondary variation over the course of a week. This could be extended over a longer period of time by considering seasonal variations; however, this view would require data collected over a number of years.

Of further interest to this argument is the question that Hauer (1990) asked about the "number of opportunities" compared to the "probability-per-opportunity" inherent in probability and statistical testing. By creating a rate, we related *all* collisions happening over a specific time frame (one day, or one year) to *every* vehicle that passed through that location over the same time frame. This relationship can be misleading, as not all vehicles have the *opportunity* of interacting over the given time frame. Thus, the rate may be over- or understated for that location. Furthermore, the interpretation of such results may lead to intervention programs at the wrong time, just as inadequate locational analysis would lead to intervention at the wrong place.

It is possible for collisions to increase during the rush-hour peaks. However, if the rate of increase in traffic flow were even greater, the rate would in effect *decrease.* By looking at temporally aggregated data, a particular intersection may be targeted for redesign to accommodate increases in flow to promote safety, when, in fact, the collision rate may exhibit high values during off-peak hours. Such a redesign may have the counter-intuitive and perverse effect of *increasing* collisions.

We decided to separate Calgary traffic flow into one-hour increments over a week. This parsed the collision rates into their respective weekly and diurnal patterns, offering a more detailed picture of activity at particular locations. While this may not completely alleviate Hauer's concern, it effectively reduces the error (in-depth research beyond the scope of this paper will be required to determine an accurate way to address such issues). Further, there is continuing concern over the quality of data used in such research. As those who study these problems are well aware, collision report forms may not be as accurate as we would wish, nor is all the relevant data present—after all, it is not the duty of the police to collect information for research purposes.

By determining the time at which excessive rates manifest themselves, we have some clues about the purpose of the journey. If the rates are high during rush hour, we can reasonably assume that they involve commuter trips to or from work; if they occur during the evening, they are more likely to involve trips to or from social activities. If one or the other is implicated, then we can perform further research to examine attitudes towards driving as it relates to different journeys. One obvious conclusion might be the indication of higher involvement of alcohol in the socially motivated journeys.

■ Time Series

Time-series data take the form of discrete measurements of a particular variable over a domain such as (but not restricted to) time. Where time is the domain, the variable is considered a function of time and is depicted as

$$Y_t, Y_{t+1}, Y_{t+2}, ..., Y_{t+n}$$

where Y is the variable and t denotes the time period (Harvey, 1981). Similar to normal statistics and the inferences made between samples and populations, time-series analysis attempts to make inferences from *realizations*, a particular time series, to the process that creates the series (Gottman, 1981). Time-series data may be used for a variety of purposes: definition, forecasting and interrupted time-series experiments. From the modelling of a time series, it is possible to predict future values of the variable. But because future values are based on the past *memory* inherent in the data, it is advisable not to predict too far into the future (Nelson, 1973).

■ Temporal Data

The data for our study were supplied by the City of Calgary Transportation Planning Division and represent traffic flow recorded at eleven separate stations. Each station is a permanently installed inductive loop counter that records every vehicle passing over it, collecting the data in fifteen-minute intervals. For purposes of this project, the fifteen-minute intervals were agglomerated into one-hour segments. This decision reduced the yearly series to a smaller size, but it still contained 8,736 observations. At each location were two sensors that recorded the traffic flow in the two opposing directions, either east/west or north/south. Twenty-two time series were produced. Unfortunately, the inductive loops are subject to failure as a result of frost damage and wear. This failure manifested itself as gaps in the data, which spanned a number of days due to the time required for repairs. Five of the eleven locations were considered unfit for use as too much data was missing, four having less than fifty percent. Of the remaining locations, only one pair was complete, while the greatest amount of loss was eighteen percent. We had to reconstruct the time series to create new values in place of the missing values.

■ Testing the Data

The data were first analyzed to determine whether a trend exists. In the case of the traffic flows under study, this trend represented the growth of traffic throughout the city. A least-squares regression line was fitted to the data to determine the extent of the trend. A slight trend was detected; however, it was inconsequential and we decided to leave the data as they stood instead of performing any statistical transformation. Fitting polynomials to the curve did not alter the definition of the trend appreciably.

Instead of transforming the data, we had to find a value to insert where observations were missing. We decided to arrange the data in weekly cycles first. This created a matrix of traffic flow values by hour and by week as illustrated in Table 17.1. Thus, for every hour of the week there were 52 separate observations, less the missing values. When performing this operation, there were no less than 36 individual observations from which to derive the average for the missing variable.

Next we had to determine whether the total traffic flow for noon on Monday of one week was similar to noon on Monday for other weeks of the year. To estimate this recurrence of cycles, we performed an autocorrelation with sufficient time lags to capture at least one week. Normally, this test would be performed to determine how one should set up moving average models to smooth the data (Gottman, 1981; Harvey 1981). Two cycles became evident. The first, and most noticeable, was the daily cycle of traffic. This cycle peaked during the two daily rush hours and dropped to low values during the night. Weekly peaks were also noticeable in the data. The findings indicated that the weekly cycle expressed a high degree of homogeneity or repetition.

☐ *Reconstruction*
The reconstruction step was set up within a spreadsheet as shown in Table 17.1. Once the 52 weeks were arranged in the matrix, it was a matter of averaging the existing values and dividing by the number of observations used. The resulting sum was inserted into the corresponding missing values. This process provided a reasonable estimate for the missing value and did not appreciably alter the parameters of the time series.

Before the averaging could continue, we tested the homogeneity across each row of data (as represented in Table 17.1). As each row in this matrix represents a particular hour of the week and each column represents the 52 weeks of the year, the following question arises. If the value for a particular hour at week 10 is missing, is it possible that it is closer in value to the surrounding weeks, 9 and 11, than it would be to weeks 40 through 52? To determine the answer, we performed regression on several rows of data, analyzing one-hour values over the fifty-two weekly observations; we also performed a residual analysis. If a pattern is recognized within the residuals, then the weighted average must be used. After performing this test, we discovered the residuals were random in pattern, which allowed us to use the simpler average.

The average resulting value was inserted into the original flow. We thought the average for all traffic flows could be combined, or averaged again, to create a single series that could be used for any city location. Hence, this series would

TABLE 17.1
Matrix of weekly traffic flow

Hour	Week 1	Week 2	...	...	Week 52
1					
2					
3					
...					
...					
168					

have to be converted to proportional values (percentages). The average of all the time series was compared to the individual series to test for statistical correlation. The results of this test indicated that the individual time series are all highly correlated to the overall average derived from them. This "super average" was used as a time-series model to be applied to any traffic flow within the city. It provided a breakdown of the AAWT flows into a weekly time series consisting of 168 hours. Figure 17.2 is a time-series plot comparing the average with a single location. At each location, two observations are provided, one for each direction of traffic.

Unfortunately, the City provides traffic-flow information in a very crude fashion, that of the AADT. This figure ignores weekend values, which had to be recreated. Once done, the average weekday traffic volume was multiplied by and added to the weekend volume to obtain a total weekly volume. The value was deconstructed into individual hourly volumes through application of the percentage values as determined by the average flow curve depicted in Figure 17.2.

The rush-hour peaks signify the daily work routine, which is a socially and economically created socio-fact. Likewise, the change in pattern exhibited over the weekend also reflects the socially and economically created work cycle. Time geographers such as Torgen Hagerstrand have explored this relationship. Cloke, Philo and Sadler (1991) describe this phenomenon as

[a] depiction of regularities in how individuals *repeatedly* draw upon—and in how different individuals *simultaneously* draw upon—the

resources of time and space. These regularities amount to "time-space structures" deeply engrained in the conduct of everyday life, and they themselves are embedded within (are shaped by; are constituted by) a more intangible realm of *structure*: the realm of economic, social, political and cultural structures as those governing the distribution of wealth and power in modern capitalistic societies. (emphasis in original; p. 109)

Those who live and work in modern cities are aware of these cycles and the daily routine of battling the morning and evening rush hours. Therefore, empirical and sociological evidence appears to support our simple assumption that social and economic forces act to create traffic flows in the city that are ubiquitous and equivalent across the city.

■ Application

The model can be used to derive hourly values for numerous locations across Calgary. As this study focusses on traffic collisions, it is important to understand the temporal distribution of such collisions, especially those resulting in injury and mortality. As all collisions recorded by the Alberta collision report form specify the time and location of the event, it will be easy to incorporate this data in a GIS.

For the purpose of illustration, I produced two maps from the GIS, one of a typical Friday at 6:00 p.m. and one for Saturday morning at 2:00 a.m. The maps depict only interchanges, even though they also contain data for different types of intersections. This study compared areas of similar design to restrict the analysis to interchanges that are not at grade. I indicated collision rates using graduated circles of the same scale between the two maps.

I noticed immediately the disparity between rates at the two times. This may be explained by the difference in the amount of traffic flow, as obviously, rush hour will have high flows while the early-morning hours will have much less traffic. Nevertheless, we are comparing rates determined in the same fashion. It appears that the late-evening and early-morning hours exhibit much higher values. Thus, as a percentage of traffic flow, these times appear to indicate greater amounts of risk.

There are some similarities as to which intersections have high values, but the Saturday values show an increase in four interchanges with the appearance of high rates at three interchanges not previously implicated at rush hour on Friday. Several interchanges indicated at the Friday 6:00 p.m. time frame disappear by Saturday morning. There also is a shift in the spatial distribution in that, by Saturday morning, there is a clustering of two groups, one in the NW sector and one in the NE sector, with a single interchange indicated in the south. The Friday map shows a slightly more dispersed pattern of higher rates

FIGURE 17.2

Time-series plot of flow 3A and 3B with overall average (AVE_FL_P signifies the average predicted flow)

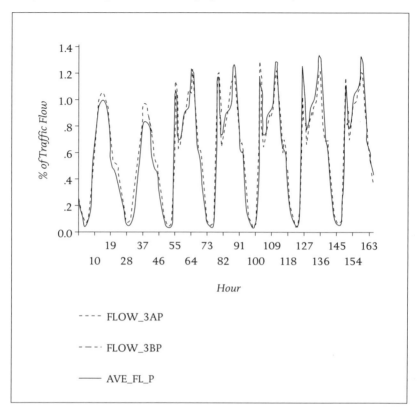

with a greater amount of interchanges along the Deerfoot Trail (the major north–south route along the east side of the city). This thoroughfare is Calgary's busiest road with extremely high rush-hour traffic flows. Even with the high traffic flows, six interchanges show up with higher rates along this route. The Saturday picture removes the emphasis from the major rush-hour routes. This shift might indicate alternate travel patterns arising from different purposes for travel. One can reasonably assume that the purpose of the trip has changed from economically to socially motivated.

This finding presents the researcher with impetus to explore the many differences that might arise from such a shift. Do we see a different mix of drivers, by age and gender? Is alcohol implicated? Is there a problem with over-supply—that is, as the traffic flows have greatly diminished by 2:00 a.m. Saturday, is there a connection between the emptier streets and riskier driving behaviour? What type of police enforcement exists at the different times and how effective is it? The ability of GIS to collect, analyze and display the data according to various criteria makes it an extremely powerful tool. This becomes readily apparent when one compares the first map, which shows a bewildering and overwhelming amount of data in the form of individual collisions, to the later maps, on which the data are organized in a clear, more focussed manner.

Comparing spatial autocorrelations across the temporal domain may yield a change in the spatial relationships over time. The change may indicate that specific areas of the city are host to various social events that are antecedent to collisions: specifically, those that include the use of alcohol. A study by the City of Hamilton Public Works and Traffic Department determined that proportionally more collisions occur during the late evening and early morning than in daytime (Solomon, 1994). Thus, even though more collisions may occur during the rush hours, they are less significant when one takes into account the volume of traffic. The volume of traffic during rush hour restricts the ability of the motorist to attain excessive speeds, whereas during late evening and early morning hours, when volumes are light, motorists can speed with little difficulty. Such information fed through the GIS format will readily allow this hypothesis to be tested.

■ Future Research

This preliminary work has developed a methodology that will be expanded in upcoming work. An expanded data set spanning five or more years will allow us to select collisions on the basis of severity. With such a large database, the remaining fatalities and injuries will be of sufficient size to be statistically significant. Furthermore, collisions in which speed is indicated as a contributing factor will also be studied.

Spatial analysis will also be performed to determine whether there is a temporal change in the distribution of collisions within the city. Global-pattern analysis can determine whether collisions are distributed randomly, clustered or distributed uniformly. If the pattern regularly changes over time, then the pattern itself may offer further insights.

Such a methodology can also be used to monitor police intervention strategies. If the police target a particular area for a particular campaign, it will be possible to see the success of such a strategy. It is also possible to determine whether there is city-wide or local change to the distribution of collisions. Thus, it can determined whether collisions increase elsewhere if they are reduced at one site.

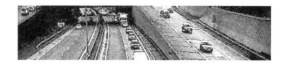

TRAFFIC STUDIES HAVE LONG BEEN CRITICIZED for their lack of solid scientific methodology, as Hearne (1981) points out:

> A casual observer might be forgiven for believing that in no other field of applied scientific work are simple methodological rules ignored so widely as in road safety work. Hypotheses are rarely clearly stated, data limitations are ignored, and very many—and not just the politicians or the publicists—commit the fallacy of *post hoc, ergo propter hoc* [after this therefore because of this] (p. 84)

Traffic researchers face a tremendous problem in that they need to collect a wide range of data on events that are by nature random. Some transportation statistics rely on annual miles driven, which is derived from the number of registered vehicles in a jurisdiction, their average mileage as derived from make and model, and fuel consumption as determined from gas sales. It is easy to see that this figure would contain many chances for the introduction, and subsequent propagation, of error. Traffic volumes are also not recorded accurately over long periods of time except at a few locations, although this trend appears to be changing with the introduction of more permanent sensors.

This project is an attempt to extend the utility of traffic-volume data without ignoring the limitations of those data. While not complicated, this work involved the logical and step-by-step creation of a model that can aid further traffic analysis. Each step uses standard, robust techniques backed up by statistical tests that lend a certain elegance to its solution. Should the methodology be extended over a longer time frame, de-trending will probably be required, but this too is a simple and robust procedure. Hakkert, Yelineck and Efrat (1991) sum up the need for such research:

> Traffic and accident patterns on urban roads are very different from those on the interurban network and therefore need a different approach. Some of the characteristics are: a dense network of roads, including intersections and parking lots requiring a spatial approach; areas of differing characteristics (business district, shopping, residential, industrial, parks, and open spaces); different types of accidents, pedestrian, intersection, etc.; problems of congestion and peak hours; a lack of detailed information on traffic volumes. (pp. 100–01)

The approach outlined in this article offers traffic researchers a holistic process that systematically analyzes city road networks. Adding the temporal dimension further refines the focus. Such refinement should improve our understanding of the cause of traffic collisions. Further, pinpointing the locations and times helps us understand the conditions that led up to the collision event. The flexibility of GIS, coupled with its ability to manage exceedingly large data sets, allows us to engage temporal analysis as well as the incorporation of other techniques such as decision support systems and spatial statistics. GIS is not an end in itself, but the marker of many new beginnings.

NOTES

1 Education campaigns are beyond the scope of this paper. The most typical enforcement strategy is to issue speeding tickets to deter speeding drivers. Hazardous location analysis can be refined to search for locations where excess speed is implicated in the high collision rate.

18

THE EVOLUTION TOWARD AN INTEGRATED SYSTEMS APPROACH TO TRAFFIC SAFETY

SANY ZEIN

TRAFFIC-SAFETY PROFESSIONALS can only prevent crashes if they understand what causes them. Traditionally, this understanding has been encompassed in the description of a traffic system that consists of three components: the driver, the vehicle and the road. A crash is described as a failure in the interaction between these three components. For example, the driver may fail to obey a red light or to adhere to safe speed for the prevailing conditions; a vehicle's brakes or steering system may fail; the road may fail to drain properly or a traffic light may malfunction. In all these cases, the direct cause of the crash appears to be a clear failure in one of the three components.

Throughout North America, the police are responsible for attending crash sites and recording the causes of crashes. Police crash data can then be aggregated to determine the most common causes. Invariably, similar aggregate results have been reported from North America, Western Europe, and Australia: driver error is involved in between 80 and 90 percent of all crashes; vehicle failure is involved in less than 10 percent of all crashes; a road-related deficiency is involved in 10 to 20 percent of all crashes. Some crashes are deemed to have more than one cause. For example, 60 to 70 percent of crashes are attributed solely to driver error, and another 20 to 30 percent may be attributed to a combination of driver error and road-related deficiency.

By collecting data and assigning causes, the police provide an invaluable service. However, the limitations of the crash causes assigned by the police are typically overlooked. In particular, the police are seeking the most direct and

immediate cause of a crash, and are trained to detect and focus on driver infractions rather than vehicle design or the road environment. Until recently, a
traditional leap in logic has unfortunately hampered the efforts towards
improved safety: the distribution of traffic-safety solutions has been *assumed* to
be similar to the distribution of crash causes among the three system components (driver, vehicle and road). In other words, it has been assumed that to
prevent the 80 to 90 percent of crashes in which driver error is a direct cause,
the majority of effort needs to be invested in creating better, error-free drivers.

■ The Human Driver

The combination of police crash data that focusses on driver error as the most
direct cause of crashes with the rush to label the causes as the solutions has lead
to many well-intentioned efforts at improving driver behaviour by providing
either better training or more severe and thorough enforcement. Some positive
results have been achieved, but we need to face one reality. Drivers are human.
Humans make mistakes. Driver error is inevitable.

In every phase of human life, pressures are brought to bear on the driver to
prevent error-free driving. At a young age (16 to 25), the driver is relatively
inexperienced, excitable, and susceptible to peer pressure and bad lifestyle
decisions (for example, speeding, drinking and driving, and driving while
fatigued). Through middle age (26 to 50), the routine pressures of life divert
the driver's mental attention: finances, family, work and the rush to succeed in
modern society. The older driver (over 50) faces a decline in physical abilities.

All of these issues are a normal part of modern life. It is the *exceptional*
driver who can overcome these challenges at every stage in life and drive error-
free. It is the *average* (rather than the incompetent or bad) driver who will be
susceptible to these challenges and commit driving errors at regular intervals.
Most errors go unnoticed. Some will result in crashes.

Attempts to design the perfect error-free driver are always well-intentioned.
These attempts have been most successful when targeted at changes in social
behaviour, such as driving after consuming alcohol. This is one area where
society's definition of *average* was successfully shifted: it used to be *normal* for
a driver to drink and drive; now only *incompetent* drivers do so. The result has
been a dramatic decline in the number of crashes caused by impaired driving,
but even this blatant driver error has not been eliminated: drinking-and-
driving crash frequencies are no longer in decline, and there appears to be a
group of drivers whose behaviour cannot be modified, probably due to overwhelming societal and personal pressures. Parallels can be drawn with the rate
of seat-belt use and, in society as a whole, with the social acceptability of
smoking. Attempts to similarly achieve overall shifts in society's tolerance of
other routine driver behaviours, such as speeding, have so far been less successful.

FIGURE 18.1
The integrated traffic-safety system

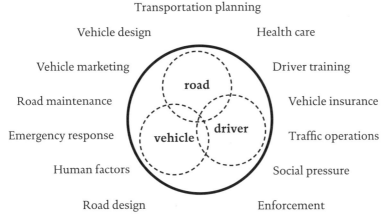

Transportation planning

Vehicle design · Health care

Vehicle marketing · road · Driver training

Road maintenance · Vehicle insurance

Emergency response · vehicle · driver · Traffic operations

Human factors · Social pressure

Road design · Enforcement

Personal/vehicular insurance

In general, interventions that define or attempt to modify driver behaviour are limited in length and effectiveness. Formal driver training lasts a matter of weeks. Most drivers learn the majority of driving habits in the early years of their experience, and these habits are generally shaped by societal factors. By the time a driver has ten years of driving experience, few of the habits learned during formal training have been retained.

Similarly, enforcement has limited impact in terms of modifying behaviour. Immediately upon receiving a speeding ticket, a typical driver response is to adhere strictly to the speed limit. This generally lasts for anywhere from two days to two months, after which societal concerns re-emerge to sweep the driver back to old habits.

■ **The Integrated Traffic-Safety System**

Drivers will always commit errors, and solutions for preventing the majority of crashes do not necessarily lie in modifying driver behaviour. These two conclusions demand that we perceive a broader, integrated traffic-safety system in order to understand the complex relationships that influence crash occurrence, as shown in Figure 18.1. Rather than a simplistic structure that highlights only the driver, the vehicle, and the road as separate entities, this model emphasizes that driver, vehicle and road are an inseparable, integrated system that is subject to a whole range of external and early influences, ranging from road planning and design to vehicle design and marketing. Prior to the driver error that may be the direct cause of a crash, there is a long sequence of events and influences that can be manipulated to reduce the crash risk.

By looking at the big picture, we can find solutions that lie beyond the obvious. In particular, the influences of vehicle design and road design on traffic safety can be explored with the understanding that, prior to a crash occurring, the driver is always in the vehicle and the vehicle is always on the road. It is difficult to design better humans. Is it not easier to design better vehicles and better roads that accommodate driver imperfections?

■ Vehicle Design to Accommodate the Imperfect Driver

In the last fifteen years, the vehicle-manufacturing industry has turned to the area of vehicle safety in an unprecedented way. Features such as driver and passenger air bags, side air bags, side-impact beams, rear-seat shoulder belts, adjustable and rear-seat head restraints, collapsible steering columns, rounded edges within the cabin and automatic emergency-centre crash notification using Geographic Positioning Systems (GPS) have all contributed to better survivability and fewer post-crash injuries.

The next wave of advancements will be in the area of design features that help to prevent crashes from occurring. Anti-lock braking and traction-control systems have been introduced, and vehicle manufacturers are starting to incorporate intelligent transportation system (ITS) technology such as forward, backward and side monitoring radar and heat sensors that warn the driver of approaching objects and impending collisions. The future in this area is promising. These preventive features are an explicit admission that drivers are imperfect and that automated tools are required to help humans drive safely.

Paradoxically and unfortunately, the marketing of new vehicles has focussed both on the new safety features and on other aspects that negate many of the same safety devices. The marketing of vehicles continues to stress power, speed and manoeuvring capabilities that are well beyond the requirements and abilities of most drivers. The marketing of anti-lock braking systems generally sent the message that drivers could travel faster and closer. And the trend towards manufacturing bigger sport-utility vehicles (SUVs) has been accompanied by marketing that promotes aggressiveness and a false sense of invincibility.

■ Road Design to Accommodate the Imperfect Driver

One area where great advances can be made in preventing crashes is road design. Since the 1950s, road design has evolved through three stages:

1. The "traditional highway" stage (1950s to 1970s) focussed on providing a safe paved roadway with little regard for the consequences when a driver unintentionally leaves the road.

FIGURE 18.2

Predictable driver error: two-lane highway

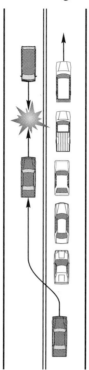

2. The "forgiving highway" stage (1970s to 1990s) expanded the responsibility of the road designer to include providing a forgiving roadside that will reduce the crash severity once a vehicle leaves the road.

3. The "caring highway" stage (1990s to the present) further broadens the responsibility of the designer to include prevention. Using positive-guidance design concepts and an understanding of human factors and driver behaviour, the caring highway attempts to provide sufficient guidance to prevent crashes, and to minimize their severity if they should happen.

In North America, the period from the 1950s to the 1970s was the golden era for road construction. Many highways still in use today were designed according to traditional concepts. As well, many of the experienced designers working today received their training and gained experience in the 1970s and 1980s, and are struggling to balance the modern, caring highway concepts among all their other responsibilities.

FIGURE 18.3

Predictable driver error: signalized intersection

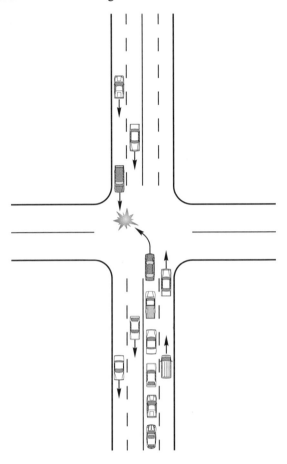

These realities have created the need for two integrated road-safety initiatives: multi-modal operational and safety reviews to improve the safety of existing roads; and road-safety audits to reduce the crash risk at the design stage of a project. Both initiatives have at their core the fundamental principle that roads need to accommodate the predictable errors that the imperfect human drivers will commit. This principle applies to both new roads that are being designed and existing roads that are in service and where crashes are occurring. By following these principles, crashes that are currently *caused* by driver error can be *prevented* by roads that are engineered and designed to anticipate and accommodate these predictable errors.

Three examples are illustrated in Figures 18.2, 18.3 and 18.4. Figure 18.2 shows a predictable driver error on a two-lane rural road. A platoon forms and

FIGURE 18.4

Predictable driver error: freeway interchange

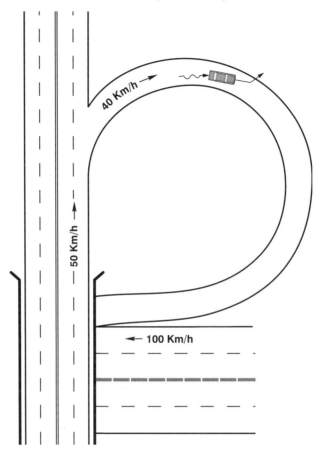

an aggressive driver attempts a dangerous overtaking manoeuvre that results in a head-on crash. Road designers and traffic analysts can predict the formation of platoons and the associated dangerous driver behaviour, and can prevent many such crashes by providing adequate passing opportunities or notices of upcoming passing opportunities.

Figure 18.3 shows a predictable driver error at an urban signalized intersection where a left-turning driver accepts an inadequate gap in oncoming traffic and causes a left-turn opposing crash. Road designers and traffic analysts can predict the supply and demand of traffic gaps, and can prevent many such crashes by providing left-turn lanes or protected left-turn signal phases, among other solutions.

FIGURE 18.5
Multi-modal operational and safety review process

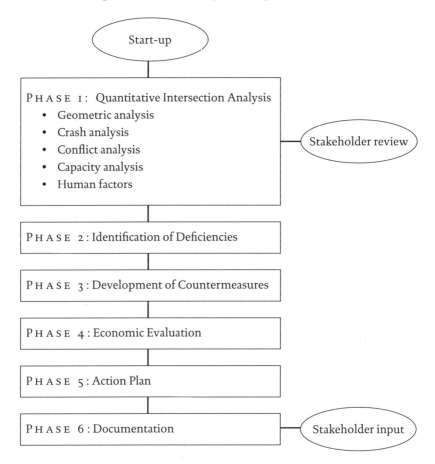

Figure 18.4 shows a predictable driver error on a freeway loop that links a 50-kph arterial with a 100-kph freeway. Due to a tight radius, the loop has a 40-kph advisory speed limit. Road designers and traffic analysts can apply human factors concepts to predict the low likelihood of drivers adhering to the advisory speed limit, and the high risk of off-road crashes. A wider turn radius, roadside barriers, rumble strips and chevrons are some of the engineering countermeasures that could be considered.

These examples show the importance of system-level thinking applied to traffic safety. Although driver error is the cause, better road design can very often be the solution, because drivers are inexorably linked to the road as part of one system.

FIGURE 18.6
Road-safety audit process

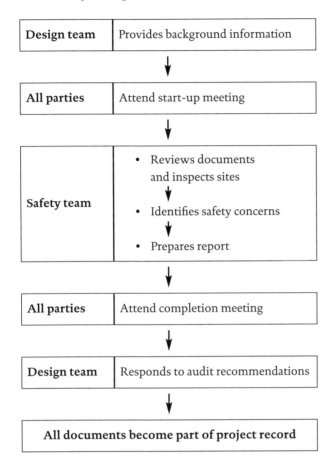

Design team	Provides background information

↓

All parties	Attend start-up meeting

↓

Safety team	• Reviews documents and inspects sites ↓ • Identifies safety concerns ↓ • Prepares report

↓

All parties	Attend completion meeting

↓

Design team	Responds to audit recommendations

↓

All documents become part of project record

☐ *Multi-modal operational and safety reviews*
By conducting integrated multi-modal operational and safety reviews at intersections and along corridors where the crash risk is known to be high, engineering countermeasures can be identified and implemented, and significant traffic-safety improvements can be achieved. The multi-modal operational and safety review is dedicated to systematically understanding the causes of crashes at a particular location, and to finding cost-effective road-engineering solutions from the range of available and proven countermeasures.

The typical systematic process involved in conducting a multi-modal operational and safety review is shown in Figure 18.5. The modern features of these studies include the following:

- combining the analysis of traffic geometry, traffic operations and human factors to analyze traffic conditions from an integrated rather than discrete perspective;
- conducting traffic-conflict surveys whereby the interaction between the drivers and the road conditions is observed and recorded by trained traffic analysts;
- focussing on multi-modal concerns and solutions, whereby the safety needs of pedestrians, cyclists, buses, people with disabilities, heavy commercial vehicles, and motorcycles as well as personal vehicles are taken into account; and
- conducting a reliability-based economic evaluation using documented effectiveness studies to quantify the potential benefits of road-engineering countermeasures as a business case for implementation.

Since 1990, multi-modal operational and safety reviews have been used in Canada and the United States to great effect, and significant benefit-to-cost ratios have been achieved when the recommendations of these studies have been implemented.

□ *Road-safety audits*
A road-safety audit is an independent review of the multi-modal safety aspects of a transportation design project by an expert team of safety analysts. Audits are a preventive tool applied prior to the construction of a project, with the intention of reducing the initial crash risk. Road-safety audits provide input to the project design team in the same way that environmental, geotechnical and socio-economic studies are often used as inputs to the design.

A typical road-safety audit process is shown in Figure 18.6. While design standards focus on road geometry and traffic analysis focusses on efficient traffic operations, road-safety audits analyze future traffic conditions from a multi-modal, integrated perspective where the driver and the road are in constant interaction as a dynamic system. Using the principle that crash risk is a function of exposure, probability and consequence, audits attempt to quantify the crash risks inherent in the design and provide safer alternatives for the consideration of the audit team.

Road-safety audits are now being successfully used in the United Kingdom, Australia, New Zealand, Canada and the US, among other countries.

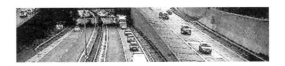

BY UNDERSTANDING THAT THE DRIVER is human and that human beings will always be prone to errors, we can improve the design of our roads to accommodate driver imperfections. Road designers and traffic analysts now have at their disposal tools such as the multi-modal operational and safety review for existing roads and road-safety audits for new transportation projects. Both of these tools approach the issue of traffic safety from an integrated, multi-modal perspective that acknowledges the dynamic system between the driver and the road, and the need to design roads that minimize crash risk by anticipating predictable driver errors. By using such tools, we move closer to an integrated systems approach to traffic safety.

19

IS USING A CELLPHONE LIKE DRIVING DRUNK?

DONALD A. REDELMEIER

& ROBERT J. TIBSHIRANI

TALKING ON A CELLULAR telephone while driving can be productive and glamorous. Is it also dangerous? Some people say yes and tell stories about using a telephone and getting into an accident. Other people say no and support their position with three arguments. First, cellphones allow drivers to call ahead when running late and travel with increased peace of mind, thereby decreasing their risk of a collision. Second, the huge growth of this technology in recent years (with the number of subscribers increasing from zero to ten percent of the population in less than a decade) has not been accompanied by a dramatic increase in collision rates. Finally, drivers face many other distractions (such as eating and talking with passengers) so that singling out cellphones seems unjustified. In this chapter, we describe a study that examined whether cellphones are hazardous.

We were motivated to do this research for several reasons. Motor-vehicle collisions are a leading cause of mortality, disability and other forms of suffering throughout the world. Cellphone conversations are one of the few driving behaviours that can be studied scientifically because an objective record of activity is produced outside of the vehicle. Moreover, even a small change in risk might have substantial public-health importance and explain why some countries have enacted regulations restricting cellphone use while driving. Some of our friends, however, cautioned us about initiating a research effort because it might threaten the enormous financial interests of private industry. The cellphone industry in North America, for example, has daily revenues of over $60 million (substantially more than the daily revenues of $25 million for the Microsoft Corporation; see Value Line Investment Survey [1997] and Cellular Telecommunication Industry Association [1996]).

We decided to go forward, and our first inclination was to conduct a case-control study. To do so, we planned to survey drivers who had car telephones and those who did not, and compare the number of collisions each person experienced during a one-year interval. A brief look at the literature, however, revealed that such a study had already been completed in 1978 to evaluate an early generation of mobile telephone (Smith, 1978). This survey of 498 individuals found that the overall frequency of traffic collisions was marginally lower among mobile telephone subscribers than among members of the general public (11 percent versus 12 percent). The difficulty in interpreting these data was the possibility of biases in favour of mobile-telephone owners. In particular, prior to the 1990s, most mobile-telephone owners were young, intelligent, urban professionals who would otherwise be expected to have very low collision rates and very safe driving patterns.

Our next idea was to consider a before-and-after trial comparing individuals' driving records in the year before purchasing a cellphone to their driving records in the year after purchasing a cellphone. Doing so would allow each person to serve as their own control and reduce confounding due to characteristics such as intelligence, personality and eyesight. Another trip to the library uncovered a study of this sort involving cellphone subscribers in 1985 (see Canete). This study of 305 individuals found a significantly lower collision rate in the year following the purchase of a cellphone (8.2 percent versus 6.6 percent). We were impressed by these data but still worried about residual confounding. People's driving might generally improve over time. Additionally, perhaps some individuals used the fact of a recent collision to justify the purchase of a new telephone. If true, the apparent protective association might be misleading.

We realized that there was only one way to eliminate confounding (Moore, 1977): namely, a controlled experiment that removed any self-selection. We again returned to the library looking for a randomized trial that assigned individuals to either use or not use a cellphone while driving. This time we found nothing, presumably because it is unethical to deliberately expose individuals to potential hazards. What we did find were studies that used driving simulators and reported worsening performances on some indirect measures. In one study (Alm & Nilsson, 1995), for example, the average participant's reaction time increased significantly when using a hands-free cellphone (1.6 ms versus 2.2 ms). However, we weren't convinced. Data obtained in artificial circumstances that involve hypothetical risks and unnatural conversations might not provide an accurate assessment of the real relationship between cellphone calls and motor-vehicle collisions.

At the library, we also noticed an interesting article on whether episodes of heavy exercise triggered heart attacks in middle-aged people (Mittleman, Maclure, Tofler et al., 1993). The design was fascinating and seemed to provide a novel method for testing the transient effects of a brief exposure on the onset of an acute condition. In that study, investigators interviewed heart-attack survivors and asked each what they were doing just before the heart-attack began. Of the 1,228 patients, more had been exercising during the hour before the heart attack than during the same hour on the day before the heart attack (54 versus 13). After taking into account self-matching, Bayes' formula and the near-equivalence of probability and odds for rare events, the investigators inferred that heavy exercise was associated with a five-fold increase in the risk of a heart attack. This design is called the case-crossover and this statistical approach is called McNemar's test (Maclure, 1991).

We decided to carry out a case-crossover study to assess whether cellphone calls were associated with motor-vehicle collisions (Redelmeier & Tibshirani, 1997). We identified drivers in Toronto between July 1994 and August 1995 who had been in a collision involving significant damage but no personal injury (persons involved in injury collisions were not accessible). In total, 5890 were screened, of which 1064 acknowledged having a cellular telephone, 742 consented to our reviewing their phone records and 699 provided accurate telephone numbers that could be linked to detailed billing records. The data showed that drivers were more likely to have made a cellphone call during the ten-minute interval immediately before the collision than during a similar interval on the day before the collision (twenty-four percent versus five percent). The summary results from this study suggested that drivers were at a 6.5-fold increased risk of a motor-vehicle collision when they were using a telephone compared to when they were not using a telephone.

These results were interesting, but we believed that the detective work needed to pursue some shaky-looking characters. In particular, we still had doubts because of the potential for residual confounding. For example, selecting the day prior to a collision for the control interval might be inappropriate if it meant comparing Monday-morning driving to Sunday-morning driving. Perhaps the individual never drove on the weekend. More generally, people drive intermittently, rather than every day at the same time. To address this issue, we re-interviewed the individuals in our study and recomputed the relative risk based only on those individuals who were confident they had been driving a motor vehicle at the time of the collision on the day before the collision. The analysis of this highly selected group revealed a relative risk of 7.0.

This result was encouraging, but we still had some concerns and wondered whether there might be another method for adjusting for driving intermittence, as a double-check.

For an alternative approach, we considered the probability that an individual would drive on two consecutive days and appealed to the logic of conditional probability. That is, if people have only a 50-percent chance of driving a vehicle at a given time on 2 consecutive days then, by random chance alone, we should expect only half as many cellphone calls in the control interval as in the hazard interval. Therefore, a crude analysis might detect a relative risk of two but an adjusted analysis would reveal a relative risk of one. We could not find a good estimate of this probability in the literature, so we conducted our own survey of drivers involved in a collision (not necessarily cellphone owners) and obtained an estimate of 0.65 for the probability of driving on the day before the collision at the same time as the collision. Adjusting the results of the primary analysis by this factor yielded a relative risk of 4.3.

Selecting the day immediately prior to the collision was still somewhat bothersome because it was arbitrary. Fortunately, we had collected several consecutive days of data on each driver and were able to test other comparison days, each adjusted for driving intermittence using the conditional-probability approach. In one analysis, we used the preceding day of the work week—that is, a collision on Monday was compared to the previous Friday. In another analysis, we used the day exactly seven days prior—that is, a collision on Monday was compared to the preceding Monday. In a third analysis, we used three consecutive days before the collision and selected whichever day yielded the most conservative estimate. In other analyses, we used other comparison days. All of the analyses yielded a relative risk of about 4, thereby giving us some faith in the robustness of our findings.

We next considered biases arising from not knowing the precise moment of every collision. We reasoned that individuals might use their cellphones immediately after a collision to make an emergency call. It would be a blunder to mislabel these calls made after the fact as having contributed to the collision. To tackle this question, we reviewed our technique for establishing the time of collision; namely, by retrieving the individuals' statement, police records and telephone listing of emergency calls. In cases when all three sources agreed (or when one source was missing but the other two agreed), we classified the collision times as exact. Otherwise, we classified the collision times as inexact and used the earliest available time in our analysis. This seemed reasonable but imperfect. When we reran our analysis on the 231 who had exact collision times, we obtained a relative risk of 4.0. When we reran our analysis based on the 272 who later made an emergency telephone call, we obtained a relative risk of 7.6. Both results were statistically significant and both were adjusted for driving intermittence.

We next explored some potential explanations for the apparent association between cellphone calls and motor-vehicle collisions. When we restricted the analysis to the 144 who had owned a cellphone for more than five years, we still obtained a relative risk of 4.1. This suggested that the association was not just a reflection of inexperience but, instead, might indicate a more basic limitation in driver performance. We then analyzed the 148 who used a hands-free cellphone and obtained a relative risk of 5.9. This suggested that hands-free cellphones offered no large safety advantage and implied that the main factor in a collision was a driver's limitations in attention rather than in dexterity. A false sense of security, however, could also have led people to have a liberal attitude towards hands-free cellphones and thereby to expose themselves to greater risk than if they had hand-held cellphones.

The apparent association seemed to incriminate not so much what drivers were doing with their hands but what they were doing with their brains. But what about vision or hearing? In the mid 1990s, voice-activated dialing was not generally available and was not directly evaluated in our study. To examine potential safety advantages, we re-analyzed the data based on only incoming cellphone calls. The results showed a relative risk of 3.0, suggesting that the act of dialing was not the main contributor to the observed association. The acoustic quality of cellphone calls in the mid 1990s was less than ideal and may have been particularly poor in hands-free units compared to hand-held units. We had no way to test this hypothesis and recognize that it may also explain the absence of a large safety advantage associated with hands-free cellular telephones if annoying noises were especially distracting.

We next wondered whether there were any circumstances when talking on a cellphone was more or less risky than average. To find out, we reran the analyses for collisions occurring in the morning, afternoon and evening, and found consistent results throughout. We concluded that no particular time of the day was especially dangerous or safe. Similarly, we recalculated the association for collisions occurring in winter and summer, and again found consistent results. We concluded that the potential hazards might apply to other regions that are warmer or colder than Canada. Finally, we compared collisions occurring at high-speed locations to collisions occurring at low-speed locations and obtained a significantly greater relative risk in locations with significantly greater relative speeds (5.4 versus 1.6). However, we formed no strong conclusions from this comparison because we did not know the actual speed of the vehicle at the time of impact or the type of roadways travelled during the control interval.

Our results suggested that cellphones may distract drivers and thereby contribute to an increased risk of a motor-vehicle collision. On this basis, we recommend that cellphones be used sparingly. That is, drivers should avoid unnecessary calls, keep the conversations brief and suspend dialogue during particularly hazardous circumstances. Late at night when roads are wet is not the time for drivers to multiply their risk of a collision by a factor of four. As one of us is a medical doctor, we also repeated established advice that all drivers should abstain from alcohol, avoid excessive speed and minimize other distractions. For people who do not have cellphones but converse with those that do, we suggest an awareness of the potentially distracting effect and encourage both parties to interrupt dialogue any time during hazardous driving circumstances.

In our study, we also directed some effort to estimating positive aspects of using a cellular telephone. For example, we were able to show that cellphones offered benefits because people could use them to make emergency calls swiftly. The technology is reasonably durable, able to withstand the initial impact of most motor-vehicle collisions and thereafter can be useful for summoning help. Overall, 39 percent of the people in our study made at least 1 emergency call immediately after the collision. Additionally, cellular telephones seemed to be convenient during the rest of the day for making calls either to home, the office, the insurance company, the repair shop or other persons. Some people in our study only used their cellphones for emergencies and never made a call otherwise. For these few individuals (14 out of 699), the technology offered some potential benefits and no potential risks.

After publishing our main results, we were approached by many journalists and learned to anticipate several common questions. As insinuated by the title of this article, some people have interpreted our research to indicate that using a cellphone is equivalent to driving drunk. This is not true. Driving with a blood-alcohol level at the legal limit is associated with a relative risk of four (Simpson, 1985), which is about the same as what we found for using a cellular telephone. However, driving with a blood-alcohol level 50 percent above the legal limit is associated with a risk factor of ten (Simpson, 1985). And greater degrees of intoxication must surely be associated with even higher relative risks. Furthermore, alcohol stays in the bloodstream for several hours whereas a typical cellphone call lasts only one or two minutes. The cumulative risks associated with intoxication are much greater than those associated with using a cellphone.

The brief duration of most cellphone calls also helps explain why the increased popularity has not been accompanied by a dramatic increase in the number of collisions. Consider a driver who has about a 1 in 50 annual chance, or 0.020, of being in a collision. The relative risk of 4 for cellphones means that if the driver was always on the telephone, the annual chance of a collision would increase to about 0.080. Spending only a third of the time on the telephone, perhaps a more realistic estimate, would amount to a 0.040 annual chance of a collision (0.33 x 0.08 + 0.67 x 0.02). And a population where 5 percent of drivers suddenly acquired cellphones would show an increase from 0.020 to 0.021 annual chance of a collision (0.05 x 0.04 + 0.95 x 0.02). The difference between 0.020 and 0.021 would be imperceptible when compared to overall trends in collision rates (Ontario Ministry of Transportation, 1996).

We have sometimes been asked for the number of drivers who were still holding their telephones at the time of impact. An exact answer is difficult because the duration of each call is not recorded to the nearest second. Some drivers in our study might have dropped their phones a moment before the crash. And a few might have been off the phone for as much as a minute before the crash. Not knowing the precise time each call ended, therefore, adds irrelevant calls. Such irrelevant calls appear in both the hazard and control intervals, with the net effect of having our analysis under-estimate the relative risk ratio. Roughly speaking, irrelevant calls dilute the apparent relative risks. Thus, the degree of under-estimation depends on when each call stops being relevant. The degree of under-estimation would be large if the effects of a call resolved immediately after it ended (and small if drivers need substantial time afterwards to return their full attention to the road).

Journalists have wondered how the relative risk associated with using a cellphone might compare to the relative risk associated with drinking coffee, applying makeup or shaving while driving. Our study involved only cellphones, and we can only speculate about these other potential distractions. Indeed, speculation may be the only insight available for a long time, given that objective records of these activities are unlikely to be available soon. One notable distinction, however, is that taking a sip of coffee only takes a moment and drivers can self-select the moment they think appropriate. In comparison, a cellphone conversation is a much more extended exposure, during which driving circumstances can change dramatically. Hence, we limit our discussion of relative risks to conversations occurring on cellphones.

We have also been asked whether a conversation with a fellow passenger is identical to a cellphone conversation. Again, scientific data won't be available soon. There are three reasons to speculate, however, why these two types of conversations may not be the same. First, a fellow passenger contributes not just to distraction but also to vigilance (by pointing out factors such as nearby pedestrians, a missed street sign or an approaching vehicle). Second, a fellow passenger is unlikely to be a major client, an immediate supervisor or a surprise visitor. Third, a fellow passenger will be somewhat sensitive to roadway conditions and understand, for example, why a driver might have stopped talking when merging into heavy traffic. None of these three factors necessarily applies to the same extent for conversations occurring on cellphones. Again, we limit our discussion only to cellphone conversations.

Many journalists have pressed on the issue of regulation even though our study emphasized individual awareness and decision-making. As scientists, we believe our role is to provide reliable estimates of the magnitude of the risks and benefits; others must decide for themselves whether the benefits outweigh the risks. The most powerful argument in favour of regulation is that bad driving imposes risks on others. The most powerful rebuttal against regulation is that cellphones also confer advantages onto others (for example, the reporting of medical emergencies, criminal activity and mechanical break-downs). Public debate is necessary since cellphones contribute directly to quality of life, work productivity and peace of mind for more than 25 percent of the population in some countries. Scientific data contribute to this dialogue but should not dominate the discussion.

The most outlandish question we were asked (three times on-camera in rapid succession!) was whether cellphones are lethal weapons. Such a question betrays an overly dramatic interpretation of our research. We did not examine collisions that resulted in death, and we do not know how the association might change across the spectrum of severity. cellphones are not a sufficient cause, given that most calls do not result in a fatal collision. Cellphones are not a necessary cause, given that the majority of fatal collisions do not involve a cellphone call. Even if one accepted that cellphones could contribute to colli-sions, the exact causal mechanism is unknown and the potential would remain for making a change elsewhere (in the driver, vehicle or environment) that could eliminate risk of death. Statistics offers evidence so that decision-makers neither neglect nor exaggerate real-world situations.

20 RED-LIGHT CAMERAS

Techno-Policing at the Crossroads

J. PETER ROTHE

THE IMPLICATIONS of techno-policing as exemplified in photo-radar and red-light cameras for researchers and citizens are vast, giving spice to our work. We cannot be detached from its rigorous analysis, because techno-policing is not just an abstract, theoretical ideal. Rather, it is a definite process that leads to a tangible product, service and gain.

The effectiveness of red-light cameras, a mainstay of techno-policing, has been the subject of many studies. It has become law enforcement's claim for its side. In some circles, it has become a passion, a compulsion to better balance intersection safety. The introduction of red-light cameras has become a vital tool in the policing arsenal, intended to reduce red-light running at intersection and decrease injury and death.

Data from research projects, when taken together, indicate a variety of methodologies, findings, assumptions about technologies and ideologies about enforcement. This chapter critically reviews relevant findings pertaining to the sensitive topic of red-light cameras. Several questions underpin my review: How effective have red-light cameras been? How has effectiveness been defined and measured? What are some weaknesses or unintentional outcomes inherent in the deployment of red-light cameras?

■ Vital Definitions

As technological wizardry, the red-light camera is situated in a context of concepts and logic that requires brief mention before we dive into the issues. Red-light cameras are automated systems designed to photograph vehicles in violation of red traffic signals. They operate under any weather, road or light conditions. Automated cameras capture red-light violators on 35-mm film. They record date, time and location on each frame in a data bar. The cameras are usually tied directly to the traffic-signal system and are active only during the red phase of a traffic signal code. They are activated when a vehicle crosses a trigger during the red phase of a signal. The device is designed to provide evidence of red-light offences, officially intended to supplement law enforcement, enhance traffic safety, deter risk and provide income (Retting et al., 1995).

Red-light running occurs when drivers, for whatever reason, fail to stop their vehicles when instructed to do so by red-light signals and continue their journey over the "Stop" line, usually travelling into and through the junction. Red-running crashes occur when drivers fail to comply with the red-light signals and, as a direct effect of those actions, collide with either pedestrians or other vehicles (Birmingham City Council, 1989). The concept of red-light running has recently been reconfigured to discriminate between drivers who unwillingly find themselves in the dilemma of having to stop quickly or run the red because of speed and drivers who willfully choose to run the red light. In most cases, red-light running occurs when a vehicle enters an intersection, the vehicle is detected by pavement sensors after the signal has been red for a minimum elapsed time of 0.4 seconds, and the measured speed of the vehicle is at least 15 mph or 0.3 seconds without a speed component (Popolizio, 1995; Retting et al., 1997a., 1997b).

■ Red-Light Cameras as Traffic Surveillance
The red-light camera is part of automated traffic enforcement defined by Turner and Polk (1998) as

> the use of image capture technology to monitor and enforce traffic control laws, regulations or restrictions. Where enabling legislation authorizes the use of automated enforcement, the image capture technology negates the need for a police officer to directly witness a traffic offense. (p. 20)

The red-light camera system does not stand in isolation before the world of suspect drivers. It is a close cousin of the controversial photo-radar system, intended to pinpoint drivers who exceed the posted speed at a defined section of the roadway and present them with a significant traffic fine.

The red-light camera follows scenarios similar to those of photo-radar cameras. As drivers enter an intersection a second after the light turns red, they are caught on camera. Later they receive a traffic ticket. Recently, some traffic-safety and enforcement agencies have suggested a double whammy: introducing both red-light and photo-radar cameras to catch drivers for speeding and running red lights (discussed in meetings with Mission Possible manager, February 2000).

As part of techno-policing, red-light cameras fall within the broad ideology of pathological deviance (Pfohl, 1985), where electronic camera systems are designed to perform a recurrent search for drivers who are defined as high-risk agents. For example, on May 17, 1995, the British Columbia Minister of Transportation said that photo radar is introduced in accordance with the strategy that "targets high-risk and bad drivers" (Hansard, p. 14359). A month later, the same politician expounded, "We will be focussing on the worst offenders" (Hansard, p. 15269), followed by the remark, "We're looking at bringing the high-risk driver down to reasonable speed" (Hansard, p. 15453).

An original proposal for the large-scale introduction of photo radar in British Columbia declared that the province has 2,400,000 drivers (British Columbia Motor Vehicle Branch, 1995). The document further stated that British Columbia police forces hand out approximately 400,000 speeding tickets by conventional means. The British Columbia Motor Vehicle Branch expects an additional 1,600,000 violation tickets per year when photo radar has been successfully implemented. When the number of conventional citations are added to the expected number of citations offered through photo radar, we get a sum of approximately 2,000,000 speeding tickets per year. Taking it to its logical conclusion, the speeding tickets handed out/expected would be for more than 80 percent of the British Columbia drivers. Previous research completed in Victoria, Australia, estimates that 80 to 87 percent of all photo-radar tickets issued go to drivers who receive only one ticket per year. If we are bold enough to translate this percentage to British Columbia, ever so conservatively, we are left with the issue of bad or high-risk drivers. According to a senior official for the British Columbia Motor Vehicle Branch, photo-radar surveillance is quickly approaching the saturation stage, the point where there are fears that the public may react against the entire program and its supporting agencies (personal discussions, June 2000). Satisfaction with enforcement may likely be replaced by the alienation of the average driver (Corbett, 1995). The reach and intensity of state control through techno-policing will likely increase, regardless of the numbers of pathologically deviant drivers (Cohen, 1985).

From Becker's (1963) perspective, traffic-safety personnel cannot assume a given act of exceeding the speed limit or crossing an intersection at the beginning of a red light to be high-risk driving simply because it is commonly regarded as such. It is incumbent on the researcher to account for the process of labelling and blaming. The push for increased techno-policing drew on many sources: research methodologies to produce supportive findings, metaphors to describe targeted drivers, legalistic language to account for the official stance and the direct involvement of moral entrepreneurs like police and other sponsoring agencies. For example, Tignor and Warren (1995), Hauer (1971), Garber and Gadiraju (1989) and Lave (1985) note that whenever speed is stressed as the leading cause of crashes, officials are implying or outright suggesting that low speed is safe driving. Higher speeds do not necessarily increase crash rates; they increase only the severity of injury (Garber & Gadiraju, 1989). The use of metaphors like "speed kills" is a form of propaganda that overrides the issue of slow drivers being as much a "public hazard as fast ones" (Lave, 1985, p. 1163). Such incessant claims depend on a rationality that equates driving quality with sources of copious quantification. As Hauer et al. (1991) concludes,

> a venerable and large body of scientific literature tells us that it is difficult to identify accident-prone drivers on the basis of their record and convictions for offenses against the traffic law. (p. 133)

A second issue for debate is how the introduction of photo-radar enforcement affects human rights, average driver dignity and economic well-being. Does it do so justly and with respect for the interest of each driver, or does it favour the interests of others? The state (Pfohl, 1985)? In Canada, the penalty from two speeding tickets costs the driver approximately $300 to $400 (AMA Insurance Brochure, 2000). Could the increase in insurance premiums arising from two speeding citations provide insurance companies with a small windfall of money, or does it justify the cost of risks? Some prominent researchers, like Lave and Elias (1994), Prahlad et al. (1992), Chang et al. (1991), Garber and Gadiraju (1992), Sidhun (1990) and Pfefer et al. (1991), have written that when the United States increased speed limits from 55 mph to 65 mph, little discernable effect on the fatality rate was noted. Once external factors were accounted for, the increase in speed did not increase the number of fatal and injury crashes.

Local jurisdictions use photo-radar cameras to benefit from the continuous stream of income derived from automated systems that are designed to catch not the recidivist hard drivers but average citizens travelling at the 85th percentile. It is in their best interest that the community accepts "official" accounts of photo-radar effectiveness to help normalize routine activation of the system. With public approval, local jurisdictions feel empowered to expand their field of techno-policing by incorporating red-light cameras into their electronic surveillance portfolio.

Are the photo-radar equipment manufacturers and marketers major benefactors? The answer is a reluctant yes. Some jurisdictions have contracts with manufacturers who agree to provide the technology cost-free. However, there is an important proviso. Each jurisdiction is expected to distribute a certain number of speeding tickets for defined periods of time. The expectation becomes an unpublicized standard for policing and a point of silence for police spokespersons.

The ideology of centralized control, profit for jurisdictions and benefit for special agencies promotes the importance of driver passivity over action, dependence over autonomy, rigidity over flexibility, closedness over openness and authoritarian demands over democratic inquiry. Enforcement officials desire that the "driver personality" change from confidence to fear. As the logic goes, the change would create lower risk-taking, which in turn leads to reduction in the number and severity of crashes. In short, it promotes traffic safety.

■ Justifying Red-Light Cameras

Justifications are socially approved accounts that assert the positive value of a claim (Lyman & Scott, 1970). In the case of red-light cameras, justifications are used to explain that driving through intersections is problematic, and hence technological countermeasures are justified. Red-light cameras are controlled by the discretion of jurisdictions like cities or towns, provinces and police detachments. Stakeholders functioning within these jurisdictions tend to emphasize two justifying techniques to condemn the critics and appeal to loyalists. Through the use of condemnation, police spokespeople acknowledge the socially sensitive nature of red-light cameras. However, they quickly assert that bad drivers run red lights at intersections—drivers who are not noticed, caught, punished and condemned. This fact overrules their concern for social sensitivity.

The appeal to loyalties justifies the implementation of red-light cameras to serve the interests of other drivers and public safety. The following typical pro-enforcement appeals to loyalty substantiate the issue of installation:

- Deliberate running of red lights is a common and serious violation that contributes substantially to fatal crashes.
- The greater the number of crashes at a designated intersection, the more evidence there is of a problem in need of solution.
- The greater the number of traffic citations issued at a designated intersection, the more evidence there is of a problem in need of solution.
- The greater the number of public complaints about red-light running at a designated intersection, the more evidence there is of a problem in need of solution.
- The greater the volumes of traffic at a particular intersection, the greater the likelihood of violations.
- The greater the speed, the greater the likelihood of a red-light violation and the more dangerous any resulting crashes.

- The lower the cost to implement red-light cameras, the more likely they will be installed.
- The more the street is in need of major repairs, the less likely the installation of cameras, to avoid the cost of re-installing components that may be damaged during such work.

Fleck and Smith (1998) reported an extreme form of justification. In October 1994, a San Francisco motorist ran a red light and injured thirteen pedestrians waiting for a bus. The mishap resulted in a public campaign for red-light camera use in the city. According to the researchers, the rally was media-driven. In response to opponents arguing about unfair intrusions into the rights of motorists, a former traffic supervisor responded, "Being hit by a 3,000-pound car is a real invasion of one's rights."

■ Scanning the Research

A review of the literature reveals differences in the intents of red-light camera research. Emphasis was placed on using research strategies that could best identify crashes, estimate cost savings resulting from the implementation of the technological devices and uncover a change in numbers of crashes, injuries and deaths resulting from the implementation of the devices. A second stream of research clarified possible interrelationships between social, medical, economic and ethical divisions. This stream has important implications for traffic-control practice, stressing the need to sense and scan critical boundaries.

□ Methodologies used in previous studies

Time of measurement is one of the most controversial issues for discerning differences between pre-existing and present trends at red-light camera inter-sections. Some researchers follow the rule that simple year-to-year compar-isons are meaningless because of anomalous years. To attain a reasonable measure of trend, a five-year time-series study is required to ensure that the years are representative. The time-series allows for accurate historical trends within larger national or international trends.

A second common issue is the assurance that red-light camera intersections are compared to control sites. There might be similar crash reductions at loca-tions not using cameras. The question then becomes, if there are control sites, do they match the criteria used at the experimental sites?

Third, researchers expanded on the thesis that traffic volumes remain con-stant to avoid changes at a designated intersection because of, for instance, a new feeder route or growing suburb. An obvious result would likely be an increase in fatalities. According to Fridstrom (1995) and Oppe (1991), the number of crashes and fatalities is a function of traffic volume. To reduce the accident toll significantly, traffic-safety personnel decrease traffic volume, because it is one of the most important systematic determinants.

Fourth is the question of intervening variables. Researchers recognized the need to account for external factors that may have influenced crash or violation rates. For example, has the media played a significant and consistent role in red-light camera coverage? Have the weather, introduction of other traffic-safety programs, technological problems with the continuous operation of the cameras, and changes in the level of tolerance interfered with the data-collection? If so, have they been documented?

☐ *Reasons for researching red-light cameras*

A dominant objective for the study of red-light cameras was "to produce a detailed and rigorous cost–benefit analysis of red-light cameras" (Hansen, 1999; see also Rochi et al. 1997a, 1997b; Hook, Knox & Portas, 1996; Hooke, Knox & Portas, 1996; Popolizio, 1995). The ideology underlying such studies suggests that researchers wanted to prove that the implementation of red-light cameras is revenue-positive: no cost to the municipalities. Researchers set out to determine if the revenue realized from payment of violations would not only offset total cost but create additional revenue. Economic interests drove such studies.

An extension of economic gain was the determination of whether a red-light camera enforcement strategy can become a "violator funded" safety program (Hansen, 1999). Data analyses were undertaken to determine how financial savings on red-light cameras would pay for the technology within certain periods, e.g., one, two, three or more years (Birmingham City Council, 1989). South et al. (1988) sought to find the cost–benefit ratio of using the cameras versus the savings per year through number of crashes occurring at the research sites.

Numerous studies were engaged to measure impact—that is, whether the red-light cameras help modify driver behaviour as illustrated in a reduction in red-light running crashes or casualties (Maisey, 1981; Hillier, Ronczaka & Schnerring, 1993; Ng, Wong & Lum, 1997; Rogers, 1998). Andreassen (1995) was the first researcher to use a consistent accident-type code for analyzing records and determining impact. Measuring red-light running violations was also a high-priority objective for studying the effectiveness of red-light cameras. According to Thompson, Steel and Gallear (1989), measurement of effectiveness through red-light camera use is less obtrusive than police-intensive techniques. The traditional presence of police cruisers reduces the probability of detection, since drivers behave more cautiously in this situation.

Kent et al. (1997) studied the nature and extent of red-running behaviour in Victoria, Australia. The researchers wanted to study the differences in red-light running between intersections that had and did not have red-light cameras by examining the effects of road cross section, speed zone, traffic volume, lane type and day of week. Their goal was to make recommendations on future direction for the red-light camera program. Their objectives eliminated interest in the economic gains.

Studies undertaken by Retting et al. (1995, 1996, 1997a, 1997b, 1998) were designed to research only red-light violations, not crashes or their outcomes. Further, the research team wanted to profile red-runners so that future red-light camera programs could be made more effective. Members of the team intended to determine the extent to which drivers and police officers favoured the use of red-light cameras. No attention was paid to crashes, mortality or morbidity.

The majority of red-light camera studies cited in this review were evaluation-based, measuring crash or violation indicators. Others were designed to evaluate red-light camera strategies that included media, information sharing and public education (South et al., 1988; Hillier et al., 1993; Agent, 1996; Tarawneh, Singh & McCoy, 1997; Fleck & Smith, 1998; Hansen, 1999). Some focussed on the social acceptance of red-light cameras (Retting et al., 1997a, 1997b; Retting & Williams, 1998). These studies, in whole or part, used surveys to establish the extent to which people were informed about red-light cameras and whether their knowledge contributed to change in their driving behaviour.

☐ *Social impact*
People's experiences of society are, first of all, experiences with other people in their everyday lives. This is their micro-world, their immediate reality. Beyond that, people inhabit a macro-world that consists of large structures and institutions. Their relationships with others are more abstract, anonymous and remote. Both worlds give meaning, and both worlds are affected by innovations. They are part of patterns that regulate the behaviour of citizens, part of the institutional order that supports moral order and the sanctions of law.

Technologically designed law-enforcement tools and policies are specific examples of the legal institution whose rules are explicitly administered by special personnel like the police, judges, attorney generals, district attorneys and other professionals. A techno-policing tool like the red-light camera will surely have a social effect beyond the direct impact on specific crash, legal and injury characteristics. This effect is an important criterion by which to report previous red-light camera research.

Hulscher (1984) featured the importance of red-light cameras and social impact. He concluded that the effectiveness of traffic regulations can be measured in terms of social acceptance, which includes drivers' general knowledge and understanding of them, and deterrent consequences of non-compliance. Social acceptance of techno-policing stratagies continued to play a vital role in the late 1990s and the new millennium. Retting et al. (1997a, 1997b) recognized the importance of social acceptance. The research team engaged in public surveys in Oxnard, California, and Fairfax, Virginia. Results of the Oxnard (1997a) surveys conducted six weeks before and six weeks after implementation of a camera enforcement program, with a six-month follow-up, indicate that nearly eighty percent of Oxnard residents supported the use of red-light cameras as a supplement to traditional enforcement of traffic signals (p. 1). The same support was reached in the Fairfax, Virginia, study (1997b, p. 1).

Social-impact research on red-light cameras included the characterization of violators and how they perceive traffic enforcement. After researching red-light running on high-speed roads, Baguley (1998) defined three types of red-runners: drivers who are caught in the dilemma zone, drivers held up by slower traffic ahead or wavering due to indecision, and drivers who are able to stop comfortably but choose to deliberately run the red. According to Mahalel and Zeidel (1985), the first two types of red-light runners are not high-risk and can be managed by extending the traffic lights' amber periods or increasing the visibility of signal lights. But drivers who deliberately run red lights pose serious dangers and require surveillance enforcement techniques. Hardens (1986) agreed with Mahalel and Zeidel's (1985) conclusion. His study showed that an increase in amber from 3 to 4 seconds produced a reduction in red-running violations from 4.8 percent to 1.8 percent. An amber light of less than three seconds significantly increased the number of violations. He confirmed that a three-second period be used to provide an adequate clearance interval for speeds up to fifty kph. Thus, time itself can overcome certain red-light problems.

One of the leading goals for red-light camera research is to determine the extent to which the findings of research can be used to launch campaigns that define running red lights as dangerous and unacceptable. For example, the Birmingham City Council 1998 study concluded that running red lights is an intentional act that can be selected and modified through education campaigns. It needs to be exposed as dangerous and socially unacceptable. Similarly Hook, Knox and Poretas (1996) recommended that greater emphasis be placed on publicity to influence driver perceptions of risk. One strategy would be to publish the number of red-light-running prosecutions in an area.

Rogers (1998) studied photo-radar and red-light cameras in London, England. He analyzed media articles at the same time as he measured red-light violations. He reported that appropriate public relations encourages local media involvement for red-light cameras and more supportive reporting. For example, the local media used to refer to red-light cameras as "police spy cameras." They stopped using this label after police teams presented their point of view (p. 8). To attain even greater public relations, police officers offered local magistrates presentations in advance of red-light camera implementation.

The police made themselves available to answer any queries from the courts, communities and press (Rogers, p. 8).

South et al. (1988) reported that publicity for the use of red-light cameras created a demonstrable change in behaviour. For example, a red-light camera was installed at a high-volume intersection in Melbourne, Australia. When the public was not aware of the presence of the camera, "about 300 offenders were photographed each week" (South et al., 1988, p. 3). The number dropped to about twenty per week after the media attention.

☐ *A matter of ethics*

Ethics plays a major role in serious discussion on techno-policing. Hans (1997) featured two realities that need to be recognized when red-light cameras are installed. First is the interest from insurance companies, who want to be notified if their policyholders receive excessive numbers of tickets. Second is the balance between the individual and social good. Hans illustrated that a large sector of citizens regard the right to safe intersections as more important than fears about government surveillance and intrusive policing.

The concept of ethics and ethical behaviour on the part of the police and government officials proved to be the number-one issue in local media coverage on red-light cameras. Different perspectives on the issue of the common good versus personal liberty were found in many of the newspaper articles. Rogers (1998) was specific:

> We have no sympathy for the attitude which treats the Road Traffic Law as if it were some kind of game with rules which should allow the offender a sporting chance to escape. Enforcement of the Road Traffic Law is to prevent as many as possible of the 5,000 deaths and 300,000 casualties each year on the roads. That objective amply justifies the police making use of the best available means within the law to deter and detect offenders. That includes using the latest technology and targeting the use of that technology as precisely as possible on those most likely to be in breach of the law. (p. 13)

As a staff writer from the *Edmonton Sun* summed it up, "There's no reason why the police shouldn't utilize all the technology that's available to them if it means saving lives" (Bradley, 1998). That objective amply justifies the police using the best available means within the law to deter and detect offenders, including the latest technology, and targeting the use of that technology as precisely as possible on those most likely to be in breach of the law.

Rogers (1998) further suggested that because of the success of red-light cameras in reducing the number of red-light-related crashes and fatalities, other applications should be considered. For example, officials in his jurisdiction are looking at the feasability of using cameras to identify other offenses, such as prohibited turning movement (yellow boxes), by using real-time cameras linked directly to Scotland Yard. By introducing a broader spectrum of operation, Rogers has stepped into the ethical fray of red-light camera use and increased techno-policing.

Red-light cameras and constitutional rights are often combined to make ethical claims. To that end, Blackburn and Gilbert (1995) provided evidence of a 1950s US court decision that still stands today. In 1958, in *People versus Pett 178 N.Y.S.2d*, the Supreme Court concluded that the use of foot patrol that recorded a vehicle's speed and photographed its licence plate was not a violation of an individual's constitutional rights. Frangos (1999) considered this to be the forerunner of today's photo radar. The court stated that, "We have passed the horse and buggy days and are living in a new era. The question is, did the defendant do it and was there sufficient proof offered to find the defendant guilty beyond a reasonable doubt" (quoted in Frangos, p. 5). After hearing testimony by police officers and viewing trial tests of the system, the Court found the system was scientifically reliable and allowed the evidence to be admitted (Pasetti, 1997).

☐ *Privacy*

Beyond a doubt, the most pronounced ethical feature concerning techno-policing is privacy. Retting et al. (1998) engaged a series of random telephone surveys of Fairfax residents to determine their awareness and opinions about red-light enforcement approximately one month before and one year after a local program was implemented. Red-light cameras were preceded by a 30-day warning period; signs advising motorists of photo enforcement were posted on major roadways at numerous locations; press packages were provided to local media; postcards announcing the program were mailed to all Fairfax City residents. Citizens were well informed. Although 61 percent of the residents were in favour of red-light cameras, a constant number of residents still opposed red-light cameras because of privacy concerns. The authors answered the group's criticism with the following logic:

> Driving is a regulated activity on public roads, and neither the law nor public opinion suggests that drivers should not be observed on the road or have their violations documented. Red-light cameras can be designed to photograph only a vehicle's rear license plate and not the vehicle occupants, as is the case in Virginia. (p. 9)

National public opinion surveys in the US sponsored by the Insurance Institute for Highway Safety (IIHS) showed high support for the implementation of the technology in large cities (83 percent). According to the Society for Safety by Education Not Speed Enforcement (SENSE), although the studies were methodologically appropriate, the ethical premises reflect bias of the insurance companies. SENSE suggests that IIHS is a powerful lobby group funded by the US insurance industry (sense.bc.ca/research.htm).

Popolizio (1995) confirmed the importance of the privacy issue after his team of researchers evaluated red-light cameras. His focus was on the driver's picture. The city of New York uses only rear photographs to reduce the chance of identifying drivers. Turner and Polk (1998) promoted legal opinion in their treatment of the privacy issue. Their legal experts concluded that the red-light camera does not violate a citizen's legal right to privacy. Unfortunately, people do not readily accept the judgement because they perceive their cars as private places. Much like their homes, their cars have windows and walls, creating a sense of privacy and anonymity.

Media have used the privacy angle as a key lead-in to red-light-related articles. For example, N. Lakritz (1999), a staff writer from the *Calgary Herald,* exemplified the major privacy issue in the red-light camera debate:

> Red-light running is a serious problem and the idiots who do it deserve to be caught and made to pay the consequences, but there are ways to deal with this kind of offence that don't involve the continued and subtle erosion of privacy to which we are, increasingly, expected to resign ourselves. (p. A9)

The author discusses how red-light cameras dehumanize average motorists more than do police officers on location, because they are under the discomforting scrutiny of ongoing video surveillance. Jenkinson (1999) of the *Edmonton Sun* responded to civil libertarians' contention that the constant monitoring of people's behaviours erodes personal freedom by arguing that freedom does not include the right to break the law without expecting punishment. It is everyone's choice to use self-control and decide not to run red lights.

☐ *Red-light camera warnings*
Some research teams suggested that fair play should help determine how and where red-light cameras are placed. For example, Hook, Knox and Poretas (1996) concluded that use of red-light cameras has wider benefits than reducing crashes and red-running violations. Anecdotal evidence indicated that local communities derive benefit from the knowledge that speeds will be reduced and accidents will decrease. Further, the research showed that the

Department of Transport's use of signage achieved a high degree of driver recognition. The research team recommended that the impact of signage be regularly reviewed to increase the probability of drivers modifying their behaviour.

South et al. (1988) undertook an evaluation of red-light cameras based on the principle of deterrence rather than detection. Their focus was on visibility of the red-light cameras. While other jurisdictions operated on the principle of detection through surreptitious devices, Melbourne used warning signs as visible symbols of enforcement and deterrent effect on red-light running. But the deterrent effect was based more on economic effect than it was on safety principles: it was designed to limit police resources for processing offence photographs.

□ *Rear-end collisions*

A much-discussed hypothesis is that the implementation of red-light cameras contributes to an increase in rear-end collisions. This hypothesis is based on the assumption that drivers who normally run amber lights and likely continue driving through the red light may now stop suddenly because they fear the red-light camera. Drivers following behind operate on the "going through" assumption and possibly hit the lead car when the driver slams on the brakes.

Hillier et al. (1993) focussed on the rear-end collision hypothesis. The research team analyzed sixteen camera sites and sixteen matched control sites that were based on accident history, traffic volume and intersection configuration. Data were collected from 1986 to 1991 (p. 9). Log-linear analysis was used to determine whether there was any relationship between four key characteristics: camera/control, degree of accident causality/non-causality, accident type, and period before/after use of cameras. The researchers concluded that, although the red-light camera intersections reduced right-angle crashes and right-turn-against crashes, they increased rear-end crashes by "25 to 60 percent depending upon the location" (p. 36). Their analysis showed that right-angle and right-turn-opposed accidents decreased by 48 percent at camera sites but decreased by only 25 percent at the control sites; rear-end accidents increased by 61 percent at camera sites but decreased by 23 percent at control sites. However, rear-end accidents had a lower incidence of casualty accidents than right-angle and right-turn-opposed crashes. And this was an environment in which drivers were aware of red-light camera enforcement! The researchers concluded that there was no significant difference between total crashes at the camera sites and control sites. They generalized that the red-light cameras may have caused an exchange in which one group of crashes decreases while another group increases.

Ng et al. (1997) reported that they analyzed casualty accidents at 42 high-accident treatment junctions with a similarly matched sample of comparison junctions in Singapore. After analyzing data over a period of three years before introduction of red-light camera implementation and three years after, the researchers reported that a net reduction in collisions was about nine percent, with more than two-thirds contribution being from the head-to-side category (p. 80). Whereas head-to-side collisions experienced a net reduction of ten percent, an increase of six percent was observed for head-to-rear collisions (p. 80). The chi-square testing, however, did not reveal statistically significant differences at the five-percent level. This was in part due to the manner in which the collision data were coded, the possibility of an underlying mismatch between treatment and comparison samples, and the possibility of an area-wide effect (p. 80).

Andreassen (1995) engaged a parallel study to Hillier et al. (1993). He examined 41 sites and compared data from 5 years (1979-1983) pre-camera to 5 years (1985-1989) post-camera installation. The purpose of the study was to determine what effect red-light cameras had on crash type and frequency. He found no significant difference in pedestrian accidents, adjacent approaches and right-through crashes; however, rear-end crashes were significantly different: the rate in the first period was significantly less than the rate in the second period. Only five out of forty-one sites showed a decrease in rear-end crashes.

Other studies (Ogden, 1996; Perth Auditor General in Rochi et al., 1997a) concluded that the introduction of red-light cameras has decreased angle collisions, but there has been no similar improvement in rear-end collisions.

□ *Other collisions*
Most of the literature indicated that red-light cameras reduced the number of collisions occurring at intersections. Hook, Knox and Portas (1996) studied ten police force areas in London, thought to be broadly representative of the city from November 1995 to March 1996. Their collision-based findings showed a drop in the collision rate by 18 percent (0.48 per site per year) at traffic-light sites. Hillier, Ronczaka and Schnerring (1993) described how the presence of red-light cameras in Sydney, Australia, decreased the number of collisions between 1986 and 1991 by 13.5 percent. Fleck and Smith (1998) reported a more modest 9.2-percent reduction of collisions between 1992 and 1997 in their San Francisco study.

□ *Medical benefits*
Rogers (1998) used two locations in the greater London area that had high casualty rates attributed to red-light non-compliance. He noted that accident data for the first 3 years of operation on the Highway Agency road network

within the demonstration area showed that fatal accidents were down 70 percent while serious crashes were reduced by 38 percent and slight accidents were down 8 percent (p. 9). Unfortunately the author did not define the severity of injury scale. Fleck and Smith (1998) attributed a decrease of 9 percent in injury collisions to a reduction of red-light violators from 1992 to 1997 in San Francisco, while Hillier, Ronczaka and Schnerring (1993) concluded that casualty accidents that include fatalities and injuries decreased by 13.5 percent. The change was the same as the reduction in overall crashes.

□ *Red-light running*
A report from the City of Edmonton Police Services and Transportation and Streets (2000) stated that, by the end of a 14-month trial period, the occurrence of red-light violations had declined from 9.6 per day to 5.4 per day at a single intersection. Credit went both to the installation of the technology and the public-awareness campaign that emphasized the dangers of red-light violations. No further breakdowns of the findings were presented. Winn's (1995) Scottish study on red-light cameras showed that a 69-percent reduction in the total number of infringements recorded at 6 sites.

Retting et al. (1988) studied the prevalence and characteristics of red-running crashes in the US by evaluating the fatality-analysis reporting system and the general estimates system. They analyzed a subset of red-running crashes, which involved just two drivers, both of whom were going straight prior to the crashes. Red-running crashes accounted for five percent of all injury crashes nationwide and seven percent of injury crashes on urban roads. Red-running crashes are more likely than other crashes to have produced some degree of injury (47 percent versus 33 percent): 15 percent resulted in fatality or incapacitation, 31 percent caused non-incapacitating injuries and 54 percent produced possible injuries with severity distribution similar for other types of crashes. Ninety-seven percent of the sample crashes involved two or more vehicles; three percent involved pedestrians or cyclists. Cities with more than 200,000 residents account for 34 percent of fatal red-running crashes. The average rate was 2.5 crashes per 100,000 residents for the 5-year period. The study in Oxnard, California, established that there was an overall reduction of 40 percent red-running violations at camera sites and 50 percent at non-camera sites; the difference was not statistically significant. However, overall violation rate across camera and non-camera sites reduced approximately 42 percent from 13.2 to 7.7 per 10,000 vehicles compared to control sites (p = 0.0118) at 4 months; overall violation rates at control sites were essentially unchanged at 7.0 per 10,000 vehicles before and 6.7 after. Red-running crashes were twice as likely to occur on urban than rural roads (urban, 86 percent versus rural, 42 percent) compared to other fatal crashes, and they were more likely to occur during the day (day, 57 percent versus night, 48 percent); both red-light running and other intersection crashes occurred primarily in good weather conditions (91 percent and 87 percent).

Kent et al. (1997) studied 120 Melbourne sites and showed that red-running rates were higher for right-turn movements compared to through movements, especially in arterial roads with 60-kph speed zones and undivided roads. Red-running was also more common during the evening peak period. There were fewer encroachments at the sites where all approaches had fully controlled right-turn phases. Furthermore, the authors reported no difference in red-light running between camera and non-camera approaches when the traffic flow and environmental influences were relatively constant.

Ng, Wong and Lum (1998), implemented a 9-year traffic accident count at 125 red-light camera junctions in Singapore. They noted trends for red-running violations. One was vehicle type: motor-taxis, buses and minibuses were found to have high indices of violation, while motorcycles and scooters remained the lowest. The second was by type of intersection: violations were higher at three-legged compared to four-legged intersections (0.25 versus 0.19 violations per camera per hour). The results were statistically significant. Observational field studies were undertaken of 7 T-intersections along a major arterial road with speed limit of 70 kph for 2 periods of 1 hour each. The overall highest violation rate was 0.0088 for no-camera intersections, compared to a one-camera intersection rate of 0.0049 and a two-camera rate of 0.0020.

Chin (1989) also completed a red-light camera study in Singapore. Twenty-three sites were selected based on reports of red-running incidents. His analysis showed that red-running was reduced at camera sites but not at non-camera sites; the average reduction in red-running was approximately 40 percent—a significant finding. It was lowest for motorcycles and highest for trucks. Chin speculated that the speed and acceleration limitations of larger vehicles may have deterred drivers from attempting to run red lights.

□ *Red-light violator characteristics*
Red-light runners do not represent a common or generalized definition. Some drivers inadvertently enter an intersection after onset of the red signal; others commit intentional acts of red-light running. Because drivers cannot predict the onset of a yellow signal, the likelihood that a driver will stop is related to speed and distance from the intersection when the signal changes (Retting, Williams & Green, 1996, p. 23). According to these researchers, traffic-safety practitioners should pay attention to drivers who choose to proceed through a red light—deliberate red-light runners.

Jones (1992) established that the three-second mark was key for red-light running. He stated that most drivers who were within three seconds of the stop line at the onset of the yellow light chose to proceed. Most drivers who were more than three seconds from the stop line at the onset of the yellow light chose to stop.

Based on database analysis, Retting et al. (1988) reported that red-light runners were more likely to be younger than age 30 (43 percent versus non-red-light runners, 32 percent) and male. They were more likely to be fatally injured at intersection crashes (fatal, 40 percent versus non-fatal, 34 percent). Deaths of drivers or passengers occurred in 55 percent of red-running vehicles and in 47 percent of non-running vehicles. Red-light runners were more likely to have been driving with suspended, revoked or otherwise invalid driver's licenses, and were more likely to have prior DWI convictions and two or more moving driving violation convictions.

Retting et al. (1996) established that red-light runners in Arlington, Virginia, were less likely to drive late-model vehicles. Only thirteen percent had cars made after 1991, compared to twenty percent of compliers; six percent of violators drove large cars, compared to ten percent of compliers. Violators were less likely than compliers to wear safety belts (67 percent versus 74 percent). There was no gender difference between violators and compliers (both 71 percent). Twenty-six percent of violators were under thirty, compared to fourteen percent of compliers. Violators were three times more likely to have multiple speeding convictions: sixteen percent had three or more convictions versus only six percent of compliers; violators were also twice as likely to have very low point balances. Finally, violators and compliers had the same proportion (13 percent) of previous crashes reported to the Department of Motor Vehicles driver abstracts.

☐ *Economic implications*

Hook, Knox and Portas (1996) proposed that the use of cameras in London, England, released officers for other duties. Rather than patrol intersections, they could contribute to the investigation and detection of other crimes. Because the report was prepared by the police research group, police interest was evident: the researchers emphasized that red-light cameras increased income and decreased the workload for the police department. They further recommended that many tasks related to red-light cameras be undertaken by civilians under police supervision to reduce costs.

Hansen (1999) described how red-light violations were originally monitored. A team approach to red-light enforcement included an officer to observe the violation from a stationary position and radio the relevant information to other officers who stopped the targeted violators. Helicopters and unmarked vehicles were used at different observation locations. By using this strategy, a single three-hour enforcement costs more than $360 in personnel alone;

hence, only frequently repeated efforts are effective. This perspective helps illustrate why economics is highly relevant to red-light camera research.

Rocchi et al. (1997) developed a cost–benefit evaluation to "determine whether an investment in a red-light camera program could be considered by the Insurance Corporation of British Columbia" (p. 15). They reported several advantageous cost–benefit ratios in other jurisdictions. For example, New York city recorded a ratio of 1.35, while the United Kingdom reported a ratio of 2.0 over 1 year and a ratio of 12.0 over 5 years. After reviewing such potential for income, it makes sense for Klauz (1998) to feature the distribution of ticket revenue. As he comments, "It is important to decide in the design stage for what purpose the revenue generated by the automated enforcement system will be used."

Consistent with the ideological component of economic gain are studies that seek to establish primary cost–benefit analysis or that include cost–benefit as one of the objectives of the study. Birmingham City Council's (1988) study in Birmingham, UK, engaged in a cost–benefit analysis to ascertain the potential financial benefit of using red-light cameras. The researcher concluded that the introduction of red-light cameras in Birmingham, a city of one million people, reduced red-running crashes by twenty percent. The researcher did not consider the saving substantial and in fact found it disappointing.

Fleck and Smith (1998) pinpointed the economic perspective by measuring the extent to which red-light cameras can be both beneficial and income neutral. Their implementation plan was based on red-running statistics already entered in the local database. They estimated that violators cost the local economy approximately $40 million per year, excluding property damage costs (p. 2). Members of the San Francisco red-light camera project invited all interested vendors to participate in the pilot project. Two parties became involved and were responsible for two intersections. The city paid each vendor $30,000 to install the necessary equipment at intersection. Vendors received $17.50 per paid citation (the fine for violators was $104 plus 1 driver's point). The equipment remained the vendor's property. According to the authors, it became evident that $17.50 per citation was inadequate to maintain the program, and one vendor withdrew. The pilot finished with five cameras at five different locations (p. 2). After discovering that a fine for $104 was not enough to finance the program, the penalty was raised to $271. Local agencies were to receive $148 from each fully paid citation. The researchers concluded that a low issuance rate and high cost of automated enforcement may not be a cost-effective initiative. They wrote that "the bottom line is that photo enforcement, in combination with education and stiff police enforcement, has shown that it can increase public safety in a revenue neutral manner" (p. 4).

Rogers (1998) estimated a savings of twenty million pounds per annum due to decreased numbers of intersection crashes. Unfortunately, he did not include a detailed process used to arrive at the figure. However, he later defined staffing resources required to operate conventional automatic 35-mm camera sites. He concluded that the remote system is cost-effective:

- No site visits are required to load and then unload cameras to collect evidence ...
- Without leaving the monitoring position, one officer can remotely enforce any traffic regulation which would normally require an attendance on the street, with the exception of those offences requiring a notice to be attached to the offending vehicle.
- CCTV outstations, being on average at a height of 8 meters or above are seldom subject to vandalism, which increases their availability for monitoring. (p. 12)

South et al. (1988) engaged in a "limited look" at traffic-collision costs and their relationships with red-light cameras. The researchers concluded that there was a 13.8-percent reduction in crashes due to the presence of the red-light cameras. The percentage equated savings to $30,253 per site per year, totalling $1,390,000. The cost of operating the red-light cameras was $520,000 and thus the cost–benefit ratio was 2.7:1.

Hansen (1999) reported that a cost analysis by the Howard County, Maryland, police department determined that using a team enforcement approach to red-light violations resulted in personnel cost of $25.40 for each red-light-violation citation issued. Because of the high cost of traditional enforcement, the administration was concerned that this approach would become a burden to the taxpayer. Hence the County suggested red-light enforcement should be "violator funded" to benefit the citizens of Maryland and should only be initiated by jurisdictions that felt it was necessary for increased safety. The administrative fine would be returned to the jurisdiction that issued the administrative notice. No research-based explanation was provided.

□ *Commodifying the law*
Popolizio (1995) provided some insight into the private interests in red-light cameras. New York sought an advantaged position in the installation of red-light cameras because of the city's fiscal restraint program. Electronic Data Systems proposed a strategy of camera installation under the premise of no cost to the city. The revenue realized from payment for violations was to offset the total contractor and city costs (Popolizia, 1995, p. 114). The basis for

revenue is a function of the total number of possible violations captured by the red-light cameras. Thus, a realistic expectation of the number of violations had to be determined for covering costs. The total contract cost was $13,900,000 over 3 years for 15 cameras. By citing the owner of the car, not necessarily the driver, the violation is treated as a parking violation and the contractor can be paid. (If it were treated as a moving violation then all the revenue, except administrative costs, would pass to the state.)

A similar system was reported for Howard County, Maryland. Contract vendors are paid solely per violation issued. For this revenue, private companies furnish and operate cameras, identify the license numbers and obtain owner information from the Motor Vehicle Administration. It is up to the vendor to track each violation through payment or court adjudication. The recorded benefit is that the vendor system has created a violator-funded program to apprehend red-light runners, improve traffic safety, encourage metropolitan cooperation and permit police to direct most of their energies toward other police functions (Walter, 1998, p. 26).

Unfortunately, this kind of information was seldom included in the research and evaluation studies. It would be important to know the extent to which such contracts effect the number of red-running violations expected over a period of time and how those numbers provide a cost–benefit ratio for private companies and local governments.

■ Critical Rejoinders

A key point is that intersection collisions attributed to red-light running were assumed to result from drivers entering the intersections after the right of way had terminated. However, these crashes could also have occurred when drivers entered the intersection on the amber light and were not provided sufficient signal time to clear the intersection prior to the release of conflicting traffic (Retting & Williams, 1996).

Studies like South et al. (1988) and Andreassen (1995), which used control and treatment sites over periods of five or more years, have not been able to isolate intervening variables or "black spot" interventions. Such variables might include major or minor changes in signal timing; road surfacing; intermittent police enforcement; new driveways built near an intersection to accommodate new businesses and parking lots; and proximity to large-scale sports, entertainment or recreation events.

As Hillier et al. (1993) pointed out, the probability of red-light running causing an accident is still largely unknown. The best we can arrive at is a general estimate. Further, we still do not know whether the probability of crashes due to red-light running varies from intersection type to intersection type or from intersection to intersection. The site selections vary greatly according to roadway engineering, traffic volume, number of lanes, number of violations, crashes, deaths and injuries, geographical proximities, and similarity of traffic signals. Any of these variables could play a role in the power to generalize from control to treatment.

An issue arising from the many studies reviewed is the amount of time allowed for data collection. The times ranged from four weeks in the pre- and post- phases of implementing red-light cameras (Chin, 1989) to five years or more. Some studies focussed entirely on a simple pre/post treatment by way of specifically timed campaigns. Unfortunately, short-term observations do not allow for the dissipation of the halo effect and for situational and time-sensitive variables like bad winters, special events, or the initiation of other traffic-safety strategies (such as publicity, media sensationalism, construction, traffic-light synchronization and so on) to normalize over a period of time. Short-term observations isolate the findings from long-term trends or cycles. Retting, Williams, Farmer and Feldman (1998) developed a three-stage data collection plan in which red-light violation data were collected immediately prior to a public-warning period and then three months and one year afterward. Still, trends over years were not recorded. It may be that there already were time-based trends that showed red-light running was already declining.

For many studies, it is hard to separate the behavioural influences of red-light cameras from the influence of widespread media attention, publicity programs and public education. For example, Agent and Wagner (1996) engaged in a survey to establish the extent to which advertising about the red-light cameras contributed to behaviour. The finding was that 65 percent of the respondents remembered seeing public-education material, and 50 percent of those who answered stated that they had seen or heard red-light-running information indicated that they had changed their driving behaviour. Most stated that they now stopped for yellow lights. According to Wagner (1996), the most effective source of information was a changeable message sign that read "In the Bluegrass, Red Means Stop." Three signs were used at eight locations in Lexington for a total of 386 days.

Wagner's findings are relevant. If drivers respond to the fear of being caught, then the strategy might be to offer greater publicity and reduce the number of cameras. But since the cameras are largely implemented on a user-pay formula, the greater the number of citations given, the better the cost–benefit ratio. As a result, publicity or deterrence becomes less important.

The assumption that greater energy be spent to enforce red-light running is limited and fragile. Other techniques have been suggested that could also advance safety. For example, many traffic signals are not appropriately timed. Inadequate yellow clearance intervals force drivers to enter on the red, depending on the driver's speed and distance from the intersection at the time the light turns yellow. According to Retting and Williams (1996), this is not deliberate red-light running. Hence, increasing the duration of the amber signal has been shown to reduce the proportion of vehicles entering intersections prior to the release of conflicting traffic (Wortmon, Witkowski & Fox, 1985; Sten, 1986). Similarly, Retting, Williams and Greene (1998) proposed that traffic signals maintained at locations with very low traffic volumes may contribute to red-light running and intersection crashes. Kay, Neudorff and Wagner (1980) have shown that low-volume intersections that were converted from signal control to stop-sign control had fewer crashes and injuries.

Finally, insufficient attention has been paid to the ethical foundation of camera use as part of traffic enforcement generally and intersections specifically. When the cost–benefit ratio approaches 12.0 over a 5-year period (Hooke, Knox & Portas, 1996), and municipalities are fighting for increased revenue, it is not difficult to imagine the possibility of electronic surveillance becoming a significant contributor to city coffers, irrespective of safety. In concert with this proposition is the fact that most of the research to date has been done by stakeholders in the venture, such as police detachments and insurance-related empiricists. It is not surprising that expanded use of electronic surveillance is now being considered for other traffic scenarios.

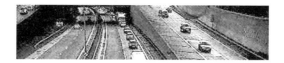

THIS REVIEW OF THE LITERATURE suggests that red-light cameras are effective in reducing red-running crashes and red-light violations. However, the installation of red-light cameras cannot be isolated from other factors. Future study should consider balancing the enforcement objectives with engineering, education and media, instead of relying entirely on techno-policing to fix everything (Turner & Polk, 1998).

Traffic Safety: Content over Packaging

J. PETER ROTHE

THE CLASSIC DEBATE in traffic safety is the basic character of traffic safety. To define it, we need to be holistic. An eye toward the future demands an appreciation of the past and a careful look at the present. In traffic safety, we have a situation where systems and sub-systems interrelate to form a completeness—a centrality of reality. Although we are a long way from exhausting all possible ways of recognizing and measuring traffic-safety reality, we are beginning to discern important conditions for broadly defining that reality.

It is often said that simple systems behave in simple ways. Unfortunately, that is not quite true. Traffic-safety systems are composed of complex behaviours that imply complex causes and entangled factors. Each system has its own experts whose lenses are focussed almost exclusively on their own subject matter. For example, a civil engineer who uses laboratories to measure asphalt wearing under different conditions, an economist who researches economic factors of transportation without much concern for geography, and a psychologist who studies cognition and driving while turning away from laws and government: all are professionals who know their area of expertise has collegially or self-imposed limitations. However, in combination, they form a complex traffic-safety reality in which systems form a web of interdependent fields.

We find ourselves approaching a crossroads. Should we continue with traditional means and methods that deal indepth with isolated phenomena but negate breadth? Or do we need new insights and explanations? I believe we need a paradigm shift, a fresh way to understand driving that combines human factors with the netted world of traffic. More and more, we feel the futility of studying elements apart from the whole of traffic safety. Thus, our resources are directed toward ideas that astonish us with regularity but leave us with many questions and concerns.

Traffic safety is not the gate to Dante's Hell or the embodiment of Camus' Sisyphus. Nature and people form patterns and are sensitively interdependent. These interdependent relationships become the new means for systems. If we take time to understand the systems of traffic safety, we can better look to the future and begin to interpret trends that will shape different systems.

■ The Future

This book is meant to contribute to energizing traffic safety in the future, a future that serves the needs of all while maintaining a sense of social dignity, equality and ethics. Based on the cybernetic lenses we used for sense-making, I suggest some possibilities for the future of traffic safety.

But first, an immediate issue. The implementation of techno-policing continues to rise. We are becoming increasingly exposed to the techno-policing advocates' rationalistic, moralistic, health-determining and cost-based decisions. More specifically, the use of red-light and photo-radar cameras has shown early successes in reducing deaths, injuries and red-running violations at intersections. However, counter arguments concerning public safety at the cost of government-based profiteering, increased control and commodification of traffic laws hang dangerously low over the heads of police administrators; insurance companies; municipal, provincial and federal politicians; and others in enforcement-related ventures.

It would be wise to ensure that techno-policing, like other enforcement strategies, be above ethical reproach. Its use on the streets should not encourage public cynicism, skepticism or anger. It should not profit from "average drivers." It would be in communities' best interests to develop municipal committees, made up of representatives from different walks of life, to analyze red-light cameras' important practical, economic, legal, moral, industrial and social assumptions, as well as their embeddedness in a democratic society. These findings should be distributed to the media and educational institutions so that everyone in the community understands the positive and negative realities of techno-policing. Such a strategy would serve the common good, not interest-driven agencies making backroom deals with enforcement officials.

Future traffic-safety endeavours suggest the concepts of authenticity and language. Many terms in traffic-safety jargon reflect democratic ideals but serve as little more than rationalizations or legitimizers. For example, how is community policing defined and used? Does community policing encourage police offices in specific regions to provide community-sensitive enforcement, education and social contact according to the needs of the community? If a paradigm shift is realized, how does the spirit and practicality of community policing relate to the increasing use of techno-policing that is anonymous, depersonalized, top-down enforcement? Similar arguments can be raised for community-development programs in traffic safety that are championed by the police. The police like to practise the ideology of "catch and penalize" while the community puts great faith in an ideology that embraces awareness, education, self-determination, information and understanding of legal issues. Enforcement plays but one role in the equation. Traffic safety's ultimate good, its altruistic intention to unconditionally save lives, is constantly being encroached upon by the ideology of cost–benefit, profit and techno-control.

To date, we have placed insufficient emphasis on community-development strategies and community-sensitive traffic-safety initiatives. We need more involvement here. Coalition groups are essential to initiate community programs that address the many traffic sub-systems. For example, local college or high-school students can be trained to observe and document "roadway conflicts." Their findings can be tabulated, interpreted and presented to municipal officers, who in turn may engage engineers, legal professionals or geography experts to review possible intervention strategies, such as crosswalk signs, flashing yellow lights and stop signs. Other community activities can be initiated to include cultural and social emphases on driving, while enforcement techniques are organized with full support of the community. Driver training upgrades, medical analysis of injuries, local emergency-room statistics, media exposure and sensitive treatment may also be included in community programs. Finally, local or grassroots initiatives particular to a community should be planned for implementation.

In many ways, our work here suggests that the "next step" in rethinking traffic safety is to figure out how to support a wider array of research and intervention strategies that encompass a cybernetic approach. We must take advantage of "opportunities" in various sectors to initiate and promote interrelated innovations that address, simultaneously, different levels of the traffic-safety reality. The next step challenges us to reconceptualize how we view labelled road users, define causation and risk, promote enforcement, design roads and vehicles, and manage traffic-safety services in order to facilitate true system participation, ethical delivery and integration.

BIBLIOGRAPHY

Aamodt, A. & Plaza, E. 1998. *Case-Based Reasoning: Foundational Issues, Methodological Variations and System Approaches.* Available on-line at www.iiia.csic.es/People/enric/AICom_ToC.html.

Abelson, R.P. 1981. Psychological status of the script concept. *American Psychologist,* 36, 715–29.

Adams, J. 1993. Risk Compensation and the Problem of Measuring Children's Independent Mobility and Safety on the Roads. In Mayer Hillman (Ed.), *Children, Transport and the Quality of Life* (pp. 48–58). London: Policy Studies Institute.

Adams, J. 1995. *Risk.* London: University College London Press.

Advocates for Highway and Auto Safety. 1999. *Stuck in Neutral: Recommendations for Shifting the Highway and Auto Safety Agenda into High Gear, A Comprehensive Report on the Major Highway and Auto Safety Issues Facing America.* A. Butler, K. Pson & B. Gill. Washington, DC: Author.

Agent, K.R. & Wagner, D. 1996. *Evaluation of Red Light Running Campaign.* Research Report KTC–96–29, Kentucky Transportation Center, Lexington, KY.

Alberta Centre for Injury Control and Research. 1998. *Injury Statistics.* Edmonton.

Alberta Motor Association. 1996. *Mission Possible: Integrated Traffic Safety Initiative for Alberta.* AMA Mission Possible policy paper presented to partners, Edmonton.

Alberta Transportation. 1997. *Alberta Traffic Collision Statistics, 1997.* Edmonton: Alberta Transportation.

Aldenderfer, M. 1996. *Anthropology, Space, and Geographic Information Systems.* New York: Oxford University Press.

Allison, E. W. & Allison, M.A. 1995. Using culture and communication theory in postmodern urban planning: A cybernetic approach. *Communication Research*, 22 (6), 627–45.

Alm, H. & Nilsson L. 1995. The effects of a mobile telephone task on driver behaviour in a car following situation. *Accident Analysis and Prevention*, 27, 707–15.

American College of Surgeons on Committee on Trauma. 1997. *Advanced Trauma Life Support for Doctors.* Instructor course manual, 417–38.

Andaluz, D., Roberts, T. & Siddall, S. 1997. GIS Adds a New Dimension to Crash Analysis. *URISA Journal*, 9 (1), 56–59.

Andersen, R. 1998 (September/October). Road to Ruin. *Extra!*, 22–23.

Anderssen, E. 2000. Inquest hears accident horror stories. *Globe and Mail*, 10 June.

Andreassen, D. 1995. *A Long Term Study of Red Light Cameras and Accidents.* Victoria, Australia: Australian Road Research Board.

Anheier, H. 2000. Can culture, market and state relate? *LSE Magazine,* 12 (1), 16–18.

Arthur, R.M. 1996. GIS Analysis of Speed Related Traffic Collisions. Unpublished master's thesis, Department of Geography, University of Calgary, Calgary, AB.

Arthur, R.M. & Waters, N.M. 1995a. *Exploratory Multivariate Analysis of Traffic Collision Data.* Canadian Transportation Research Forum, Annual Conference Proceedings, 618–32.

Arthur, R.M. & Waters, N.M. 1995b (November). GIS to Maximize Photo Radar Deployment Effectiveness. *GIS/LIS Annual Conference and Exposition,* pp. 20–28.

Arthur, R.M. & Waters, N.M. 1997. Formal Scientific Research of Traffic Collision Data Utilizing GIS. *Transportation Planning and Technology*, 21 (2), 121–37.

Baguley, C.J. 1988. Running the red at signals on high-speed roads. *Traffic Engineering Control*, 29, 7.

Bahro, M., Silber, E., Box, P. & Sunderland, T. 1995. Giving up driving in alzheimer's disease—An integrative theraputic approach. *International Journal of Geriatric Psychiatry*, 10, 871–74.

Baker, S.P., O'Neill, B., Ginsburg, M.J. & Goyhu, L. 1992. *The Injury Fact Book* (2nd Ed.). Oxford: Oxford University Press.

Ballard, J. 1973. *Crash*. New York: The Noonday Press.

Barbone, F. et al. 1998. Association of road–traffic accidents with benzodiazepine use. *The Lancet*, 352, 1331–36.

Barnhart, C.L. & Barnhart, R.K. (Eds.) 1983. *The World Book Dictionary*. Chicago: World Book.

Barss, P., Smith, G., Baker, S. & Mohan, D. 1998. *Injury Prevention: An International Perspective. Epidemiology, Surveillance, and Policy*. New York: Oxford University Press.

Bateson, G. 1972. *Steps to the Ecology of Mind*. New York: Ballantine Books.

Bateson, G. 1979. *Mind and Nature: A Necessary Unit*. New York: E.P. Dutton.

Becker, H. 1964. *The Other Side: Perspectives on Deviance*. New York: Free Press.

Becker, H. 1966. *Social Problems: A Modern Approach*. New York: J. Wiley & Sons.

Beirness, D., Mayhew, D. & Simpson, H. 1997. *DWI Repeat Offenders: A Review and Synthesis of the Literature*. Ottawa: Health Canada.

Benekohal, R.F. 1997. *Traffic Congestion and Traffic Safety in the 21st Century: Challenges, Innovations and Opportunities*. Proceedings of the Conference Sponsored by the American Society of Civil Engineers, ASCE, New York.

Berger, J. 1972. *Ways of Seeing*. London: British Broadcasting Corporation and Penguin.

Berger, K.T. 1988. *Zen Driving*. New York: Ballantine Books.

Berger, P. & Berger, B. 1975. *Sociology: A Biographical Point of View*. New York: Basic Books.

Berger, P.L. & Luckmann, T. 1966. *The Social Construction of Reality*. Harmondsworth: Penguin.

Bergqvist, C. & Findlay, S. 2000. Representing Women's Interests in the Policy Process: Women's Organizing and State Initiatives in Sweden and Canada, 1960s–1990s. In L. Briskin & M. Eliasson (Eds.), *Women's Organizing and Public Policy in Canada and Sweden* (pp. 119–46). Kingston & Montreal: McGill-Queen's University Press.

Bierness, D.J. & Simpson, H.M. 1988. Lifestyle Correlates of Risky Driving and Accident Involvement Among Youth. *Alcohol, Drugs, and Driving*, 4 (3–4), 193–204.

Birmingham (UK) City Council. 1989. *Red-Light Running: Accidents and Surveillance Cameras*. AA Foundation Report Series, AA Foundation for Safety Research, Fanum House.

Blackburn, R.R. & Gilbert, T.A. 1995. Photographic Enforcement of Traffic Laws. *Synthesis of Highway Practice*, 219.

Blazer, D., George, L.K., Landerman, R., Pennybacker, M., Melville, M.L., Woodbury, M., Manton, K.G., Jordan, K. & Locke, B. 1985. Psychiatric disorders: Rural–urban comparison. *Archives of General Psychiatry*, 42, 651–56.

Blincoe, L.J. 1994. *The Economic Cost of Motor Vehicle Crashes, 1994*. National Highway Traffic Safety Administration. Washington, DC: US Department of Transportation.

Bloom, B.S. (Ed.) 1956. *Taxonomy of Educational Objectives: The Classification of Educational Goals. Handbook I: Cognitive Domain.* New York: David McKay.

Bonzano, A., Cunningham, P. & Meckiff, C. 1996. ISAC: A CBR System for Decision Support in Air Traffic Control. In Smith and Faltings (Eds.).

Bowron, D. 1996. *A Portable Residential Speed Limit Warning Sign System for Controlling Speed on Urban Roadways.* Unpublished master's thesis, Department of Civil Engineering, University of Calgary, Calgary, AB.

Bradley, K. 1998. "Red light Spy-Cam Tops Cops. *Edmonton Sun,* 7 November.

Bradsher, K. 1997. Collision Odds Turn Lopsided As Sales of Big Vehicles Boom. *New York Times,* 19 March.

Bradsher, K. 1997. A Deadly Highway Mismatch Ignored. *New York Times,* 24 September.

Briskin, L. 1999. Mapping Women's Organizing in Sweden and Canada. In L. Briskin & M. Eliasson (Eds.), *Women's Organizing and Public Policy in Canada and Sweden* (pp. 3–50). Montreal & Kingston: McGill-Queen's University Press.

Brody, J.E. 1994. Personal Health. *New York Times,* 19 January.

Bronfenbrenner, U. 1977. Toward an Experimental Ecology of Human Development. *American Psychologist,* 518.

Broome, M.R. 1985. *The Implication of Driver Stress.* Proceedings Seminar NPTRC, Summer Meeting Vol. P270.

Brown, I. 1994. Driver Fatigue. *Human Factors,* 36, 298–314.

Brubacher, J.W., Case, C.W. & Reagan, T.G. 1994. *Becoming a Reflective Educator.* Thousand Oaks, CA: Corwin.

Burgess, A.R., Dishinger, P.C., Oquinn, T. & Schmidhauser, C.B. 1995. Lower–Extremity Injuries in Drivers of Air–bag Equipped Automobiles: Clinical and Crash Reconstruction Correlations. *Journal of Trauma-Injury and Critical Care,* 38 (4), 509–16.

Burneko, G. 1991. It happens by itself: The tao of cooperation, systems theory and constitutive hermeneutics. *World Futures,* 31, 139–60.

Caine, R.N. & Caine, G. 1991. *Making Connections: Teaching and the Human Brain.* Alexandria, VA: Association for Supervision and Curriculum Development.

Cameron, B. & Gonäs, L. 1999. Women's Response to Economic and Political Integration in Canada and Sweden. In L. Briskin & M. Eliasson (Eds.), *Women's Organizing and Public Policy in Canada and Sweden* (pp. 51–86). Montreal & Kingston: McGill-Queen's University Press.

Cameron, M. 2000. Workers' Compensation Board press conference, MISSION POSSIBLE @ Work launch, Edmonton, AB.

Canete, D.W. 1985. *AT&T cellular phone safety study: A survey of cellular phone owners located in the Baltimore/Washington, DC. Metropolitan Area.* Parsipany, NJ: AT&T Consumer Products.

Carlsson, G. 1997a (November 26). *Cost-effectiveness of information campaigns and enforcement and the costs and benefits of speed changes.* European Seminar in Luxembourg, Luxembourg.

Carlsson, G. 1998 (June 8–10). "Vision Zero" in Perspective of Global Generalization. In *"Vision Zero" in Perspective on Global Generalization.* Eighth PRI World Conference, Lisbon, Portugal.

Carr, W. & Kemmis, S. 1986. *Becoming Critical: Education, Knowledge and Action Research.* London: Falmer.

Carroll, B. & Solomon, R. 2000. Understanding Drinking and Driving Reforms: A Profile of the Ontario Statistics. *Injury Prevention,* 6, 96–101.

Carskadon, M. & Dement, W.C. 1981. Cumulative effects of sleep restriction on daytime sleepiness. *Psychophysiology,* 18, 107–13.

Carskadon, M. & Dement, W.C. 1987. Daytime sleepiness: quantification of a behavioral state. *Neuroscience Biobehavioral Review,* 11, 307–17.

Catalano, V. & Schoen, J. 1997. Neighborhood Traffic Management in Tucson, Arizona. In Benekohal, pp. 21–33.

Cellular Telecommunication Industry Association. 1996. *U.S. wireless industry survey results.* News Release of the Cellular Telecommunication Industry Association, March 25, Washington, DC.

Chang, G.L., Carter, E. & Chen, C.H. 1991. *Safety Impacts on the 65-MPH speed Limit on Interstate Highways.* AAA Foundation for Traffic Safety.

Checkland, P.B. 1981. *Systems Thinking, Systems Practice.* Chichester, UK: Wiley.

Chen, D.W. 1999. Suit Accusing Shopping Mall of Racism Over Bus Policy Settled. *New York Times,* 18 November.

Chin, H.C. 1989 (April). Effect of automatic red light cameras on red-running. *Traffic Engineering and Control,* 30 (4), 175–79.

Christie, J. 2000. Alliance Advocates Need for Safe Sport. *Globe and Mail,* 23 June.

Cicourel, A. 1974. *Cognitive Sociology: Language and Meaning in Social Interaction.* New York: Free Press.

Clark, A.W. & Prolisko, A. 1979. Social role correlates of driving accidents. *Human Factors,* 27 (5), 555–76.

Clark, A.W. 1975. A social role approach to driver behavior. *Perceptual and Motor Skills,* 42, 325–26.

Claybrook, J. 1984. *Retreat from Safety.* New York: Pantheon.

Clayton, D. & Waters, N.M. 1999. Distributed Knowledge, Distributed Processing, Distributed Users: Integrating Case-Based Reasoning and GIS for Multicriteria Decision Making. In J.-C. Thill (Ed.), *Spatial Multicriteria Decision Making and Analysis: A Geographic Information Sciences Approach* (pp. 247–74). Aldershot and Brookfield, USA: Ashgate.

Cloke, P., Philo, C. & Sadler, D. 1991. *Approaching Human Geography: An Introduction to Contemporary Theoretical Debates.* New York: Guilford Press

Cochran-Smith, M. & Lytle, S. 1993. *Inside/Outside: Teacher Research and Knowledge.* New York: Teachers College.

Cohen, S. 1985. *Visions of Social Control.* Cambridge, UK: Polity Press.

Collingwood, R.G. 1956. *The Idea of History.* New York: Galaxy.

Commoner, B. 1990. *Making Peace with the Planet.* New York: Pantheon.

Cooley, C.H. 1922. *Human Nature and Social Order.* New York: Scribner's.

Corbett, C. 1995. Road Traffic Offending and the Introduction of Speed Cameras in England: The First Self-Report Survey. *Accident Analysis and Prevention,* 27 (3), 345–54.

Coren, S. 1992. *Left Hander: Everything You Need to Know About Lefthandedness.* London: John Murray.

Coussins, N. 1983. *The Healing Heart.* New York: W.W. Norton.

Crandall, R.W. et al. 1986. *Regulating the Automobile.* Washington, DC: The Brookings Institute.

CRASH. 1999. *Report on Big Truck Safety by Province: April 1999.* Ottawa: Citizens for Responsible and Safe Highways.

Crawford, B. 2000. 401 Inquest: Day 1—"Clearly not typical fog." *Windsor Star,* 8 June.

Cross, P.K. 1981. *Adults as Learners.* San Francisco: Jossey-Bass.

Culyer, A.J. (Ed.) 1983. *Health Indicators.* Oxford: Martin Robertson.

Dalkie, H.S. 1993. *The Development and Application of a Model to Investigate Road Safety Issues.* PhD Thesis, University of Manitoba.

Darkenwald, G.G. & Merriam, S.B. 1982. *Adult Education: Foundations of Practice.* New York: Harper and Row.

Davies, D.I. & Herman, K. 1971. *Social Space: Canadian Perspectives.* Toronto: New Press.

Davies, J.C. & Manning, D.P. 1994a. Data collected by MAIM intelligent software: The first fifty accidents. *Safety Science,* 17 (3), 219–26.

Davies, J.C. & Manning, D.P. 1994b. MAIM: The concept and construction of intelligent software. *Safety Science,* 17 (3), 207–18.

Davis, R. 1992. *Death on the Streets: Cars and the Mythology of Road Safety*. North Yorkshire, UK: Leading Edge Press.

Dembert, M.L. 1984. The accident injury matrix and its use in diving injury investigations. *Aviation Space & Environmental Medicine*, 55 (12), 1143–47.

Dick, R. 2000. *Action Research Resources*. Available on-line at www.scu.edu.au/schools/gcm/ar/arhome.html.

Diemer, U. 2000. Contamination: The poisonous legacy of Ontario's environmental cutbacks. *Canadian Dimension*.

Dinges, D. 1995. An overview of sleepiness and accidents. *Journal of Sleep Research*, 4, 4–14.

Dow, E. 1998. *Marketing Road Safety: A Brief Case History December 1989 to December 1997*. Paper presented at the Traffic Safety Summit '98, Kananaskis, AB.

Drachman, D.A. 1988. Who may drive? Who may not? Who shall decide? *Annals of Neurology*, 24, 787–88.

Driver Behaviour at Right–Turn–on–Red Locations. 1999. *ITE Journal*, 62 (4), 18.

Drohan, M. 2000. Recent News Begs the Question: Why Not Take the Train? *Globe and Mail*, 13 June.

Ducheks, J.M., Hunt, L., Ball, K., Buckles, V. & Morris, J.C. 1998. Attention and driving performance in Alzheimer's disease. *Journal of Gerontology*, 53B, 130–41.

Dyck, D. 1999. *Wrapping Up the Wellness Package*. Available on-line at www.benefitscanada.com/content/1999/01-99/ben46.html.

Dym, B. 1987. The cybernetics of physical illness. *Family Process*, 26, 35–48.

Edmans, J.A. 1987. The frequency of perceptual deficits after stroke. *Clinical Rehabilitation*, 1, 273–81.

Edmonton Transportation and Street Department. 2000. *Intersection Photo Enforcement: The Edmonton Experience*. A report presented by the Edmonton Police Service and Transportation and Streets.

Edwards, J.R. 1992. A cybernetic theory of stress, coping, and well being in organizations. *Academy of Management Review*, 17 (2), 275–98.

Eisenhandler, S.A. 1990. The asphalt indentikit: Old age and the driver's license. *International Journal of Aging and Human Development*, 30 (1), 1–14.

Ellis, A. & Grieger, R. 1977. *Handbook of Rational Emotive Therapy*. New York: Springer Pub. Co.

Elvik, R. 1997. Effects on Accidents of Automatic Speed Enforcement in Norway. In *Transportation Research Record #1595 Highway Safety, Traffic Law Compliance, Speed Management and Heavy Trucks* (pp. 14–19). Washington, DC: Transportation Research Board, National Academy Press.

Elvik, R., Kolbenstvedt, M. & Stangeby, I. 1999. Walking or Cycling? *Nordic Road & Transport Research,* 3

Engel, G. 1980. The clinical application of the biopsychosocial model. *American Journal of Psychiatry,* 137, 535–44.

Engwicht, D. 1993. *Reclaiming Our Towns and Cities: Better Living with Less Traffic.* Philadelphia: New Society Publishers.

Erchak, G.M. 1984. The escalation and maintenance of spouse abuse: A Cybernetic Model. *Victimology: An International Journal,* 9 (27), 247–53.

Ericsson, K.A. & Simon, H.A. 1984. *Protocol Analysis: Verbal Reports as Data.* Cambridge, MA: MIT Press.

Erikson, E.H. 1968. *Identity Youth And Crisis.* New York: W.W. Norton.

Espejo, R. 1994. What is systemic thinking? *System Dynamics Review,* 10 (2–3), 199–212.

Evans, L. 1988. Older driver involvement in fatal and severe traffic crashes. *Journal of Gerontology,* 43, S189.

Fabrega, H. 1974. *Disease and Social Behavior.* Cambridge, MA: MIT Press.

Fleck J.L & Smith, B.B. 1998 (November). *Can We Make Red Light Runners Stop/ Red Light Photo Enforcement in San Francisco, California.* Report submitted to the City of San Francisco Department of Public Health.

Florman, S.C. 1981. *Blaming Technology: The Irrational Search for Scapegoats.* New York: St. Martin's Press.

Forrest, S. 1988. Suicide and the rural adolescent. *Adolescence,* 23 (90), 341–47.

Foucault, M. 1979. *Discipline and Punish.* New York: Vintage Books.

Francescutti, L.H. 1997. Injury Control: Are You Accountable? *Canadian Journal of CME,* 109–19.

Frangos, G.E. 1999 (January 10–14). *Automated Enforcement: Applied ITS technology.* Transportation Research Board 78th Annual Meeting, Washington, DC.

Frascara, J. 1997. *User-Centred Graphic Design: Mass Communications and Social Change.* London & Washington: Taylor & Francis.

Frascara, J. 1998. *Profiling the Alberta Road User.* Prepared for the Traffic Safety Summit 1998, organized by the Mission Possible coalition. Funded by the Alberta Neurotrauma Fundation.

Frascara, J. et al. 1992. *Traffic Safety in Alberta/Casualty Collision and the 18–24 Year Old Male Driver: Criteria for a Targeted Communication Campaign.* Alberta Motor Association/Alberta Solicitor General, Edmonton, AB.

Freund, P. & Martin, G. 1993. *The Ecology of the Automobile.* Montreal: Black Rose Books.

Freund, P. & Martin, G. 1997. Speaking about Accidents: The Ideology of Auto Safety. *Health*, 1 (2), 167–82.

Freund, P.E. & McGuire, M.B. 1999. *Health, Illness, and the Social Body: A Critical Sociology* (3rd Ed.). Upper Saddle River, NJ: Prentice-Hall.

Freund, P. & Martin, G. 1993. *The Ecology of the Automobile*. Montreal: Black Rose Books.

Fridstrom, L. 1995. Measuring the Contribution of Randomness, Exposure, Weather, Daylight to the Variation in Road Accident Counts. *Accident Analysis and Prevention*, 27 (1), 1–20.

Gabe, J. 1996. Health, Medicine and Risk: The Need for a Sociological Approach. In J. Gabe (Ed.), *Medicine, Health and Risk* (pp. 2–17). Oxford: Basil Blackwell.

Galbraith, J.K., Conceicao, P. & Ferreira, P. 1999. Inequality and Unemployment in Europe: The American Cure. *New Left Review*, 237, 28–51.

Gallagher, M. et al. 1989. Effects of the 60 MPH Speed Limit on rural Interstate Fatalities in New Mexico. *Journal of the American Medical Association*, 262, 2243–45.

Garber, N.J. & Gadiraju, R. 1992. Impact of Differential Speed Limits on the Speed of Traffic and the Rate of Accidents. *Transportation Research Record,* 1375.

Garber, N.J. and Gadiraju, R. 1989. Factors Affecting Speed Variance and Influence on Accidents. *Transportation Research Record*, 1213, 69.

Gennarelli, T.A., Champion, H.R., Copes, W.S. & Sacco, W.J. 1994. Comparison of mortality, morbidity, and severity of 59,713 head injured patients with 114,447 patients with extracranial injuries. *Journal of Trauma*, 37 (6), 962–68.

Goffman, I. 1974. *Frame Analysis: An Essay on the Organization of Experience.* Cambridge, MA: Harvard University Press.

Goleman, D. 1995. *Emotional Intelligence*. New York: Bantam Books.

Gooder, P. & Charny, M. 1993. The difficulties of investigating motor vehicle traffic accident mortality in a district. *Public Health*, 107 (3), 177–83.

Gottman, J. 1981 *Time Series Analysis: A Comprehensive Introduction for Social Scientists.* Cambridge, MA: Cambridge University Press.

Green, R.N., German, A., Nowak, E.S., Dalmotas, D. & Stewart, D.E. 1994. Fatal injuries to restrained passenger car occupants in Canada: crash modes and kinematics of injury. *Accident Analysis and Prevention*, 26 (2), 207–14.

Gregersen, N.P., et al. 1997. Road Safety Improvement in Large Companies. An Experimental Comparison of Different Measures. *Accident Analysis and Prevention*, 28 (3), 297–306.

Grossman, D.C., Kim. A., Macdonald, S., Klein, P., Copass, M. & Maier, R.V. 1997. Urban–rural differences in prehospital care of major trauma. *Journal of Trauma: Injury, Infection, and Critical Care*, 42 (4), 723–29.

Guastello, S.J. & Guastello, D.D. 1986. The relation between the locus of control construct and involvement in traffic accidents. *Journal of Psychology*, 120 (3), 293–97.

Gulian, E., Glendon, A.I., Matthews, G., Davies, D.R. & Debney, M. 1988. Exploration of driver stress using self report data. In T. Rothengatter and R. deBruin (Eds.), *Road User Behaviour: Theory and Research* (pp. 342–47). Assen/Maastricht, The Netherlands: Van Gorcum.

Gunnarsson, S.O. 1998. *Designing a Safer Traffic Environment.* Paper presented at the Traffic Safety Summit '98, Kananaskis, AB.

Gusfield, J. 1992. Foreword. In Ross, L.H. *Confronting Drunk Driving: Social Policy for Saving Lives.* New Haven: Yale University Press.

Gusfield, J.R. 1981. *The Culture of Public Problems: Drinking, Driving and the Symbolic Order.* Chicago: University of Chicago Press.

Gusfield, J.R. 1990. Concept, Context and Community: Sociological Perspectives on Traffic Safety. In J. Peter Rothe (Ed.), *Challenging the Old Order: Toward New Directions in Traffic Safety Theory.* New Brunswick, NJ: Transactions Publishers.

Haigh, K.Z. & Veloso, M. 1995. Route Planning by Analogy. In Veloso and Aamodt (Eds.), pp. 169–80.

Hakamies–Blomquist, L.E. 1997. Validity of medical screening as a tool for selecting older drivers. In T. Rothengatter & E.C. Vaya. (Eds.), *Traffic and Transport Psychology: Theory and Application* (pp. 445–48). New York: Pergamon.

Hakkert, A.S., Yelinek, A. & Efrat, E. 1991. Police Surveillance Methods and Police Allocation Models. In M.J. Koornstra and J. Christensen (Eds.), *Enforcement and Rewarding: Strategies and Effects: Proceedings of the International Road Safety Symposium in Copenhagen, Denmark, Sept. 19–21* (pp. 98–101). Leidschendam, The Netherlands: SWOV, Institute for Road Safety Research.

Handy, C. 1995. *The Empty Raincoat: Making Sense of the Future.* Reading, MA: Arrow.

Hansen, G. 1999. *Use of Automated Traffic Enforcement Technology to Modify Driving Behaviour.* Report presented to the Transportation Research Board, 78th Annual Meeting.

Hansen, T.D. & McIntire, W.G. 1984. *Rural Stress: Myths and Realities.* Report No. RC–015–198. Orono, ME: University of Maine. ERIC Document Reproduction Service No. ED 214 0181.

Hanson, S. 1995. Introduction. In Susan Hanson (Ed.), *The Geography of Urban Transportation* (pp. 3–25). New York: Guilford Press.

Harders, J. 1981. Untersuchungen uber die zweckmassigste Dauer der Gelbzeit in Lichtsinalanlagen. *Zeitschrift fur Verkehrssicherheit*, 27, 1.

Harper, G. & L'Huillier, L. 1990. Road Safety Campaign. In *Effective Advertising* (pp. 191–205). Advertising Federation of Australia.

Harre, R. 1984. *Personal Being.* Cambridge, MA: Harvard University Press.

Harries, K. 2000. Bring back photo radar, 401 inquest urges. *Toronto Star*, 29 June.

Harrison, T. & Laxer, G. (Eds.). 1995. *The Trojan Horse: Alberta and the Future of Canada.* Montreal: Black Rose Press.

Harvey, A.C. 1981. *Applied Time Series Models.* Hemel Hempstead, England: Philip Allan.

Hauer, E. & Ahlin, F. 1982. Speed Enforcement and Speed Choice. *Accident Analysis and Prevention*, 3 (1), 1–14.

Hauer, E. 1971. Accidents, Overtaking and Speed Control. *Accident Analysis and Prevention*, 3, 7.

Hauer, E., Bhagwant, N., Smiley, A. & Duncan, D. 1991. Estimating the Accident Potential of an Ontario Driver. *Accident Analysis and Prevention*, 23 (2–3), 133–52.

Hauer, E. 1990. The Engineering of Safety and the Safety of Engineering. In J. Peter Rothe (Ed.), *Challenging the Old Order: Towards New Directions in Traffic Safety Theory* (pp. 39–71). New Brunswick, NJ: Transaction Publishers.

Hauer, E. 1996. Statistical Test of Difference Between Expected Accident Frequencies. *Transportation Research Record* 1542.

Hearne, R. 1981. Car and Truck Speeds Related to Road Traffic Accidents on the Irish National Road System. In *Proceedings of the International Symposium on the Effects of Speed Limits on Traffic Accidents and Fuel Consumption* (pp. 81–88). Dublin, Ireland: Road Research Programme of the Organization for Economic Co-Operation and Development (OECD).

Hegel, G. 1967. *Philosophy of Right.* Translated by T. Knox. Oxford: Oxford University Press.

Hennessy, D.A. 1999. *The interaction of person and situation within the driving environment: Daily hassles, traffic congestion, driver stress, aggression, vengeance and past performance.* PhD thesis, York University, Toronto.

Hennessy, D.A. & Wiesenthal, D.L. 1997. The relationship between traffic congestion, driver stress and direct versus indirect coping behaviors. *Ergonomics*, 40, 348–61.

Hickmann, G. & Kaser, K. 1988. *Trau keinem uber tempo 30.* Stuttgart: Grunen im Landtag von Baden Wurttemberg.

Hilakivi, I. & Veilahti, J. 1989. A sixteen-factor personality test for predicting automobile driving accidents of young drivers. *Accident Analysis and Prevention*, 21, 413–18.

Hillier, W., Ronczka, J. & Schnerring, F. 1993. *An Evaluation of Red Light Cameras in Sydney.* New South Wales: Road Safety Bureau.

Holtz Kay, J. 1997. *Asphalt Nation: How the Automobile Took over America and How We Can Take It Back*. New York: Crown Publishers.

Homans, G.C. 1950. *The Human Group*. New York: Harcourt, Brace and World.

Hooke, A., Knox, J. & Portas, D. 1996. *Cost Benefit Analysis of Traffic Light and Speed Cameras*. London: Home Office Police Research Group Publication.

Horne, J.A. & Reyner, L.A. 1995. Sleep related vehicle accidents. *British Medical Journal*, 310, 565–67.

Hu, P.S. & Young, J.R. 1999. *Summary of Travel Trends*. Washington, DC: US Department of Transportation.

Hulscher, F.R. 1984 (March). The Problem of Stopping Drivers After the Termination of the Green Signal at Traffic Lights. *Traffic Engineering and Control*.

Hummel, R. 1994. *The Bureaucratic Experience: A Critique of Life in the Modern Organization*. New York: St. Martin's Press.

Hummer, J. 1994. Traffic Accident Studies. In H.D. Robertson, J.E. Hummer & D.C. Nelson (Eds.), *Manual of Transportation Engineering* (pp 191–218). Upper Saddle River, NJ: Prentice Hall.

Hunt, L.A , Murphy, C.F., Carr, D., Duchek, J.M., Buckles, V. & Morris, J.C. 1997. Reliability of the Washington University Road test: A performance-based assessment for drivers with dementia of the Alzheimer type. *Archives of Neurology*, 54, 707–12.

Hunt, L.A., Morris, J.C., Edwards, D. & Wilson, B.S. 1993. Driving performance in persons with mild senile dementia of the Alzheimer type. *Journal of the American Geriatrics Society*, 41, 747–53.

IBI Group, Knowles, V., Persaud, B., Parker, M. & Wilde, G. 1998. *Safety, Speed and Speed Management: A Canadian Review*. File No. ASF 3261–280. Ottawa: Transport Canada.

Inference Corporation. 1995. *CBR Express for Windows: Designing Case Bases*. El Segundo, California: Inference Corporation.

Injury Prevention Centre. 1993. *Injury Prevention Workshop Facilitator Handbook*. Edmonton: University of Alberta.

James, L. 1987. Traffic Violence: A Crisis in Community Mental Health. *Innercom* (Newsletter of the Mental Health Association in Hawaii). Available on-line at www.aloha.net/~dyc/violence.html.

James, L. 1996. *Traffic Psychology Research at the University of Hawaii*. Available on-line at www.soc.hawaii.edu/leonj/leonj/leonpsy/traffic/tpintro.html.

James, L. 1997a. *Aggressive Driving and Road Rage—Dealing With Emotionally Impaired Drivers. Text of Congressional Testimony on Aggressive Drivers*. Available on-line at www.aloha.net/~dyc/testimony.html.

James, L. 1997b. *Creating An Online Learning Environment That Fosters Information Literacy, Autonomous Learning and Leadership: The Hawaii Online Generational Community–Classroom.* Available on-line at www.soc.hawaii.edu/~leonj/leonj/leonpsy/instructor/kcc/kcc97.html.

James, L. 1998. *Aggressive Driving: The Effect of Age, Gender, and Type of Car.* Available on-line at www.aloha.net/~dyc/surveys/survey2/interpretations.html.

James (Jakobovits), L.A. & Nahl, D. 1987. Learning the library: Taxonomy of skills and errors. *College and Research Libraries,* 48 (3), 203–14.

James, L. & Nahl, D. 1999. *Socio-Cultural Methods of Managing Driving Behaviour in Society.* Available on-line at www.aloha.net/~dyc/drivingpsy.html.

James, L. & Nahl, D. 2000. *Road Rage and Aggressive Driving.* Amherst, NY: Prometheus Books.

Jenkinson, M. 1999. Don't Run a Red. *Edmonton Sun,* 25 May.

Jeron, J. 1996. *Co-operative Inquiry: Research into the Human Condition.* Thousand Oaks, CA: Sage.

Jones, G. 1992. *Driver Behavior at Signalized Intersections.* Unpublished master's thesis, University of Toronto, Ontario.

Kalischuk, R.G. 1999. Healing within families following youth suicide: A rural health focus. In W. Ramp, J. Kulig, I. Townshend & V. McGowan (Eds.), *Health in Rural Settings: Context for Action.* Lethbridge, AB: University of Lethbridge Printing.

Kampis, G. 1991. Different forms of causation in dynamical systems: Determinism, pattern generation, and information. *World Futures,* 30, 221–37.

Karr, A.R. 1995. Maybe the Traffic Safety Experts Missed Too Much Sleep Studying. *Wall Street Journal,* 19 January.

Kay, J.L., Neudorff, L.G. & Wagner, F.A. 1980. *Criteria for removing traffic signals.* Report DOT–FH–11–9524. US Department of Transportation.

Keegan, D. 1997. *Informal vs. Formal Traffic Laws.* PDE Publications Inc. Available on-line at www.drivers.com.

Keeny, B.P. 1983. *Aesthetics of Change.* New York: Guilford Press.

Kent, S., Corben, B., Fildes, B. & Dyte, D. 1995. Red Light Running Behavior at RedLight Camera and Control Intersections. *Monash University Accident Research Centre, Report #73.*

Kissane, D.W. & Bloch, S. 1994. Family grief. *British Journal of Psychiatry,* 164, 728–40.

Knowles, M. 1980. *The Modern Practice of Adult Education.* Chicago: Follett Press.

Kohlberg, L. 1976. Moral stages and moralization. In T. Lickona (Ed.), *Moral Development and Behaviour* (pp. 31–53). New York: Holt, Rinehart & Winston.

Komanoff, C. 1999. *Killed by Automobile.* New York: Right of Way.

Kong, L.B., Lekawa, M., Navarro, R.A., McGrath, J., Cohen, M., Margulies, D.R. & Hiatt, J.R. 1996. Pedestrian–motor vehicle trauma: an analysis of injury profiles by age. *Journal of the American College of Surgeons*, 182 (1), 17–23.

Koscielny, A.J., Tomich, D.J., Clark, J.E. & Lundgren, T.J. 1997. TRAFVU: A Graphics Processor for Traffic Simulation Models. In Benekohal, pp. 584–90.

Krathwohl, D.R., Bloom, B.S. & Masia, B.B. 1964. *Taxonomy of Educational Objectives: The Classification of Educational Goals. Handbook II: Affective Domain.* New York: David McKay.

Krech, D., Crutchfield, S. & Ballachey, E. 1963. *Individual in Society.* Tokyo: McGraw-Hill Kogakusha.

Kroj, G. & Utzelmann, H.D. 1997. The role of driver selection, improvement and rehabilitation in the field of traffic psychology. In T. Rothengatter & E.C. Vaya. (Eds.), *Traffic and transport psychology. Theory and application,* (pp. 431–34). New York: Pergamon.

Kullgren, A., Lie, A. & Tingvall, C. 1995. Crash pulse recorder—validation in full scale crash tests. *Accident Analysis and Prevention, 27* (5), 717–27.

Lafleur, C.D. 1990. *Complementarity as a program evaluation strategy: A focus on qualitative and quantitative methods.* Paper presented at the Canadian Evaluation Society Annual Conference, Toronto, ON.

Lafleur, C.D. 1995. Towards a culture of inquiry: A new research paradigm for Ontario education. *Orbit*, 26 (4), 16.

Laird, G. 1998. *Slumming It at the Rodeo.* Vancouver/Toronto: Douglas & McIntyre.

Lakritz, N. 1999. City Doesn't Need More Video Cameras. *Calgary Herald*, 23 May.

Langewiesche, W. 1998. The Lessons of ValuJet 592. *The Atlantic Monthly*, 281 (3), 81–98.

Lave, C. & Elias, P. 1994. Did the 65 MPH Speed Limit Save Lives? *Accident Analysis and Prevention*, 26 (1), 49–62.

Lave, C. 1985. Speeding, Coordination, and the 55 MPH Limit. *American Economic Review*, 75 (5), 1159–64.

Lave, C.A. & Lave, L.B. 1990. Barriers to Increasing Highway Safety. In J. Peter Rothe (Ed.), *Challenging the Old Order: Toward New Directions in Traffic Safety Theory* (pp. 77–93). London: Transaction Publishers.

Leake, D.B. (Ed.) 1996. *Case-Based Reasoning: Experiences, Lessons and Future Directions.* Cambridge, MA: MIT Press.

Leonard, J.D. & Davis, W.J. 1997. Urban Traffic Calming Measures–Conformance with AASHTO and MUTCD Guidelines. In Benekohal, pp. 14–20.

Litke, P.A. 1999. *Weasel Factor: Moral Imperatives in PSA Design.* Paper presented at the Department of Psychology Annual Student Conference, Calgary, AB.

Lonero, L. & Clinton, K. 1997. *Objectives For Behavioural Driver Safety Programs: An understanding of driver's cognitive and motivational influnces is needed for a successful approach to behaviour change.* PDE Publications Inc. Available on-line at www.drivers.com.

Lonero, L.P. et al. 1994. *The Roles of Legislation, Education, and Reinforcement in Changing Road User Behaviour.* Toronto: Ontario Ministry of Transportation.

Loo, G.T., Seigel, J.H., Dishinger, P.C., Rixen, D., Burgess, A.R., Addis, M.D., Oquinn, T., McCammon, L., Schmidhauser, C.B., Marsh, P., Hodge, P.A. & Bents, F. 1996. Airbag protection versus compartment intrusion effect determines the pattern of injuries in multiple motor vehicle crashes. *Journal of Trauma-Injury and Critical Care*, 41 (6), 935–51.

Luger, S. 2000. *Corporate Power, American Democracy and the Automobile Industry.* Cambridge, MA: Cambridge University Press.

Lum, K.M. & Wong, Y.D. 1998. Unmanned, Red-Light Surveillance Camera Systems Help to Reduce Accident Counts at Intersections. *ITE Journal.*

Lupton, D. 1999. Monsters in Metal Cocoons: 'Road Rage' and Cyborg Bodies. *Body and Society*, 5, 57–92.

Luria, A. 1961. *The Role of Speech in the Regulation of Normal and Abnormal Behaviour.* New York: Liveright.

Lyman, S. & Scott, M. 1970. *The Sociology of the Absurd.* New York: Appleton-Century Crofts.

Lynd, R. & Lynd, H. 1929. *Middletown.* New York: Harcourt Brace.

MacGregor, D. 1998. *Hegel and Marx After the Fall of Communism.* Cardiff: University of Wales Press.

Maclure, M. 1991. The case-crossover design: A method for studying transient effects on the risk of acute events. *American Journal of Epidemiology*, 133, 144–53.

Mad, Bad and on the Road. 1997. *The Economist*, 26 July.

Mahalel, D. & Zaidel, D. 1985. Safety evaluation on a flashing-green light in a traffic signal. *Traffic Engineering and Control*, 29 (7).

Maisey, G.E. 1981. *The Effect of Mechanical Surveillance Device on Urban Signalized Intersection Accidents.* Research and Statistics Report #17, Road Traffic Authority, Perth, Australia.

Marottoli, R.A., Mendes de Leon, C.F., Glass, T.A., Williams, C.S., Cooney, L.M., Berkman, L.F., & Tinetti, M.E. 1997. Driving cessation and increased depressive symtoms: Prospective evidence from the New Haven EPESE. *Journal of the American Geriatrics Society*, 45 (2), 202–06.

Martin, D. 1996. *Geographic Information Systems: Socioeconomic Applications.* London: Routledge.

Martin, G.T. & Freund, P. 1997. Speaking about accidents: the ideology of auto safety. *Health: An Interdisciplinary Journal for the Social Study of Health, Illness and Medicine*, 1 (2), 167–82.

Maturana, H.R. 1978. Biology of language: The epistemology of reality. In G.A. Miller and E. Lenneberg (Eds.), *Psychology and Biology of Language and Thought* (pp. 27–33).

Maynard, F.M. & Krasnick, R. 1988. Analysis of recreational off-road vehicle accidents resulting in spinal cord injury. *Annals of Emergency Medicine*, 17 (1), 30–33.

McKnight, A.J. & Adams, B.B. 1970. *Driver education task analysis.* Alexandria, VA: Human Resources Research Organization, 1970–1, Volumes I, II, III.

Meichenbaum, D. & Goodman, S. 1979. Clinical use of private speech and critical questions about its study in natural settings. In G. Zivin (Ed.), *The Development of Self-Regulation Through Private Speech.* New York: Wiley.

Michon, J.A. 1985. A critical view of driver behaviour models: What do we know, what should we do? In L. Evans and R.C. Schwing (Eds.), *Human Behaviour and Traffic Safety* (pp. 485–520). New York: Plenum Press.

Micik, S. & Miclette, M. 1985. Injury Prevention in the Community: A Systems Approach. *Pediatric Clinics of North America*, 32 (1), 251–65.

Midha, R. 1997. Epidemiology of brachial plexus injuries in a multitrauma population. *Neurosurgery*, 40 (6), 1182–88.

Miller, C.K. & Luloff, A.E. 1981. Who is rural? A typological approach to the examination of rurality. *Rural Sociology*, 46 (4), 608–25.

Miller, T.R. & Galbraith, M. 1995. *Traffic Safety and Health Care: State and National Estimates of Employer Costs.* National Highway Traffic Safety Administration. Washington, DC: US Department of Transportation.

Miller, W.R. & Rollnick, S. 1991. *Motivational Interviewing, Preparing People to Change Addictive Behavior.* New York: Guilford Press.

Miltner, E. & Salwender, H.J. 1995. Influencing Factors on the Injury Severity of Restrained Front Seat Occupants in Car-to-Car Head-On Collisions. *Accident Analysis and Prevention*, 27 (2), 143–50.

Miltner, E., Wiedmann, H.P., Leutwein, B., Hepp, H.P., Fischer, R., Salwender, H.J., Frobenius, H. & Kallieris, D. 1992. Liver and Spleen Ruptures in Authentic Car-to-Car Side Collisions With Main Impact at Front Door or B-Pillar. *American Journal of Preventive Medicine*, 13 (1), 2–6.

Mischel, W. 1991. Personality dispositions revised and revised: A view after three decades. In L.A. Pervin (Ed.), *Handbook of Personality Theory and Research* (pp. 111–34). New York: Guilford Press.

Mission Possible. 1998. *Provincial Speed Management: Discussion Paper.* Presented in Red Deer at the Provincial Speed Management Workshop.

Mitler, M.M. et al. 1997. The Sleep of Long-Haul Truck Drivers. *New England Journal of Medicine,* 337, 755–61.

Mittleman, M.A., Maclure, M., Tofler, G.H., et al. 1993. Triggering of acute myocardial infraction by heavy exertion. *New England Journal of Medicine,* 329, 1677–83.

Mohan, D. 1997. Discussion. In T. Fletcher and A.J. McMichael (Eds.). *Health at the Crossroads* (pp. 138–40). New York: John Wiley.

Moore, D. 1977. *Statistics: Concepts and Controversies* (4th Ed.). New York: W.H. Freedman Co.

MSN MoneyCentral. 1999. *Auto insurance for twentysomethings.* Available on-line at www.moneycentral.msn.com/articles/insure/auto/5113.asp.

Murray, C.J.L. & Lopez, A.D. (Eds.) 1996. *The Global Burden of Disease.* Cambridge, MA: Harvard University Press.

Myersw, R.J. & Haggerty, R.J. 1962. Streptococal infection in families: Factors altering individual susceptibility. *Pediatrics,* 29, 539–49.

Näätänen, R. & Summala, H. 1976. *Road-User Behaviour and Traffic Accidents.* Amsterdam: North Holland Publishing Co.; New York: American Elsevier Publishing Co. Inc.

Nader, R., Milleron, N. & Conacher, D. 1993. *Canada Firsts* (2nd Ed.). Toronto: McClelland and Stewart.

Nahl, D. 1993. *CD-ROM Point-of-Use Instructions for Novice Searchers: A Comparison of User-Centered Affectively Elaborated and System-Centered Unelaborated Text.* PhD Dissertation, University of Hawaii. Available on-line at www2.hawaii.edu/~nahl/articles/phd/phdtoc.html.

Nahl, D. 1997. Information Counseling Inventory of Affective and Cognitive Reactions while Learning the Internet. *Internet Reference Services Quarterly,* 2 (2/3), 11–33.

Nahl, D. 1998. Novices' First Use of Web Search Engines: Affective Control in Cognitive Processing. *Internet Reference Services Quarterly,* 3 (2), 51–72.

Nahl, D. 1999. *What is Driving Informatics?* Available on-line at www.aloha.net/~dyc/informatics.html.

Nahl, D. & James, L. 1996. *Achieving Focus, Engagement, and Acceptance: Three Phases of Adapting to Internet Use.* Available on-line at www.lib.ncsu.edu/stacks/e/ejvc/aejvc-v4no1-contents.txt.

Nash, J.E. & James, M.C. 1996. *The Meanings of Social Interaction.* Dix Hills, NY: General Hall Publishers.

Nathens, A., Jurkovich, G., Cummings, P., Rivara, F. & Maier, R. 2000. The Effect of Organized Systems of Trauma Care on Motor Vehicle Crash Mortality. *Journal of the American Medical Association*, 283 (15), 1990+.

National Committee for Injury Prevention and Control. 1989. Injury Prevention, Meeting the Challenge. *American Journal of Preventive Medicine*. New York: Oxford University Press.

National Highway Traffic Safety Administration 1998. *Traffic Safety Facts A Compilation of Motor Vehicle Crash Data from the Fatality Analysis Reporting System and the General Estimates System Motor Vehicle Traffic Crashes.* Washington, DC: US Department of Transportation.

National Safety Council. 1992. *Accident Facts*. Itasca, IL.

National Sleep Foundation. 1997. *Use of Continuous Shoulder Rumble Strips: consensus report.*

Neff, J.A. & Husaini, B.A. 1985. Stress buffer properties of alcohol consumption: The role of urbanicity and religious identification. *Journal of Health and Social Behaviour*, 26 (3), 207–22.

Nelson, C. 1973. *Applied Time Series Analysis for Managerial Forecasting.* San Francisco: Holden–Day Inc.

Ng, C.H., Wong, Y.D. & Lum, K.M. 1999. The Impact of Red-Light Surveillance Cameras on Road Safety in Singapore. *Road and Transport Research,* 6 (2), 72–81.

NHTSA. 1999. *Early Assessment of 1999 Crashes, Injuries, and Fatalities.* Available on-line at www.nhtsa.dot.gov/search97cgi/s97_cgi.exe.

Niemcryk, S.J., Kaufmann, C.R., Brawley, M. & Yount, S.I. 1997. Motor vehicle crashes, restraint use, and severity of injury in children in Nevada. *American Journal of Preventive Medicine*, 13 (2), 109–14.

Nikkel, K. 1998. BMW's Safety Breakthrough: Head Airbags. *Motor Trend*, 50 (1), 28.

Norman, D. 1992. *Turn Signals Are the Facial Expressions of Automobiles.* New York: Addison-Wesley.

Norman, D.A. 1993. *Things That Make Us Smart.* Reading, MA: Addison-Wesley.

Nouri, F.M. & Lincoln, N.B. 1992. Validation of a cognitive assessment: predicting driving performance after stroke. *Clinical Rehabilitation*, 6, 275–81.

Novaco, R.W. 1991. Aggression on Roadways. In R. Baenninger (Ed.), *Targets of Violence and Aggression* (pp. 253–327). New York: Elsevier.

Novaco, R.W., Stokols, D., Campbell, J. & Stokols, J. 1979. Transportation, stress and community psychology. *American Journal of Community Psychology*, 18, 231–57.

Ogden, K.W. 1996. *Safer Roads: A Guide to Road Safety Engineering.* An Avebury Technical Report, Aldershot, Australia.

Oldfield, R.C. 1971. The assessment and analysis of handedness: The Edinburgh Inventory. *Neuropsychologia*, 9, 97–113.

Ontario Ministry of Transportation. 1996. *Ontario road safety annual report 1994*. Downsview, ON: Safety Research Office, Ministry of Transportation.

Oppe, S. 1991. The Development of Traffic and Traffic Safety in Six Developed Countries. *Accident Analysis and Prevention,* 23 (5), 401.

Oppe, S. 1992. A comparison of some statistical techniques for road accident analysis. *Accident Analysis and Prevention,* 24 (4), 397–423.

Osberg, J.S. & Di, S.C. 1992. Morbidity among pediatric motor vehicle crash victims: the effectiveness of seat belts. *American Journal of Public Health*, 82 (3), 422–25.

Owsley, C., Ball, K., McGwin Jr., G., Sloane, M.E., Roenker, D.L., White, M.F. & Overley, E.T. 1998. Visual processing impairment and crash risk among old adults. *Journal of the American Medical Association*, 279, 1083–88.

Panitch, L. 2000. The New Imperial State. *New Left Review, Second Series,* 2, 5–20.

Parasuraman, R. & Nestor, P.G. 1991. Attention and driving skills in aging and Alzheimer's disease. *Human Factors*, 33, 539–57.

Passetti, K.A. 1997. *Use of Automated Enforcement for Red Light Violations.* CVEN 677 Advance Transportation Systems, Texas A & M University.

Pastore, A.L. & Maguire, K. 1996. Utilization Project. *Sourcebook of Criminal Justice Statistics*. Albany, NY: University of Albany.

Perrow, C. 1984. *Normal Accidents: Living with High-Risk Technologies.* New York: Basic Books (reprinted in 1999 by Princeton University Press, Princeton, NJ).

Persson, D. 1993. The elderly driver: Deciding when to stop. *The Gerontologist*, 33 (1), 88–91.

Petrie, H.G. 1981. *The Dilemma of Enquiry and Learning.* Chicago: University of Chicago Press.

Pfeffer, R.C., Stenzel, W.W. & Doo Lee, B. 1991. Safety Impact of the 65-MPH Speed Limit: A Time Series Analysis. *Transportation Research Record*, 1318, 22–33.

Pfohl, S. 1985. *Images of Deviance and Social Control, A Sociological History.* New York: McGraw-Hill.

Pharoah, T. & Apel, D. 1995. Case Studies: London. In T. Pharoah and D. Apel (Eds.), *Transport Concepts in European Cities* (pp. 27–55). Aldershot: Avebury.

Phelps, M. 2000. Canada Does Poorly on Child Poverty. *Globe and Mail*, 13 June.

Picard, R. 1997. *Affective Computing.* Cambridge, MA: MIT Press.

Pimble, J. & O'Toole, S. 1982. Analysis of accident reports. *Ergonomics*, 25 (11), 967–79.

Popolizio, P.E. 1995. *New York City's Red Light Camera Demonstration*. Report in 1995 Compendium of Papers, Institute of Transportation Engineers, 65th Annual Meeting.

Prahlad, D., Pant, A.A. & Niehaus, J. 1992. Effects of the 65-MPH Speed Limits on Traffic Accidents in Ohio. *Transportation Research Record*, 1375.

Prior, L. 1995. Chance and Modernity: Accidents as a Public Health Problem. In R. Bunton, S. Nettleton and R. Burrows (Eds.), *The Sociology of Health Promotion* (pp. 133–44). London: Routledge.

Probst, J. & Lewis, J. 1987 (March). *Planning for Court Monitoring*. SRA Technologies, Final Report to NHTSA, Contract No. DTNH–22–85–R–07255.

Probst, J., Lewis, J., Asunka, K., Hersey, J. & Oram, S. 1987 (March). *Assessment of Citizen Group Court Monitoring Programs*. SRA Technologies, Final Report on Contract No. DTNH22–85–C–07255 to NHTSA.

Ramp, W. 1999. Introduction, rural health: context and community. In W. Ramp, J. Kulig, I, Townshend & V. McGowan (Eds.), *Health in Rural Settings: Context for Action*. Lethbridge, AB: University of Lethbridge Printing.

Redelmeier, D.A. & Tibshirani, R.J. 1997. Association between cellular-telephone calls and motor vehicle collisions. *New England Journal of Medicine*, 336, 453–58.

Redmond, P., Barton, D., McQuillan, R. & O'Higgins, N. 1990. An audit of road traffic accident victims requiring admission to hospital. *Irish Medical Journal*, 83 (4), 133–36.

Reed, C. 1998. Lethal Weapon? *The Guardian*, 8 June.

Regina vs. *Schrader* 1999. Ontario Court. Provincial Division.

Reinarman, C. 1998. The Social Construction of an Alcohol Problem: The Case of Mothers Against Drunk Driving and Social Control in the 1980s. *Theory and Society*, 17, 91–120.

Retting, A., Williams, A., Farmer, C. & Feldman, A. 1997a. *Evaluation of Red Light Camera Enforcement in Oxnard, California*. Report of the Insurance Institute for Highway Safety, Arlington, VA.

Retting, A., Williams, A., Farmer, C. & Feldman, A. 1997b. *Evaluation of Red Light Camera Enforcement in Fairfax, Virginia*. Report of the Insurance Institute for Highway Safety, Arlington, VA.

Retting, R. & Green, M.A. 1994. *Characteristics of Red Light Violators: Results of a Field Investigation*. Arlington, VA: Insurance Institute for Traffic Safety.

Retting, R. & Green, M.A. 1995. *The Influence of Traffic Signal Timing or Running and Potential Vehicle Conflicts at Urban Intersections*. Arlington, VA: Insurance Institute for Traffic Safety.

Retting, R. & Williams, A. 1996. Characteristics of red light violators: Results of a field investigation. *Journal of Safety Research*, 27, 10.

Retting, R., Williams, A. & Greene, M. 1998. "Red light running and sensible countermeasures." *Transportation Research Record*, 1640, 23–26.

Rhodes, R. 1999. *Why They Kill*. New York: Alfred Knopf.

Rice, D.P., Mackenzie, E.J. & Assoc. 1989. *Cost of Injury in the United States*. Report to Congress. San Francisco: University of California in San Francisco, Institute of Health and Aging, and the Johns Hopkins University, Injury and Prevention Center.

Rice, F.P. 1995. *Human Development: A Life Span Approach* (2nd Ed.). Englewood Cliffs, NJ: Prentice Hall.

Rimer, S. 1998. Status for Retirement—Villagers, A (Still!) Valid Driver's Licence. *New York Times Magazine*, 15 November, 78–79.

Road Safety and Motor Vehicle Regulation Directorate. 1987. *Smashed*. Ottawa: Transport Canada.

Robertson, L.S. 1981. Patterns of teenaged driver involvement in fatal motor vehicle crashes: implications for policy choice. *Journal of Health Politics, Policy, and Law*, 6, 303–14.

Robertson, L.S. 1992. *Injury Epidemiology*. New York: Oxford University Press.

Rocchi, S., Hemsing, S., Yee, H. & Coffin, A. 1997a. *Benefit–Cost Review of Red Light Cameras. Technical Memorandum # 1–State of the Art Review*. Prepared by G.D. Hamilton Associates for the Insurance Corporation of British Columbia.

Rocchi, S., Hemsing, S., Yee, H. & Coffin, A. 1997b. *Benefit–Cost Review of Red Light Cameras. Technical Memorandum # 2*. Prepared by G.D. Hamilton Associates for the Insurance Corporation of British Columbia.

Rogers, J.H. 1998. *Traffic Signal Design: Techniques and Programs, Automatic Enforcement Cameras and Traffic Systems Control Unit*. A PTRC Report submitted March 25, London, England.

Rolling the Dice. 1997. *The Guardian,* 5 December.

Rosenberg, J. 1986. *Policy forum: The Personal Stress Problems of Farmers and Rural Americans*. Rockville, MD: National Institute of Mental Health.

Rosenfield, I. 1988. *The Invention of Memory*. New York: Basic Books.

Rosman, D.L., Knuiman, M.W. & Ryan, G.A. 1996. An evaluation of road crash injury severity measures. *Accident Analysis and Prevention*, 28 (2), 163–70.

Ross, H.L. 1994. *Confronting Drunk Driving: Social Policy for Saving Lives*. New Haven: Yale University Press.

Rothe, J.P. 1981. *Complementarity: A concept and a case*. Paper presented at the Annual Conference of the Australian Association for Research in Education, Adelaide, Australia.

Rothe, J.P. 1987. Erlebnis of Young Drivers Involved in Injury Producing Crashes. In J. Peter Rothe (Ed.), *Rethinking Young Drivers* (pp. 47–120). Vancouver: Insurance Corporation of British Columbia.

Rothe, J.P. 1991a. Traffic sociology: Social patterns of risk. In *The Second International Conference on New Ways for Improved Road Safety and Quality of Life Proceedings.* Tel Aviv, Israel.

Rothe, J.P. 1991b. *The Trucker's World: Risk, Safety and Mobility.* New Brunswick, NJ: Transaction Publishers.

Rothe, J.P. 1993a. *Novice Driver Education: A Social Psychological Perspective.* Paper presented at the Novice Driver Education, Edmonton, AB.

Rothe, J.P. 1993b. *Qualitative Research: A Practical Guide.* Heidelberg, ON: RCI/PDE Publications.

Rothe, J.P. 1994. *Beyond Traffic Safety.* New Brunswick, NJ: Transaction Publishers.

Rothe, J.P. 1996. *The Influence of Dispatching on Truck Driver Safety.* Report Submitted to Coordinator of Highway Safety, Research Grant Office Safety Research Office Safety Policy Branch. Toronto: Ontario Ministry of Transportation.

Rothe, J.P. 2000. *Undertaking Qualitative Research: Concepts and Cases in Injury, Health and Social Life.* Edmonton: University of Alberta Press.

Rothe, J.P. (Ed.) 1987. *Rethinking Young Drivers.* New Brunswick, NJ: Transaction Publishers.

Rothe, J.P. (Ed.) 1990. *Challenging the Old Order: Towards new directions in traffic safety theory.* New Brunswick, NJ: Transaction Publishers.

Rothe, J.P. (Ed.) 1990. *Rethinking Young Drivers.* New Brunswick, NJ: Transaction Publishers.

Rothe, J.P. & P.J. Cooper (Eds.). 1992. *Motorcyclists, Image and Reality.* New Brunswick, NJ: Transaction Publishers.

Royal Commission on Environmental Pollution. 1994. Transportation and the Environment. London: HMSO.

Rutenberg, J. 1999. SUVs are Hell on Wheels. *New York Daily News,* 18 February.

Sagan, S.D. 1993. *The Limits of Safety.* Princeton, NJ: Princeton University Press.

Sancton, T. & Macleod, S. 1998. Mystery in the Details. *Time,* 152 (10), 36–39.

Sauvé, J. 1999. *Impaired Driving in Canada,* 1998, Juristat, Catalogue 85–002, Vol.19, No. 11, Canadian Centre for Justice Statistics, Statistics Canada.

Schmidt, S.L., Oliveira, R.M., Krahe, T.E. & Filgueiras, C.C. 2000. The effects of hand and gender on finger tapping performance asymmetry by the use of an infra-red light measurement device. *Neuropsychologia,* 38, 529–34.

Schmidt, S.L., Oliveira, R.M., Rocha, F.R. & Abreu-Villaça, Y. 2000. Influences of handedness and gender on the grooved pegboard test. *Brain and Cognition*, in press.

Searle, J.R. 1969 *Speech Acts*. Cambridge, England: Cambridge University Press.

Seigel, J.H., Masongonzalez, S., Dishinger, P.C., Cushing, B., Read, K., Robinson, R., Smialek, J., Heatfield, B., Hill, W., Bents, F., Jackson, J., Livingston, D., Clark, C.C., Norwood, S.H., Parks, S.N., Hawkins, M.L., Reath, P.B. & Gregory, J.S. 1993. Safety Belt Restraints and Compartment Intrusions in Frontal and Lateral Motor–Vehicle Crashes–Mechanisms of Injuries, Complications, and Acute Care Costs. *Journal of Trauma-Injury and Critical Care*, 34 (5), 736–59.

Senge, P. & Lannon-Kim, C. 1991. *The Systems Thinker Newsletter*, 2 (5).

Senge, P., Kleiner, A., Roberts, C., Ross, R. & Smith, B. 1999. *The Dance of Change: The Challenges to Sustaining Momentum in Learning Organizations*. New York: Doubleday.

Shafer, C. (Ed.) 1998. *PARnet*. Available on-line at www.parnet.org/otherwebsites.cfm.

Shah, A.J. 1994. *Public Health and Preventive Medicine in Canada*. Toronto: University of Toronto Press.

Sharma, J.A. 1999. Analysis, Design, and Development of a Sustainable Community Fire Station–Based Injury Control and Research Centre. Master of science thesis, University of Alberta, Edmonton, AB.

Shinar, D. 1990. *Impact of Court Monitoring on DWI Adjudication*. Final Report, DOT HS 807 678 to NHTSA.

Sidhu, C. 1990. Preliminary Assessment of the Increased Speed Limit on Rural Interstate Highways in Illinois. *Transportation Research Record,* 1281, 78–83.

Siegfried, D. 1991. *Gute Argumente: Verkehr*. Munich: C.H. Beck.

Simpson, H. 1985. Polydrug effects and driving safety. *Journal of Alcohol Drugs and Driving*, 1, 17–44.

Singer, P. 1995. Hegel, Georg Wilhelm Friedrich 1770–1831. In Ted Honderich, *The Oxford Companion to Philosophy* (pp. 339–43). Oxford: Oxford University Press.

Sjogren, H. & Bjornstig, U. 1991. Injuries to the elderly in the traffic environment. *Accident Analysis and Prevention*, 23 (1), 77–86.

Skolimowski, H. 1994. *The Participatory Mind*. London: Penguin.

Slattery, P. 1995. A postmodern vision of time and learning. *Harvard Educational Review*, 65 (4), 612–33.

Smith, I. & Faltings, B. (Eds.) 1996. *Advances in Case–Based Reasoning*. Lecture Notes in Artificial Intelligence, No. 1168. New York: Springer–Verlag.

Smith, N. 1990 (October). *Accidents Before and After 65 MPH Speed Limit in California*. California Department of Transportation, Division of Traffic Operations.

Smith, V.J. 1978. What about the customers? A survey of mobile telephone users. In *Proceedings of the 28th IEEE Vehicle Technology Conference*. New York: The Institute of Electrical and Electronics Engineers Inc.

Solomon, H.L. 1994. *1994 Hamilton-Wentworth Collision Report*. Prepared for the Transportation/Environmental Services Department of the Regional Municipality of Hamilton-Wentworth and The Hamilton-Wentworth Regional Police Department. Hamilton: The City of Hamilton Public Works and Traffic Division.

South, D.R., Harrison, W.A., Portans, I. & King, M. 1988. *Evaluation of the Red Light Camera Program and the Owner Onus Legislation*. Special Report: 1981–1986. Hawthorn, Australia: Road Traffic Authority.

Spring, G.S. & Hummer, J. 1995. *Identifying Hazardous Locations Using Geographic Information Systems*. Report for the Southeastern Transportation Center.

Staats, A. 1975. *Social Behaviourism*. Homewood, IL: The Dorsey Press.

Staats, A.W. 1996. *Behaviour and Personality: Psychological Behaviourism*. New York: Springer.

Stacy, A.W., Newcomb, M.D. & Bentler, P.M. 1991. Personality, problem drinking, and drunk driving: Mediating, moderating, and direct–effect models. *Journal of Personality and Social Psychology*, 60, 795–811.

Steier, F. 1985. Reflections on a meeting: Scenes from a courtship. Unpublished manuscript.

Stein, H.S. 1986. Traffic signal change intervals: Policies, practices and safety. *Transportation Quarterly*, 40, 3.

Stenhouse, L. 1967. *Culture and Education*. London: Nelson.

Stoop, J.A. 1995. Accidents–In–depth analysis; towards a method AIDA? *Safety Science*, 19 (2–3), 125–36.

Strange, S. 1989. Towards a Theory of Transnational Empire. In E.-O. R. Czempiel, *Global Changes and Theoretical Challenges* (p. 169). Lexington: University of Kentucky Press.

Strauss, A. & Corbin, J. 1994. Grounded theory methodology: An overview. In N.K. Denzin & Y.S. Lincoln. (Eds.), *Handbook of Qualitative Research* (pp. 273–85). Thousand Oaks, CA: Sage.

Strauss, M.A. 1973. A general systems theory approach to a theory of violence between family members. *Social Science Information*, 12 (3), 105–25.

Student Reports. 1997. *Generational Curriculum, Traffic Psychology at the University of Hawaii*. Available on-line at www.soc.hawaii.edu/leonj/leonj/leonpsy/traffic/tpintro.html.

Sultan, K. 1999. *Women's Role In Road Rage Up, Statistics Show.* Available on-line at www.womanmotorist.com/sfty/female-roadrage.shtml.

Summala, H. 1985. Modeling driver behaviour: A pessimistic prediction? In L. Evans & R. Schwing (Eds.), *Human Behaviour and Traffic Safety* (pp. 43–58). New York: Plenum Press.

Tarawneh, T.M., Singh, V.A. & McCoy, P. 1997. *Evaluation of Media Advertising and Police Enforcement in Reducing Red Light Violations.* Paper presented at the 87th Annual Meeting of the Transportation Research Board, Washington, DC.

Taylor, R.L. & Watson, J. 1989. *They Shall Not Hurt: Human Suffering and Human Caring.* Boulder, CO: Colorado Associated University Press.

The Value Line Investment Survey. 1997. Part 3: Ratings and Reports, 52 (26), 2219.

Thia, L. 1996. Effects of Parental Involvement on Pedestrian Safety Awareness in Five and Six-year-olds. Unpublished thesis, University of Calgary, Calgary, AB.

Thompson, S.J., Steel, J.D. & Gallear, D. 1989. Putting Red Light Violators in the Pictures. *Traffic Engineering and Control,* 30, 122–25.

Transport Association of Canada. 1999. *Canadian Guide to Traffic Calming.* Ottawa: Transportation Association of Canada.

Transport Canada. 1998a. *Alcohol Use by Drivers Fatally Injured in Motor Vehicle Accidents in Canada in 1996 and the Previous Nine Years.* Ottawa: Government of Canada.

Transport Canada. 1998b. *Road Safety Vision 2001.* Ottawa: Government of Canada.

Tremblay, S. & Kemeny, A. 1998. *Drinking and Driving: Have We Made Progress?* Canadian Social Trends, Summer. Statistics Canada — Catalogue 11–008–XPE.

Turner, S. & Polk, A. 1998. Overview of automated enforcement in transportation. *ITE Journal.*

Urry, J. 2000. *Sociology Beyond Societies: Mobilities for the Twenty-First Century.* New York: Routledge.

US Department of Transportation. 1999. *Traffic Safety Facts 1998.* Washington, DC: US Government.

UMTR Institute. 1995. The safety and mobility of oler drivers: What we know and promising research issues." *UMTRI Research Review,* 26 (1), 4–6.

Vahl, H.G. & Giskes, J. 1990. *Traffic Calming Through Integrated Urban Planning.* Paris: Amarcande.

Veloso, M.M. 1994. *Planning and Learning by Analogical Reasoning.* Lecture Notes in Artificial Intelligence, No. 886. New York: Springer-Verlag.

Veloso, M.M. and Aamodt, A. (Eds.) 1995. *Case-Based Reasoning Research and Development.* Lecture Notes in Artificial Intelligence, No. 1010. New York: Springer-Verlag.

Vilenius, A.T., Ryan, G.A., Kloeden, C., McLean, A.J. & Dolinis, J. 1994. A method of estimating linear and angular accelerations in head impacts to pedestrians. *Accident Analysis and Prevention*, 26 (5), 563–70.

Von Glaserfeld, E. 1983. *Deviation of the American System of Cybernetics*. Washington, DC.: The American Society of Cybernetics.

Wade, B. 1999. Driving Yourself to Distraction. *New York Times*, 12 December.

Wallace, A.F.C. 1965. Driving to Work. In M.E. Spiro (Ed.), *Context and Meaning in Cultural Anthropology* (pp. 277–92). New York: The Free Press.

Walter, C.E. 1998. The case for red light cameras. *ITE Journal*.

Waters, N.M. 1988. Expert Systems and Systems of Experts. In W.J. Coffey (Ed.), *Geographical Systems and Systems of Geography: Essays in Honour of William Warntz* (pp. 173–87). London, ON: Department of Geography, University of Western Ontario.

Waters, N.M. 1989. Expert Systems within a GIS: Knowledge Acquisition for Spatial Decision Support Systems. In *Proceedings of the National Conference for Geographic Information Systems* (pp. 740–59). Ottawa: Canadian Institute for Surveying and Mapping.

Waters, N.M. 1996. Internet Search Engines Abound. *GIS World*, 9 (9), 62.

Waters, N.M. 1999. Transportation GIS: GIS-T. In Paul Longley, Michael Goodchild, David Maguire & David Rhind (Eds.), *Geographical Information Systems: Principles, Techniques, Applications and Management* (2nd Ed.). New York: John Wiley & Sons.

Watson, D.L. & Tharp, R.G. 1985. *Self-Directed Behaviour: Self-Modification for Personal Adjustment*. Monterey, CA: Brooks/Cole.

Watzlawick, P., Weakland, J.H. & Fisch, R. 1974. *Change: Principles of Problem Formation and Problem Resolution*. New York: W.W. Norton & Co.

Wiener, N. 1948. *Cybernetics: Or Control and Communication in the Animal and the Machine*. Cambridge, MA: MIT Press.

Wildavsky, A. 1989. *Searching for Safety*. New Brunswick, NJ: Transaction Publishers.

Wilde, G.J.S. 1988. Risk homeostasis theory and traffic accidents: Propositions, deductions and discussion of dissension in recent reactions. *Ergonomics*, 31 (4), 441–68.

Wilde, G.J.S. 1994. *Target Risk*. Toronto: PDE Publications. Available on-line at psyc.queensu.ca/target/index.html#contents.

Williams, R. & Williams, V. 1993. *Anger Kills*. New York: Harper Perennial.

World Health Organization. 1998. Averting the three outriders of the transport apocalypse: Road accidents, air and noise pollution. *World Health Organization Press Releases*, WHO 57. Geneva: Author.

Wortman, R.H., Witkowski, J.M. & Fox, T.C. 1985. *Traffic Characteristics During Signal Change Intervals.* Transportation Research Record No. 1027, Washington, DC: Transportation Research Board.

Wynn, R. 1995. *Running the Red an Evaluation of Strathclyde Police's Red Light Camera Intiative.* Glasgow: The Scottish Office Central Research Unit.

Yang, Q. & Koutsopoulos, H.N. 1996. A Microscopic Traffic Simulator for Evaluation of Dynamic Traffic Management Systems. *Transportation Research C,* 4 (3) 113–29.

Zhang, J., Fraser, S., Lindsay, J., Clarke, K. & Mao, Y. 1998. Age-specific patterns of factors related to fatal motor vehicle traffic crashes: focus on young and elderly drivers. *Public Health,* 112, 289–95.

Zielbauer, P. 1999. Highways as Speedways: Drivers Push the Limits. *New York Times,* 27 December.

Zuckerman, M. 1983. A biological theory of sensation seeking. In M. Zuckerman (Ed.), *Biological Bases of Sensation Seeking, Impulsivity, and Anxiety* (pp. 37–76). Hillsdale, NJ: Lawrence Erlbaum Associates.